# Resilience

"Professors Southwick and Charney have nailed it. After serving for over 30 years as a SEAL leader, I see resilience as the one thing you never think of or learn about until you need it the most: then it becomes one of the most important things you wish you could master. Who we are is defined not only by what we achieve, but also by how we handle life's curveballs. Every parent, coach, and organizational leader should read this now, and pass it on to those they care about the most."

Rear Admiral Navy SEAL Scott Moore (retired)

"*Resilience: The Science of Mastering Life's Greatest Challenges* is a book for our time. At some point, all of us have to deal with stress and anxiety. Drs Southwick and Charney review the science, much of which has been conducted by them, that will enable all of us to not only get through tough times, but to also get stronger."

Steven Hyman, Harvard University Distinguished Professor of
Stem Cell and Regenerative Biology and Former Director
of the National Institute of Mental Health

"How thrilling to read top-flight research that is both inspiring and pragmatic! Charney and Southwick are seasoned guides on the path to resilience. Their hopeful news is that each of us can build resilience in ourselves and across our communities. Our brains are wired for it."

Jerry White, Professor of Practice, University of Virginia,
author of *Getting Up When Life Knocks You Down*

"*Resilience* is one of the most impactful books I've ever read in my life. It gave me a more informed understanding of my own life experiences and an even deeper appreciation for the ability to overcome adversity. This book was both personal and relatable: as my own resilience has not only been the difference between success and failure, but it has also been the difference between life and death. Thank you Dennis and Steven for the years of study it took to write this book."

Curtis Martin – NFL Pro Football Hall of Famer 2012

"This special book is for everybody. We all face adversity in our lives. The authors, who are world-renowned experts, provide a roadmap for resilience and well-being in the face of both physical and emotional challenges .They do this through inspiring stories of incredible people and the latest science. This book has my highest recommendation."

Deepak Chopra MD

# Resilience

## The Science of Mastering Life's Greatest Challenges

### SECOND EDITION

**Steven M. Southwick**
Yale University School of Medicine

**Dennis S. Charney**
Icahn School of Medicine at Mount Sinai

# CAMBRIDGE
## UNIVERSITY PRESS

University Printing House, Cambridge CB2 8BS, United Kingdom

One Liberty Plaza, 20th Floor, New York, NY 10006, USA

477 Williamstown Road, Port Melbourne, VIC 3207, Australia

314–321, 3rd Floor, Plot 3, Splendor Forum, Jasola District Centre, New Delhi – 110025, India

79 Anson Road, #06–04/06, Singapore 079906

Cambridge University Press is part of the University of Cambridge.

It furthers the University's mission by disseminating knowledge in the pursuit of education, learning, and research at the highest international levels of excellence.

www.cambridge.org
Information on this title: www.cambridge.org/9781108441667
DOI: 10.1017/9781108349246

First published by Cambridge University Press 2012
Second edition Cambridge University Press 2018

Printed in the United States of America by Sheridan Books, Inc.

*A catalog record for this publication is available from the British Library.*

*Library of Congress Cataloging-in-Publication Data*
Names: Southwick, Steven M., author. | Charney, Dennis S., author.
Title: Resilience : the science of mastering life's greatest challenges / Steven Southwick, Yale University School of Medicine, Dennis Charney, Mt. Sinai School of Medicine.
Description: Second edition. | Cambridge, United Kingdom ; New York, NY : Cambridge University Press, 2018. | Includes bibliographical references and index.
Identifiers: LCCN 2017061573 | ISBN 9781108441667 (alk. paper)
Subjects: LCSH: Resilience (Personality trait) | Adaptability (Psychology)
Classification: LCC BF698.35.R47 S68 2018 | DDC 155.2/4–dc23
LC record available at https://lccn.loc.gov/2017061573

ISBN 978-1-108-44166-7 Paperback

# Contents

# Preface

The cover image of this book is taken from a painting by the great American artist Winslow Homer. *The Life Line*, painted in 1884, depicts an unconscious woman being rescued from a shipwreck by a courageous man during a treacherous storm. Homer's painting is a portrait of resilience complete with adversity, stoicism, and profound courage. The viewer's eye is drawn to the center of the painting where a red wind-blown scarf obscures the face of the rescuer. By choosing to keep the rescuer anonymous, Homer presents an act of selfless heroism: where the act, and not the actor, seems most important. In the authors' experience, veterans, first responders, firefighters, and police officers often adopt a similar stance. They don't like to be called heroes. They believe that their acts of bravery are simply part of their job and are directed toward someone in need and not toward honor and praise for themselves.

But resilience is not reserved for soldiers or first responders. Most of us are far sturdier than we know. Even though we may never be called upon to rescue someone at sea, we will be challenged again and again during our lives, and – like the anonymous rescuer – we can choose to step up and squarely face adversity with heart and soul.

## Further Reading

Khan Academy. Homer, The Life Line (video). A conversation with Kahn Academy's Dr. Beth Harris and Dr. Steven Zucker. Accessed February 2, 2018 at www.khanacademy.org/humanities/art-americas/us-art-19c/realism-us/v/winslow-homer-the-life-line-1884

# Acknowledgments

This book would not have been possible without the generous contributions of the many inspiring individuals who granted us permission to interview them and share portions of those interviews with our readers. These courageous men and women told us about extremely painful and trying experiences in their lives. Talking with us in depth about these experiences was extraordinarily difficult, but they chose to speak so that their stories and their insights might help others. Their stories and their advice make up the heart and soul of this book. It has been an honor and a privilege for us to interview and learn from these remarkable individuals. They have become our role models just as we hope they will become yours. They have taught us to look for light at the end of the tunnel; to view adversity as an opportunity for growth and wisdom; to live by our own highest moral and ethical standards; to foster strong personal relationships in which we both give and receive support; to rigorously train our physical, emotional, cognitive, and spiritual selves; and to assume responsibility for our own growth and resilience. They have shown us how to seek the very best in ourselves, and they have taught us that we are each far stronger and more resilient than we think.

We also wish to thank the editors and writers who helped to shape this book. Specifically, we acknowledge and express thanks to Lisa Berger, who partnered us in our early efforts to write about resilience. Lisa is an outstanding writer and editor. In addition, Cathy Shufro, Kara Baskin, and Marcia Southwick provided expert guidance in writing style and editing. We were also very fortunate to work with Elsa Peterson, who is an extremely talented scholar, writer, and editor. Elsa made enormous contributions to every aspect of the book – research, writing, and editing.

Many of our friends and colleagues helped us as we formulated ideas about resilience. They also reviewed drafts of the book and provided valuable suggestions and edits. We wish to thank Jeanne Stellman and Christina Baker, who reviewed and edited the book. Paul Morrissey, Ron Duman, Eric Jackson, Jo Ann Thorp, Robb Pietrzak, Ann Graber, Catherine Chiles, Brian Iacoviello, Eric Nestler, and Lori Davis provided guidance and edits on specific chapters. We extend special thanks to Bernadette Lowthert for her depth of insight and for her creative approach to conceptualizing, organizing, and integrating all sections of the book.

Finally, we wish to thank the many professionals at Cambridge University Press who edited and published this book.

SMS and DSC

# CHAPTER 1

# What Is Resilience?

Most of us at some point will be struck by one or more major traumas: violent crime, domestic violence, rape, child abuse, a serious automobile accident, the sudden death of a loved one, a debilitating disease, a natural disaster or war. If you are very lucky, then you have never encountered any of these misfortunes; but most likely you will someday. It is estimated that up to 90 percent of us will experience at least one serious traumatic event during our lives (Norris & Sloane, 2007).

Indeed, since the first edition of this book the authors have experienced traumatic events in their own lives. One of us (Dennis Charney) lost a father and was the victim of a shooting with a shotgun that involved intensive rehabilitation. The other (Steven Southwick) lost both of his parents, helped his brother recover from the amputation of his leg, and is currently dealing with his sister's cancer and his own cancer. Both of us have found the approaches to resilience outlined in this book to be very helpful. We hope you, the readers, do as well. Traumatic events throw our lives into turmoil in unpredictable ways; no two people will respond to them in exactly the same manner. For some, the stress of the event will become chronic, lasting for years. They may undergo a dramatic change in outlook, becoming sullen, demoralized, withdrawn, cynical, and angry. Some will become depressed or develop posttraumatic stress disorder (PTSD). Horrific, intrusive memories and nightmares will haunt them for days, months, or even years, and they will feel unsafe in the world – hypervigilant – as if another serious danger lurks just around the corner. Some will take up drinking or drugs to numb their pain and dull their memories.

Nevertheless, many people will find ways to meet the challenge and continue with purposeful lives. For a period after their ordeal, they may become distressed, but in time they will bounce back and carry on. For some, it will be almost as if the trauma had never occurred. For others, the distress will persist, but they will find healthy ways to cope. Some survivors will even grow stronger and wiser because of their trauma. These survivors may report that their tragedy has helped them to appreciate life more, to become closer to family and friends, to find greater meaning, and sometimes to embark on a new mission in life. In the words of Elisabeth S. Lukas (1984), a protégée of the neurologist, psychiatrist, and Holocaust survivor Viktor Frankl, "The forces of fate that bear down on man and threaten to break him also have the capacity to ennoble him."

## Resilience After 9/11

On the clear, balmy morning of September 11, 2001, 45-year-old Jimmy Dunne was playing golf in New York's suburban Westchester County, looking forward to qualifying for the US Mid-Amateur Championship tournament. Along with the other golfers, he was stunned to learn that planes had crashed into the World Trade Center. Dunne's shock was intensified by the fact that his own company, the financial services firm Sandler O'Neill, was located at Two World Trade Center (the "South Tower"). As details of the damage became available, his fears were confirmed: the plane that struck the South Tower burst into flames on the 78th through 84th floors, trapping hundreds on the floors above (Dwyer *et al.*, 2002). Sandler O'Neill was on the 104th floor.

While Dunne watched television in disbelief, thousands of employees, visitors, police, firefighters, emergency medical personnel, and concerned bystanders were fighting to save lives while they struggled to understand what was happening. One Sandler O'Neill survivor, Karen Fishman, had arrived at her office in the South Tower about 8:45 that morning – moments before the first plane struck the North Tower and sent a massive, blinding ball of flame shooting through the air outside her office window. Shaking, she got up from her desk, stepped out into the hallway, and quickly found herself headed for the stairs with two colleagues who had announced, "We're getting the hell out of here" (Brooker, 2002, p. 56).

"I don't know why I left," Fishman said later. "I don't know that it was a conscious decision. It was instinct. So much depended on who you saw right at that moment." Several other Sandler O'Neill employees left, but others stayed in the office and made phone calls assuring family members and business associates that they were all right. Still, the horrors in the neighboring building had everyone so upset that CEO Herman Sandler told his workforce, "Whoever wants to leave can leave."

Fishman had reached the 64th floor when she heard an announcement that only the North Tower was affected and there was no need to evacuate the South

Tower. But by then the stairwell was crowded, and turning back would have meant going against the tide of people headed down, so she continued.

Fishman was on the 62nd floor at 9:03 when United Airlines Flight 175 crashed into the South Tower. Forty-two stories above her, a Sandler O'Neill assistant was on the phone with her husband – "Oh, my God" were the last words he heard her say. A trader called his wife: "There is smoke everywhere. People are dying all around me" (Brooker, 2002, p. 57).

Survivors described how the building shook and twisted when the plane struck, causing paneling, duct work, and electrical wires to fall out of the walls and ceilings. The lights went out, and the building's sprinkler system activated in some areas, sending cascades of water down the pitch-dark stairwells as people groped their way down. Of course, neither Karen Fishman nor anyone else knew that the building was about to collapse. In a sense this was fortunate, for the evacuation was generally orderly and unhurried – some even commented later that they had paced themselves, aiming to lessen the risk of having to walk down dozens of flights with a sprained ankle (Clark, 2006).

Karen Fishman and another Sandler O'Neill employee, Mark Fitzgibbon, had reached street level and were making their way uptown at 9:59, when the South Tower collapsed. They were far enough away from the burning towers that the surrounding skyscrapers partially obscured their view. Like many who witnessed the event, they had no idea that the entire building was gone; they thought that they were seeing smoke from an explosion or a collapse affecting only the floors above the fire line. Fitzgibbon called to Karen, "Look. The top of our building is gone." But she didn't look back (Brooker, 2002, p. 57).

A huge wave of ash and dust burst from the ruins and covered the area like a snowfall. Stunned survivors fled by themselves or in groups, some running, some walking purposefully, others wandering as if in a fog. By 10:28, when One World Trade Center and the adjoining Marriott Hotel collapsed, news organizations had begun to report a possible terrorist connection, and other landmark buildings such as the United Nations were evacuated. Not knowing whether further attacks were imminent, New York Mayor Rudy Giuliani ordered the evacuation of lower Manhattan. This released a swelling tide of pedestrians into the streets as people attempted to get home. Transportation was severely crippled: the subway service was suspended, as were the PATH trains connecting Manhattan with New Jersey. Commuter buses stopped running, as all bridges and tunnels connecting Manhattan with the outer boroughs and with New Jersey were closed to non-emergency traffic. One survivor described taking a ferry homeward to New Jersey:

> . . .as we got parallel [to the World Trade Center site] we could look over and see that both towers were gone. It was just a surreal feeling. Disbelief. How could this happen? Of course, at the time we knew nothing about the planes being hijacked, nothing about the Pentagon, nothing about the plane going down in Pennsylvania, or the FAA getting

all planes out of the air. We were completely in the dark. But we could look off to the Trade Center on our right and see that this building I had worked in for 27 years was gone. It was a staggering thought. There was silence. People just couldn't believe it.

(Clark, 2006)

While these events were transpiring, Jimmy Dunne was on the phone, calling first his wife and then a series of friends and associates. He tried repeatedly to reach Chris Quackenbush, his business partner and closest companion; the two had been friends since childhood. And he kept trying to call his boss and mentor Herman Sandler, but could not reach him either. Had Chris and Herman made it out of the South Tower alive? After four or five hours without word on the whereabouts of Chris or Herman, Jimmy began to fear the worst. As painful as it was to imagine, perhaps his best friends and colleagues had been murdered by the terrorists. Perhaps he would never see them again.

Still, like so many others on that chaotic day, Jimmy held out hope and maintained what he referred to as a "we are going to find them" state of mind. As he recalls, "There was a hope that there were people who had gotten out, gotten to a hospital, gotten somewhere and maybe they just couldn't make a phone call."

His hopes received a massive boost when he was told that a junior trader in the firm had been found.

There was an intern who worked with us. He was terrific. His name was Kevin Williams. After I left the golf course I spoke to his father, who told me they found Kevin. And I was euphoric. I remember physical euphoria when I learned that Kevin was alive. It also meant that if they found Kevin, maybe they would find Chris and Herman and the others. I was euphoric. Absolute joy.

By mid-afternoon, Jimmy learned that surviving employees of his firm were gathering in a small office that Sandler O'Neill maintained in midtown. He decided to take the train into Manhattan and meet with them.

I left for the train station with great hope. But on the way, I received a call that I will never forget as long as I live. It was Kevin's father. He said, "Jimmy, Jimmy, they found Kevin Williams – but not our Kevin Williams." And I remember physically slouching down, almost collapsing. Fortunately, there was a chair right there. I've never had anything like that happen before.

By the time the train arrived in Manhattan, however, Jimmy was surging with energy. He ran from Grand Central Station, headed toward the midtown office.

And then I remember thinking, as soon as I get there everybody's gonna be looking at me, everybody's gonna be looking for direction from me. I want to set a very different tone, one of total calm. I remember I stopped running and I walked about four blocks before I got to the office.

Under normal circumstances, Jimmy saw himself as somewhat pessimistic. "I'm like the French Foreign Legion: I prepare for the worst and hope for the best."

But on September 11, coming to terms with the news that the World Trade Center attack had been perpetrated by terrorists whose goal was to kill as many Americans as possible and create a sense of mass hysteria among the living, he remembered something his father had told him decades earlier. Jimmy and his father had been sitting together watching an Army–Notre Dame football game, and Notre Dame was crushing Army 40–7.

That's when Jimmy's father turned to him and said, "Now is the time that I would like to be a lineman on the Army squad."

Jimmy didn't understand.

> Why would anyone want to be on Army? They're being beaten 40–7! And we liked Notre Dame better than Army. Plus, being a lineman for Army, you'd be outweighed by something like 80 pounds. I can't think of a less desirable position to be in. So, I asked my father, "Why?" And I remember what he said like it was yesterday: "Because the guy on the other side of the line is gonna find out what I'm made of. I would wreak holy hell on that guy."

In his own way, after the destruction of September 11, that's what Jimmy did.

> The moment I heard what the terrorists wanted, I decided to do exactly the opposite. Osama Bin Laden wanted us to be afraid. I would show no fear. He wanted us to be pessimistic. I would be incredibly optimistic. He wanted anguish. I would have none of it.

The determination to "show them what I'm made of" served him well in the hours and days after the attacks, as the scope of the catastrophe became clear. As hard as he may have tried to prepare himself to face severe losses, the damage was unimaginable. Of 171 Sandler employees, 66 died (Kroft, 2001). Among them were Jimmy's close friends and fellow managing partners, Chris Quackenbush and Herman Sandler. In all, the deaths of the firm's workers left 46 widows and widowers, and 71 children under age 18 who had lost a father or mother. Furthermore, Sandler O'Neill was a small enough firm that its operations had been concentrated in the Two World Trade Center office. All of the company's paperwork and computer systems were destroyed. As *Fortune* magazine reported, "Every phone number of every person Sandler's traders had done business with over the years was vaporized" (Brooker, 2002, p. 60). Even more devastating was the loss of corporate memory.

Suddenly Dunne, who previously had shared responsibilities with Quackenbush and Sandler, was thrust into the role of chief executive and decision maker. The firm was so terribly crippled – should he simply dissolve it? If not, how could he possibly guide it to survival? Would an attempt to stay in business merely prolong the agony? How could so many traumatized employees manage to function and conduct business when they were grieving for their lost colleagues?

One of the first crucial decisions Dunne made was to "do right by the families" of those who had died (Nocera, 2006). He personally attended dozens of funerals and delivered eulogies for many. Despite the financial burden, comprising a third of the firm's working capital, Sandler O'Neill paid the salaries of the deceased employees through December 31, 2001 (McKay, 2002). The company paid bonuses and extended family health-care benefits for five years. In addition, the firm set up a fund for the education of the children who had lost a parent, and it provided five years of psychological counseling for all family members and for surviving employees.

Another of Dunne's crucial decisions was that he would find a way to carry on with business. If the firm failed, it could no longer support his colleagues and their families. Failure would also mean success for the terrorists. Although there were rumors – including a CNBC report – that the firm was closing, Sandler's operations never came to a halt. As much as Dunne felt the profound pain of his colleagues, he knew that the firm's only chance for survival was to rebuild immediately.

> Early on we got everyone together and they were in various levels of their pain. I said, "Look, everybody is re-evaluating their lives after 9–11." And I said, "That's fine. You can go ahead and re-evaluate your life. That's OK. And some of you may decide that coming to the city every day and chasing the dollar is not worth it, and that you should work in the post office and teach lacrosse. That's great. Some of you may want to go take a trip around the world. That's fine too. But I can tell you what I am gonna do. I'm gonna put on my Brooks Brothers suit every day and I am gonna come to work, and I am gonna rebuild this firm, and I am gonna pay for these benefits, and I am not gonna give in. That is what I have decided to do. Now for those of you who want to be doing the same thing, we have to be doing it *now*. And those of you who want to re-evaluate things and think differently, I wish you well. Go do it."

By September 17, the day the New York Stock Exchange reopened, the firm was set up in temporary office space donated by Bank of America and prepared to resume trading. Dunne and the other managers saw rebuilding the firm as a moral imperative. They were determined to honor their lost colleagues and make the trades that their colleagues no longer could. Several weeks later, after his first visit to Ground Zero, accompanying a colleague's widow who wished to view the site, Dunne commented to a co-worker, ". . .if I was determined before, I'm on fire now" (Brooker, 2002, p. 53). As founding partner Tom O'Neill told CBS's *60 Minutes*, "I don't think we appreciated the depth of [the terrorists'] hatred, but I think for every percentage that we might have underestimated them, I think they very much underestimated us" (Kroft, 2001). By the first anniversary of the attack, Sandler had hired 81 new employees and closed 59 deals, including 15 mergers worth $2.7 billion.

Although immersing himself in work was a healing influence for Dunne in many ways, the emotional toll was still vast. A year after the attacks, Dunne told National Public Radio's Scott Simon, "I'm better when I'm busy, but the very first thing I think about when I wake up in the morning and the very last thing I think about at night are those planes" (Simon, 2002). Then-Chief Operating

Officer Fred D. Price, who had been away at a conference in Seattle on September 11, agreed:

> When you are busy and active you don't think about it, but when it's quiet, when you are driving alone, or on weekends when you get up in the morning, that is when I vividly miss [my colleagues]. . . Some days, I feel bad and some days I feel good and I never know why. . . Weekends are tougher, and Sunday is my ugliest day. It's when I've got time on my hands. (Wayne, 2002)

The grief that Jimmy felt was unlike anything that he had experienced. Reflecting on the loss of his lifelong friend Chris Quackenbush and his mentor Herman Sandler, he likened it to the utter despondency that history tells us Thomas Jefferson experienced upon the death of his beloved wife Martha in 1782:

> It was absolute grief, the kind of grief that Thomas Jefferson talks about, grief without a point. I felt that kind of grief at Chris's funeral after I spoke, and when I went to see [Herman's widow] Suki Sandler. When other people talk about their grief, sometimes you don't even know what they're talking about. You don't really know what real grief is. Now I think I know. I think I have a sense about absolute grief. Those are the times I just broke down.

Five years later, *New York Times* reporter Joe Nocera interviewed Dunne and noted that "his eyes would well up while his voice would start to crack" when he talked about his partners (Nocera, 2006). Yet, far from being a sign of weakness, Dunne's heartfelt emotion was the driving force in his rescue of the firm. Jimmy Dunne personifies resilience in his unwavering determination to bounce back from the brink of despair, and to grow in the process, becoming a more compassionate, dedicated leader than he had been in the past.

# How We Became Interested in Resilience

Our interest in resilience evolved during nearly 20 years of treating and studying trauma survivors who came to us for help with conditions such as depression and PTSD. In our research, we examined the psychological, neurobiological, social, and spiritual impact of having lived through overwhelming traumas such as combat, child abuse, physical and sexual assault, and disasters including the World Trade Center disaster and Hurricane Ike (Charney *et al.*, 1993, 1996; Bremner *et al.*, 1993, 1999; Southwick *et al.*, 2006, 2007; Stellman *et al.*, 2008). We, and many other researchers, discovered alterations in psychological view of self and others, in the brain circuits that respond to frightening situations, and in feelings about one's purpose, meaning and place in the world. These alterations often had profound negative effects on the lives of our patients.

As we worked with traumatized individuals, we often wondered about survivors who seemed to somehow cope effectively with the negative effects of stress, those who did not develop stress-related symptoms, or who, if they developed symptoms, carried on successfully nevertheless. The term "resilient" (meaning having the capacity to bend without breaking, to return to an original shape or condition) described these survivors well. They had been "bent" by their traumatic experiences, but not broken.

# Defining Resilience

What is resilience? In the physical sciences, materials and objects are termed resilient if they resume their original shape upon being bent or stretched. In people, resilience refers to the ability to "bounce back" after encountering difficulty. The American Psychological Association defines it as "the process of adapting well in the face of adversity, trauma, tragedy, threats and even significant sources of stress – such as family and relationship problems, serious health problems, or workplace and financial stresses."[1] In his book *Aging Well*, Harvard University psychologist George Vaillant (2002) describes resilient individuals as resembling "a twig with a fresh, green living core. When twisted out of shape, such a twig bends, but it does not break; instead, it springs back and continues growing" (p. 285).

Resilience is complex, multidimensional and dynamic in nature (Bonanno, 2004, 2005; Carver, 1998; Layne *et al.*, 2007; Luthar *et al.*, 2000; Rutter, 1985). While experts define resilience in a variety of ways (Southwick *et al.*, 2014), a common thread in their definitions is the ability to weather adversity. This does not mean being impervious to adversity – a resilient person may be deeply affected by a traumatic event, and may experience psychological symptoms such as depression, recurrent intrusive memories, or hypervigilance – but it does mean being able to carry on with the important facets of one's life in spite of painful and distressing symptoms or even full-blown PTSD. In some definitions, resilience also entails the ability to grow from adverse events and find meaning in them.

---

[1] American Psychological Association Help Center. Accessed October 13, 2017 at http://www.apa.org/helpcenter/road-resilience.aspx. It is worth noting that researchers have identified a coping style called hardiness which involves a constellation of personality characteristics associated with high performance under stressful conditions. These characteristics include commitment (the tendency to engage fully in life activities), perceived control (belief in one's ability to exercise control over life circumstances), and challenge (the tendency to view adversity as a challenge). See, for example: Kobasa (1979), Kobasa *et al.* (1982), Bartone (1999), Maddi (2005), and http://www.hardiness-resilience.com

When faced with adversity, people may be more competent in some domains of their lives than in others, and during some, but not all, phases of their lives. For example, an individual may be remarkably sturdy in responding to adversity at work, but not so much in handling family or other interpersonal stresses. Or a person may demonstrate resilience to stress at a young age, but not as he or she grows older. It is important to note that healthy adaptation to stress depends not only on the individual, but also on available resources through family, friends, and a variety of organizations, and on the characteristics of specific cultures and religions, communities, societies, and governments – all of which, in themselves, may be more or less resilient (Southwick *et al.*, 2011).

Researchers have developed various tests to measure resilience; among them are the Connor–Davidson Resilience Scale (Connor & Davidson, 2003) and the Response to Stressful Experiences Scale (Johnson *et al.*, 2008).

These tests are self-report instruments with a five-point Likert scale (strongly agree, agree somewhat, etc.) and include statements such as the following:

- During and after life's most stressful events, I tend to find opportunity for growth.
- I have at least one close and secure relationship that helps me when I am stressed.
- When there are no clear solutions to my problems, sometimes fate or God can help.
- During and after life's most stressful events, I tend to calm and comfort myself.

Additional tests of resilience include the Dispositional Resilience Scale-15, which focuses on three dimensions – being fully engaged, having a sense of control over events, and being able to view adversity as a challenge – and the Resiliency Scale for Children and Adolescents, which assesses an array of attributes related to mastery, relatedness, and emotional reactivity (Bartone, 2007; Prince-Embury, 2008).

# What Makes Some People Resilient?

When we began our research, we had many questions. Why do some survivors appear relatively unscathed by their trauma, while others develop debilitating disorders such as PTSD, depression and alcohol dependence? (For more information about PTSD, please see Appendix 1.) And why do some survivors who develop trauma-related psychological symptoms continue to function well in spite of their symptoms? Do they differ genetically? Is there something unique about their nervous system? Have they been raised in a special manner? What about their personalities? Do they use specific coping mechanisms to deal with stress? And if we learn more about how they dealt with stress and trauma, will these lessons be helpful to PTSD patients and to the general public? Can the average person learn to become more resilient?

These were the questions that we asked ourselves as we began to investigate social, biological, psychological, and spiritual factors associated with resilience to stress. And, of course, we also wondered whether these lessons would be helpful to us. Could we, ourselves, learn to become more resilient? We had many unanswered questions.

So, we made a decision to search actively for answers to our questions about resilience. We knew that our task would be daunting, because anyone who has spent time studying human behavior, or investigating the nervous system and brain, understands that thoughts, feelings, and behaviors are the complex products of genetic, biological, psychological, and social forces. Resilience is far more than a simple psychological trait or biological phenomenon. To truly understand it, researchers must approach it from multiple perspectives and examine it through a number of different scientific lenses. We did this by reviewing the available scientific research and popular literature on resilience, by initiating our own psychological and neurobiological research on the topic, and by conducting in-depth interviews with a large number of highly resilient individuals (Southwick *et al.*, 2005).

To conduct these interviews, we needed to step out of our traditional clinical and research settings, and to go into the community and recruit people who had clearly demonstrated resilience in the face of extreme stress. We turned to three groups of highly resilient individuals: former Vietnam prisoners of war (POWs), Special Forces instructors, and civilian men and women who had not only survived enormous stress and trauma, but had somehow endured or even thrived.

# We Interviewed Former Vietnam POWs

We began by conducting detailed and lengthy interviews with more than 30 former Vietnam POWs. We chose to study former POWs for several reasons. First, the traumatic experiences they endured were extreme and of long duration; for some, the ordeal lasted for more than 8 years. Second, because their captivity took place decades ago, we could examine how their lives had unfolded over many years after the trauma. Third, we believed that the former POWs were good role models and that their methods of coping with stress and trauma would be highly instructive for anyone facing or recovering from their own stressors.

Most of these former POWs were pilots who were captured when their planes were shot down over North Vietnam. After ejecting from disabled burning fighter jets flying at speeds of greater than 400 miles per hour, they parachuted into the jungle. There they were captured by North Vietnamese.

The North Vietnamese treated American prisoners as war criminals, not as POWs protected by the Geneva Conventions. Often captured Americans were paraded through crowds of hostile villagers before being imprisoned, interrogated, beaten, and tortured. The largest and most infamous facility where POWs were held was Hoa Lo Prison in Hanoi, which the Americans sarcastically nicknamed the "Hanoi Hilton." Here prisoners were subjected to interrogation techniques like the "rope trick," in which both arms are tied behind the back and then gradually lifted higher and higher until one or both shoulders are pulled out of their sockets. At other times, guards wrapped a rope around the prisoner's throat, stretched the rope behind his back, and tied it to his ankles, so that if he relaxed his arched back, he would choke.

POWs were also starved. Typically, they were given meager portions of barely edible food: swamp grass or cabbage soup, a chicken head floating in grease, pumpkin soup, a piece of bread covered with mold, the hoof of a cow, an occasional tiny piece of pig fat, or a handful of rice that might be full of rat feces, weevils, or small stones. Even prisoners in solitary confinement rarely dined alone. Colonel Larry Guarino (1990, p. 45) describes his "dinner guests":

> A new civilian guard brought food, and as he set it down on the far bunk, a horde of hungry ants rushed out from the block mounts of the leg irons and swarmed into the tin plates. . . . While eating, I was startled by two lightening-fast brown rats who darted around the cell and between my feet looking for food . . . I had more visitors. Arriving under the door were two huge scorpions . . . The scorpions came in with raised stingers, but when they sensed my presence, they backed out into the cement channel where the pickings were presumably better . . . Mosquitoes by the hundreds lived under the cement bunks, where it was very damp. I sat swinging my legs and swatting mosquitoes until my hands were swollen. Suddenly, I saw a huge gray-white, web-footed rat poking his head under the door. He was so big he couldn't get under the door to enter the cell. He sniffed about, showing me inch-long white fangs, then swirled his head under the door, still trying to get in. His tail was over an inch thick! No doubt this rat and his friends were the producers of the huge turds that covered the outside yard. What a disgusting and frightening creature. My heart pounded so, it was difficult for me to breathe, even as I told myself to calm down and take it easy.

In *Glory Denied: The Saga of Vietnam Veteran Jim Thompson, America's Longest-Held Prisoner of War*, Captain Thompson describes one of his "accommodations":

I was put into a horizontal cage maybe two feet wide, two feet high, and five feet long. There I was kept for four months, chained hand and feet. The leg irons were a nasty device, a U-bolt with a rusted rod through the back, much too small for American legs. Every time they put the thing on it took a chunk of flesh. This cage sat in the back room of a house in complete darkness. They had a bamboo wall around it so I saw nothing. I was not let out for exercise. For ten minutes a day I could use the latrine and wash up. Then they would stick me back in and put the leg irons back on.

(Philpott, 2002, p. 147)

In this environment, it is not surprising that many POWs developed serious illnesses and were sick during much of their time in prison. They described skin infections, malnutrition, extreme weight loss, open untreated wounds, broken and dislocated bones, dysentery, malaria, depression and symptoms of posttraumatic stress, such as terrifying nightmares. Plagued by dysentery and needing to defecate dozens of times each day, some prisoners became severely dehydrated. Others described boils and skin diseases, where pus and blood attracted jungle flies and mosquitoes, and where maggots thrived.

All of the POWs we interviewed were deeply affected by their prison experience. A substantial number developed trauma-related depression and/or PTSD and experienced difficulty adjusting to civilian life. However, despite their wartime experiences, these former POWs went on to live productive lives after their release. In fact, many of them reported having a greater appreciation of life, closer connections with family, and a newfound sense of meaning and purpose because of their prison experience.

# We Interviewed Special Forces Instructors

The second group of people we interviewed were members of the Special Forces (SF). The Special Forces is an elite command within the US Army. The Army selects these soldiers and trains them to be among the hardiest, most resilient men and women on the planet. In the world today, there are perhaps no groups that are better conditioned to handle stress than are SF troops and Navy Seals. They benefit from the US Military's constant refinement of its combat and training programs. SF soldiers are rigorously trained to deal with hardship and life-and-death situations. They are intelligent, agile, resourceful, and exceptionally well-prepared for covert missions related to reconnaissance, counter-intelligence, unconventional warfare, and foreign internal defense.

All of the SF members we interviewed were instructors. To become an instructor, one must first serve as an SF soldier. After completing tours of duty stationed around the globe, the instructor's job is to assess and train the next generation of elite soldiers. We chose to interview instructors in order to learn about their philosophy of training and about the actual principles and techniques they use to enhance resilience. These men had all served as instructors at the rigorous SERE course (Survival, Evasion, Resistance, Escape), which is designed to teach soldiers survival fieldcraft so that they can maneuver in enemy-controlled areas, escape detection, and return unharmed to friendly forces. They participate in a grueling war game with a well-equipped "enemy" while they have no food, water, or weapons. They learn how to live for several days with nothing but a knife and canteen and to overcome food aversions so they can eat snakes, insects, worms, and dead animals. During the last segment of the course, trainees are taken captive and held in a mock POW camp. Here they are stripped of their uniforms and identity, and deprived of food and sleep. As SERE graduates who teach soldiers in this course, the SF instructors are real-life experts in how to cope with high levels of emotional and physical stress; in how to become emotionally and physically stronger.

Retired four-star general Henry Hugh Shelton, former Chairman of the Joint Chiefs of Staff, also talked with us about resilience. Early in his military career, he trained as an Army Ranger and later served as head of the Special Operations Command for all of the Armed Forces. He told us that his Ranger training gave him the tools that he needed to overcome the personal and professional traumas in his adult life.

Special Forces instructor Bruce Norwood described a mission that particularly stood out in his memory. He and his wife were living in Puerto Rico when his beeper went off one night and he was told to drive to his office immediately. Thirty minutes later, he and four team members were on board a Black Hawk helicopter, flying to Venezuela. As they approached their destination, in heavy rain and violent gusts of wind, the pilot directed the chopper's searchlight to the road below. There they could see scores of people being swept away by the torrential flood waters.

Once the pilot located a cluster of terrified survivors, Norwood and his colleagues slid down a rope while the Black Hawk hovered above. Norwood's left boot struck a firm but spongy object as he stepped onto the slippery terrain. It was an infant girl who had died in the flood.

> We worked for forty straight hours and saved hundreds of people, maybe as many as 1500. Most people don't know it, but at least 50 percent of our missions are humanitarian. They call us the Peace Corps with guns. Even when we're on a foreign international defense mission, the SF medics will go out to the front gate and treat whoever shows up. Some poor campesinos bring their dead baby that they carried across the mountains for three days, and they've never seen a doctor before. The SF medics will be out there five, six, seven hours a night on their off-time treating the locals. The engineers will go down to the nearest town and see what they can do for the schools, the churches. They'll put a new roof on. They'll build a new school, a new church.

# We Interviewed Resilient Civilians from Many Walks of Life

The third group we interviewed consisted of civilian men and women who have gone on to lead productive and accomplished lives after experiencing severe psychological traumas, such as congenital medical problems, childhood sexual abuse, death of parents at an early age, abduction and rape, loss of a limb, and cancer.

Eleanor Jensen, for example, lost her parents in an automobile accident when she was eight. Eleanor remembers sitting with her sister on the front porch of their house, waiting to find out where and with whom they would live. After temporary placement with relatives, they were adopted by a childless couple who lived in another region of the country.

Soon Eleanor's new stepfather began to show "special" interest in her and started to touch her. One night, when her stepmother was out of the house, Eleanor's stepfather came into her room and asked her to sit with him.

> He started feeling me, French kissing me. And I didn't know what was happening...
> I was still. Dead. A robot.

The situation became chronic.

> My stepmother put a lock on my door, a screw and hook, and I could hear him come up the steps and scratch at the door. He would work on the lock with this little ruler until it opened. Then my stepmother tried a slide lock, and he'd work on it until he eventually got in, then a bolt lock, then a twist lock. There were about 4–5 locks on the door. I'd always be afraid to be home alone. One time when the dog got away and ran down the road and I was running after it, he drove in the car after me and told me to get in and I froze. I could not move my muscles. He said, "I'm sorry, I'm sorry, I won't touch you, I promise. Get in the car, I'll take you home." There was always this tension in being alone, and I'd panic.

As a teenager, Eleanor was sent to a boarding school where she was safe. Although the memories of abuse haunted her for years, she was eventually able to forgive her stepfather. Eleanor went on to become a highly respected nurse practitioner and psychotherapist specializing in treating PTSD.

Additional examples of ordinary people who found constructive ways to cope with their trauma include, among others:

- Deborah Gruen, who, despite a serious congenital neurological condition, won bronze medals in swimming in the 2004 and 2008 Paralympics, competed as a member of the Yale University Women's Varsity Swim Team and graduated summa cum laude from Yale with a major in economics, attended Georgetown University Law School and went on to a career with a prestigious law firm.

- Angela Diaz, who grew up in an impoverished, fragmented family in the Dominican Republic, emigrated to the United States as a teenager, was accepted to Columbia Medical School, became Director of the Adolescent Health Center at Icahn School of Medicine at Mount Sinai, and donated a kidney to a friend's husband.
- Elizabeth Ebaugh, who was kidnapped, raped, and thrown over a bridge into a freezing river only to survive and, over the ensuing years, build a thriving clinical social work practice that focuses on holistic approaches to helping survivors of trauma and tragedy.
- Jerry White, who lost his leg to a landmine while hiking in Israel as a college student, and then slipped into depression. Years later he co-founded Landmine Survivors Network and played a leading role in the International Campaign to Ban Landmines coalition, which was awarded the Nobel Peace Prize in 1997.

## What We Found: Ten Resilience Factors

During our interviews, we kept hearing a number of recurrent themes. Although their circumstances differed greatly, the resilient people we interviewed tended to use the same or similar coping strategies when confronted with high levels of stress. By conducting a detailed analysis of the interviews, we identified ten coping mechanisms that proved to be effective for dealing with stress and trauma. Throughout the book, we refer to these coping mechanisms as "resilience factors." In response to stress, all of the individuals we interviewed confronted their fears, main-tained an optimistic but realistic outlook, sought and accepted social support, and imitated sturdy role models. Most also relied upon their own inner moral compass, turned to religious or spiritual practices, and found a way to accept that which they could not change. Many attended to their health and well-being, and trained intensively to stay physically fit, mentally sharp, and emotionally strong. And most were active prob-lem solvers who looked for meaning and opportunity in the midst of adversity and sometimes even found humor in the darkness. Finally, all of the resilient people we interviewed accepted, to an impressive degree, responsibility for their own emotional well-being, and many used their traumatic experiences as a platform for personal growth.

We recognize that this list of what we call "resilience factors" (i.e. realistic optimism, facing fear, moral compass, religion and spirituality, social support, resilient role models, physical fitness, brain fitness, cognitive and emotional flexibility, and meaning and purpose) is by no means definitive or complete and that other factors certainly contribute to stress hardiness. We focus on the above-mentioned resilience factors because they were the ones most often described as crucial, and sometimes even life-saving, for the individuals we interviewed. In upcoming chapters, we will discuss each of these factors in greater detail.

Most of us will never become a prisoner of war or step on a landmine, but we will inevitably face our own stressors, traumas, and tragedies. Today, for example, many people throughout the world face prolonged unemployment, financial distress, poverty, homelessness, separation from loved ones, medical and mental illness, and a host of other challenges. Fortunately, to withstand, overcome, and grow from these experiences, we don't need to have superior genes, take a "tough as nails" approach to life, or train with the Special Forces. But we do need to prepare ourselves, for life has a way of surprising us with adversity when we least expect it. As journalist Diane L. Coutu learned from her research on resilience for a *Harvard Business Review* article, top-level business executives invariably prize resilience in people they seek to hire. One CEO underscored its importance this way: "More than education, more than experience, more than training, a person's level of resilience will determine who succeeds and who fails. That's true in the cancer ward, it's true in the Olympics, and it's true in the boardroom" (Coutu, 2002, p. 47). We know of no better way to learn about tried-and-true methods for becoming more resilient than to listen to, be inspired by, and follow the advice of resilient people who have already "been there."

## How Resilient Are We?

Where are we today? How resilient are we as individuals, communities, and societies? In the world today, as throughout history, millions of people who are exposed to stress and trauma respond with extraordinary resilience. Recent inspiring examples include individual, family, community, national and even international responses to tragedies such as the World Trade Center terrorist attack of 9/11; the 2004 Indian Ocean earthquake and tsunami; Hurricane Katrina; the Japan earthquake, tsunami, and resulting nuclear crisis; the Boston Marathon bombing; and the mass shooting at the Pulse nightclub in Orlando.

Despite such impressive displays of strength and hardiness, some social critics point to recent trends in attitudes and behaviors that raise questions about the value that some societies place on building and maintaining resilience.

Consider these lifestyle statistics in the United States:

- 80 percent of American adults don't get the recommended amount of exercise (at least 2.5 hours of moderate-intensity aerobic exercise each week or 1.25 hours of vigorous-intensity activity, or a combination of both; as well as muscle-strengthening activity like weight-lifting or push-ups at least twice per week). About 40 percent of American adults engage in no regular physical exercise, and about half of the 60 percent who do exercise say their exercise is only moderate, as opposed to vigorous (Saad, 2008).
- More than one-third of American adults are obese (body mass index [BMI] 30 or higher), and another third are overweight (BMI 25–29.9) (Ogden *et al.*, 2014). Among children and adolescents, 17 percent are obese (Ogden *et al.*, 2014).
- The 2014 United States Report Card on Physical Activity for Children and Youth gave them a D–. For sedentary behaviors they got a D, spending over 7 hours per day at sedentary activities. A 2003 study found that school physical education classes provide an average of just 25 minutes per week of vigorous activity for third-graders. The study recommended 60 minutes of moderate-to-vigorous physical activity per day, but only one-quarter of youth ages 6–15 met those guidelines.
- Approximately one-third of Americans have abused or been dependent on alcohol at some time in their lives (Hasin *et al.*, 2007).
- For many years, the American Academy of Pediatrics (2001, 2013) has recommended no more than 1–2 hours a day of total entertainment screen time (television, computer, etc.) for children aged 2 and older, and no screen time for children under age 2; but a 2010 Kaiser Family Foundation report found children spending an average of 7.5 hours per day watching television, playing video games, and using computers. Further, that same report found that children and teens said their parents had "no rules" about how much time they spent with electronic devices.
- A 2009 study found that 70 percent of US children have insufficient levels of vitamin D, the "sunshine vitamin," which we get from being outdoors and which has a protective effect against cardiovascular problems (Kumar *et al.*, 2009).

The lack of resilience is so striking that it has been framed as a national security weakness. In 2009 and 2010, a nonpartisan nonprofit national security organization of retired generals, admirals, and other military leaders released reports titled *Ready, Willing, and Unable to Serve*, and *Too Fat to Fight*, citing a startling statistic: Approximately 75 percent of Americans age 17 to 24 are no longer eligible to join the military. The three most common reasons for ineligibility are poor physical fitness (e.g., obesity), failure to graduate from high school, and a criminal record. Military leadership is concerned that our country's military readiness will be at risk unless we find a way to increase resilience in American youth.

In his 2003 book *The Progress Paradox: How Life Gets Better While People Feel Worse*, Brookings Institution fellow Gregg Easterbrook points out that while in material terms the Western standard of living has improved greatly in recent decades, our subjective well-being and happiness have declined. Psychologists Jean Twenge and W Keith Campbell address an attitudinal change in *The Narcissism Epidemic: Living in the Age of Entitlement* (2009), pointing to a societal increase in a "me first" attitude, a lack of caring relationships, and a need for attention and material wealth that is somehow never satisfied.

Other authors – Robert Putnam in *Bowling Alone*, Christopher Lasch in *The Culture of Narcissism*, and David Riesman in *The Lonely Crowd*, to name a few – have expressed concern about the lack of social connections and community spirit in today's society. Dutch researcher Geert Hofstede, among other social psychologists, has categorized the United States as a highly individualistic society, where becoming a "self-made" man or woman is more highly valued than contributing to the common good. While this individualistic spirit may have roots extending back to the early days of the American republic, it seems to be enacted in a more literal way today than in the past. According to the US Census Bureau (2006), the proportion of single-person households increased from 17 percent in 1970 to 26 percent in 2005. In 2005, only 1 in 10 of the nation's households contained five or more people, down from 1 in 5 in 1970. The decrease in household size has been accompanied by dwindling membership in service clubs, religious congregations, and workers' organizations. Psychologist Shigehiro Oishi (2010) refers to "duty-free friendships" as a byproduct of our decreased investment in interpersonal relationships. As *New York Times* columnist Roger Cohen wrote in 2010:

> Community – a stable job, shared national experience, extended family, labor unions – has vanished or eroded. In its place have come a frenzied individualism, solipsistic screen-gazing, the disembodied pleasures of social networking and the à-la-carte life as defined by 600 TV channels and a gazillion blogs. Feelings of anxiety and inadequacy grow in the lonely chamber of self-absorption and projection.

So how resilient are we? Are we becoming too self-absorbed and too ready to complain about the unfairness of life instead of equipping ourselves to take action to improve our lives and the lives of those around us? Are we adequately preparing ourselves, our families, our children, and our communities to weather the inevitable storms ahead and to thrive in times of stress and hardship?

## Applying the Science of Resilience

In this book, we want to share with readers what we have learned from our interviews and from academic research about resilience. We believe that this book can benefit readers from all walks of life, including those who are currently coping with a trauma and those who have a loved one coping with a trauma; teachers, counselors, therapists, and medical professionals; and anyone who understands the need to prepare for the inevitable stresses and traumas of life.

We have organized the book into chapters focusing on specific resilience factors: facing fear, optimism, social support, and so on. Although these resilience factors overlap and interact with one another, we found it helpful to examine each one separately. The factors are described through the experiences and personal reflections of the highly resilient survivors whom we interviewed. Survivors also describe real-life methods for implementing, practicing, and benefiting from the resilience factors. In addition to providing excerpts and insights from our interviews, we interweave the latest relevant scientific research on the topic. The evidence we cite comes from the fields of psychology, sociology, neurobiology, and medicine. This evidence lends support to the strategies and recommendations for enhancing resilience that our interviewees described. It also helps to demystify the process of physical, cognitive, and emotional strengthening. There is a science behind resilience training, and by learning and practicing what is currently known, people can increase their ability to cope well in the face of stress and adversity.

## Resilience and Human Physiology

Since resilience is fundamentally related to the experience and management of stress, throughout this book we refer to various parts of the brain, the nervous system, and the endocrine system: critical components of the stress response. We will discuss the following key brain regions:

- The amygdala, which is associated with fear and alarm; it plays a central role in fear conditioning and in triggering raw emotions and the "fight or flight" response.
- The prefrontal cortex, which is often referred to as the brain's "executive center," facilitates planning and rational decision-making; it helps to

regulate emotions and acts to keep the amygdala (the "fear and alarm center") in check.

- The hippocampus, which plays a critical role in learning, forming new memories, and regulating the stress response; more so than many other brain structures, it is vulnerable to the effects of chronic stress.
- The anterior cingulate cortex, which plays an important role in our ability to focus attention, detect and monitor errors and conflicts, assess the importance of emotional and motivational information, and regulate emotions; it is connected both to the prefrontal cortex and the amygdala.
- The anterior insula, which is located in the fold of the cerebral cortex that marks the boundary between the frontal and temporal lobes; it is involved in functions related to emotions, and aids in the brain's awareness of the body's internal physical state.
- The nucleus accumbens, sometimes referred to as the "pleasure center," plays a central role in the brain's reward circuitry; in association with the ventral tegmental area, it mediates the experience of reward and punishment, and is associated with the pleasurable effects of food, sex, and drug abuse.

We occasionally also mention the limbic system. This term refers to the inner portion of the brain – located beneath the cortex – which is involved in emotion, memory, and other functions. It includes the amygdala, hippocampus, and a number of other structures and regions. Although the limbic system is technically neither a system nor a structure, the term provides a useful shorthand for referring to this area of the brain.

In addition to these brain regions, there are several other major systems in the body that respond to stress. One is the autonomic nervous system, which is composed of two parts: the sympathetic nervous system (SNS), which mobilizes the body under conditions of stress; and the parasympathetic nervous system (PNS), which conserves resources and maintains functioning under normal nonstressful conditions. For healthy functioning, it is beneficial for the SNS to have a robust response to stress and challenge, but also for the SNS to return to baseline rapidly after the stressful event is over. Another major system is the hypothalamic–pituitary–adrenal axis (HPA axis), which responds to stress with a complex set of reactions involving the hypothalamus, the pituitary gland, and the adrenal glands.

Throughout the book we will also refer to various hormones and neurotransmitters that are involved in the stress response and resilience (McEwen, 2007; Southwick *et al.*, 2008):

- Cortisol is a stress hormone released through activation of the HPA axis. It produces energy by converting food into fat and glucose (a form of sugar). It also temporarily bolsters the immune system.

- Epinephrine, also known as adrenaline, is part of the SNS. It is released by the adrenal glands under conditions of stress and accelerates heart rate, constricts blood vessels and dilates air passages as part of the SNS fight-or-flight response.
- Norepinephrine, also known as noradrenaline, is also part of the SNS. It facilitates alerting and alarm reactions in the brain and is critical for responding to danger and for remembering emotional and fearful events.
- Serotonin is involved in the regulation of mood, as well as sleep, appetite, and other functions.
- Dopamine is associated with pleasurable feelings and plays a key role in the reward systems of the brain. For this reason, it is an important factor in cravings and addictive behaviors.
- Neuropeptide Y (NPY) is associated with decreasing anxiety and hastening return to baseline after the nervous system reacts to stress.
- Oxytocin is associated with maternal behaviors, pair bonding, social communication, trust, social support, and anxiety reduction.
- Brain-derived neurotrophic factor (BDNF) acts to support the nervous system through the repair of existing neurons and growth of new ones.

# Genetics

Genes play a central role in how we respond to stress. In a longitudinal study involving 7,500 adult twins – both identical (monozygotic) and fraternal (dizygotic) – Ananda Amstadter, John Myers, and Kenneth Kendler of Virginia Commonwealth University (2014) assessed resilience and response to stressful life events (SLEs). They found that genes and environmental events each contributed to resilience; in fact, the magnitude of their respective contributions was approximately equal. "Roughly half of the contribution of variation in the latent level of resilience could be accounted for by [events and actions taken by the individual] that had an enduring effect" (p. 278). In addition, mildly stressful experiences ("certain doses of stress" [p. 279]) can have the effect of building resilience, similar to how physical exercise builds muscle.

DNA research is beginning to investigate how variations in our genes affect the way that we respond to stress. Researchers have found preliminary evidence that certain genes are associated with resilience, including genes related to the SNS and to the HPA axis. For example, there is evidence that the SNS response to stress in the form of noradrenaline is influenced by variations of the alpha-2 adrenoreceptor gene. In a study of healthy volunteers, Alex Neumeister and colleagues (2005) found that some individuals inherit a specific variation of the alpha-2 adrenoreceptor gene (i.e. alpha-2cDel322–325-AR). People with this gene variation, compared with other people, had higher levels of norepinephrine at baseline, a greater increase in norepinephrine and anxiety when stressed, and a slower return of norepinephrine to baseline after termination of stress. The unusually robust activity of norepinephrine, and the slow return to baseline, in individuals with this genetic variation could make them more vulnerable to stress and thus less resilient.

The norepinephrine response to stress may also be affected by variations in the neuropeptide Y gene. In one study, individuals with a particular variation in this gene, a variation that is associated with low production of neuropeptide Y, experienced greater activation of the amygdala and greater anxiety when exposed to threat-related stimuli compared to subjects without this gene variation (Zhou *et al.*, 2008). As noted above, neuropeptide Y is associated with decreasing anxiety and restoring calm after stress. When stress is high, neuropeptide Y is released; this helps to inhibit the further release of norepinephrine so that the SNS does not "overshoot" and instead rapidly returns to baseline.

Israel Liberzon and colleagues at the University of Michigan (Liberzon *et al.*, 2014) reported a pair of longitudinal studies comprising nearly 3,000 subjects that identified a specific gene–environment interaction related to PTSD. Two different variants of a gene called *ADRB2* were found to have different effects on how people responded to and recovered from childhood adversity (physical abuse, sexual abuse, emotional abuse, and witnessing violence between parents). *ADRB2* is a gene for producing the beta-2 adrenergic receptor in the SNS, a major transducer of the fight-or-flight response. People who had inherited one variation of this gene, and who were exposed to childhood adversity, had increased likelihood of developing PTSD after experiencing a trauma in adulthood. Conversely, people who had inherited the other type were more resistant to developing PTSD, displaying greater resilience after exposure to trauma in adulthood, even if their childhood adversity was significantly worse than that of people in the "vulnerable" group. The "resilient" variant of the gene helps to prevent overaction of norepinephrine in the fight-or-flight response, a key component of PTSD.

Continuing in this line of research but focusing on the HPA axis, Laura Watkins and our research team at the National Center for PTSD (2016) assessed more than 1500 military veterans who reported a history of child abuse. They found that variants of a gene called *FKBP5* had similar effects: individuals with the "resilient" variant of this gene were less likely to develop PTSD after a trauma in adulthood, compared to those with the "vulnerable" variant. The *FKBP5* gene is involved in regulating the HPA axis and is related to the rate at which cortisol returns to normal after a stressor. Apparently the "resilient" gene variant helps people to turn down their stress response and recover more quickly after a stressful experience.

In addition to gene variants that affect the SNS and HPA axis, variants affecting the serotonin and dopamine systems have also been investigated in relation to traumatic stress and resilience. Gene variants related to these systems may affect the relative efficiency of the stress response (Mehta *et al.*, 2011; Skelton *et al.*, 2011). In general, an optimal stress response activates rapidly in response to threat, rises high enough to respond appropriately to danger but not so high as to cause incapacitating anxiety and fear, and then deactivates in a timely fashion. Hypoactive or hyperactive neurobiological stress systems tend to be maladaptive (Feder *et al.*, 2009).

It is important to emphasize that resilience to stress and susceptibility to develop PTSD undoubtedly result from complex interactions between multiple genes and multiple environmental factors rather than any single gene variant (Norrholm & Ressler, 2009).

# Epigenetics

In recent years researchers have made gains in understanding exactly how the environment influences our genes through the study of epigenetics. A variety of internal and external environmental events (e.g. stress, social support, fears) can trigger biochemical reactions (e.g. methylation) that then turn genes on or turn them off. These processes are dynamic and potentially reversible.

When a gene is "turned on" it directs the making of gene products (e.g. proteins). However, when a gene is "turned off" these gene products are no longer produced. In other words, various stimuli in our internal and external environment can initiate biochemical processes that either activate our genes or silence them.

For example, recent animal studies (Zhang, 2012) have shown that if a mother rat provides only low levels of licking and grooming to her pups – the equivalent of neglectful parenting in the rat world – the pups will exhibit increased susceptibility to stress throughout their lives. On the other hand, attentive maternal care, as reflected by high levels of licking and grooming, can contribute to later stress resilience. The effects of maternal licking and grooming appear to be mediated, in part, by epigenetic changes in gene expression. In research conducted in the laboratory of Michael Meaney, variations in maternal care have been associated with variations in expression of glucocorticoid receptors and hippocampal sensitivity to stress (Zhang, 2012). Similar epigenetic effects of maternal care – and other lifetime experiences – on later vulnerability or resilience to stress are likely to "hold up in humans" (Nestler, 2012).

A variety of environmental events, including stress, social interactions, and drug use, can cause epigenetic changes in gene expression (Dudley, 2011).

Although much remains to be learned, the rapidly expanding field of epigenetics may soon help us to better understand the origins of stress vulnerability and discover ways to manage it (Nestler, 2012). It may also help us to better understand resilience and the mechanisms by which training can enhance factors associated with resilience (e.g. exercise, social support, cognitive reframing). And as noted by psychopharmacologist Steven Stahl (2011), "psychotherapy can now be conceptualized not only by its classic psychodynamic principles, but also indeed as a neurobiological probe capable of inducing epigenetic changes in brain circuits, not unlike the ultimate actions of psychotropic drugs."

# Neuroplasticity

In several chapters of the book, we mention neuroplasticity. Neuroplasticity refers to "the ability of the nervous system to respond to intrinsic or extrinsic stimuli by reorganizing its structure, function and connections" (Cramer *et al.*, 2011). While many of us think of the brain as an organ that remains essentially unchanged during adulthood, neuroscientists have found that brain structure changes from moment to moment, hour to hour, day to day. Brain structure is neither fixed nor static but instead highly plastic, and like muscles in the body, the brain can be strengthened or weakened depending on how it is used. When cells in the brain are actively used, they transmit their messages more efficiently and form more connections with other cells. On the other hand, when brain cells are not stimulated, they die and are pruned away. As with other regions of the body, the well-known adage "use it or lose it" also applies to the brain.

In research dating back to the mid-1990s, neuroscientists have found strong evidence of plastic changes in the brain among professional musicians and others with extensive musical training (Münte, Altenmüller & Jäncke, 2002). For example, Elbert and colleagues (1995) found that in professional players of string instruments (violin, viola, cello, and bass) "the cortical representation of the digits of the left hand (the fingering hand) was larger" than in control subjects, whereas the right hand (which holds the bow and is not involved in fingering) did not display such differences. Studying brain activity in string players as well as keyboard players and nonmusicians, Rüber, Lindenberg, and Schlaug (2015) found differences in the structure of not just gray-matter motor areas, but white-matter fibers that connect brain areas. In string players, these were larger in the right hemisphere (controlling the left hand), but in keyboard players they were larger in both brain hemispheres. Choi *et al.* (2015) studied wind instrument players and found enlargement in areas of the brain responsible for lip movement. Further, the greater the number of years of musical training, the more pronounced were the brain changes.

Another line of research involves mindfulness-based stress reduction, a practice related to the mindfulness meditation that is part of some traditional Eastern religions. Omar Singleton and colleagues (2014) used magnetic resonance imaging (MRI) to examine the brains of volunteers before and after an eight-week program of mindfulness-based stress reduction, "defined as the nonjudgmental awareness of experiences in the present moment" (p. 1). They found an increase in the size of certain brain regions that produce neurotransmitters such as serotonin and norepinephrine; these are critically involved in regulating arousal, attention, mood, reward, and learning. In addition, the volunteers scored higher on an assessment of psychological well-being after the eight-week program.

Each of us, to some degree, has the power to change the structure and function of his or her brain. As noted by well-known author Deepak Chopra, MD and Harvard University neuroscientist Rudolph Tanzi, Ph.D. "Neuroplasticity is better than mind over matter. It's mind turning into matter as your thoughts create new neuronal growth" (Chopra & Tanzi, 2012, pg 52). The key is activity. By repeatedly activating specific areas of the brain, we can strengthen those areas. In other words, by systematically following the advice of the POWs, Special Forces instructors, and other resilient women and men in this book, virtually anyone can become more stress-resilient. That's what we have tried to do. Both of us love challenges, and now when we find ourselves doubting our ability to overcome major obstacles, we often remember a conversation that we had with one of the former POWs, Special Forces instructors, or civilians whom we interviewed. And then we try to follow their advice by repeatedly imitating a specific attitude, style of thinking, emotion, or behavior that helped them overcome their own stress and trauma. It helps us.

# Bouncing Back Is a Choice – but the Choice Is Easier for Some

When we began this project, we assumed that highly resilient people were somehow special, perhaps genetically gifted. We assumed that resilience was relatively rare, reserved for a select group of unique individuals. But we were wrong. Resilience is common (Masten, 2001). It can be witnessed all around us, and for most people it can be enhanced through learning and training. Millions of people all over the world exhibit resilience in their responses to challenging events and circumstances of all kinds. Most of us have been taught to believe that stress is bad. We have learned to see stress as our enemy, something that we must avoid or reduce. But the truth is, when stress can be managed, it tends to be very good and even necessary for health and growth. Without it, the mind and body weaken. If we can learn to harness stress it can serve as a catalyst for developing greater strength and even greater wisdom.

And yet we need to acknowledge that building resilience and bouncing back is easier for some than for others. Individuals who are temporarily (or, in some cases, permanently) unable to think clearly or regulate their moods will have difficulty putting into practice the advice in this book. For example, someone who is experiencing an episode of major depression will be handicapped by the profound sadness and sense of hopelessness, lack of energy, and loss of interest in life that characterize this disorder. As another example, someone who has suffered a traumatic brain injury may have particular difficulties with cognitive strategies and/or emotional challenges. People with these kinds of serious conditions who want to practice the skills associated with resilience would certainly be advised to work with a professional who is trained in helping with their specific condition.

Even for people who do not suffer from severe medical and/or psychological conditions, the path to bounce back is steeper for some than for others. Those of us with resources such as financial security, a high level of education, an interesting and rewarding career, and strong social networks are able to leverage those resources, whereas people who lack resources may fall into what psychologist Stevan Hobfoll (2001) calls a "loss spiral." For example, if a family already under financial strain loses its primary breadwinner, the surviving family members may be forced to scramble for basic necessities such as food and a place to live at the same time that they are grieving; further, this struggle may potentially lead to additional traumas such as those associated with living in a high-crime neighborhood. In contrast, a financially secure family will have the resources to address their grief and loss in various ways (e.g. by paying for counseling, hosting a funeral to honor the loved one, and perhaps taking time off from work or school to re-evaluate their life priorities). One family that loses its home in a hurricane will have no place to live, while another family has the option to move in with relatives, and still another family will be fortunate enough to own a second house.

On October 1, 2015, 16-year-old Cheyeanne Fitzgerald was attending her fourth day of classes at Umpqua Community College in Roseburg, Oregon when a student brandishing a high-powered rifle entered her classroom and shot 16 people before taking his own life. Cheyeanne, one of nine survivors, was shot in the back; she suffered a punctured lung and pierced kidney – which had to be removed (Healy & Holson, 2015) – in addition to injuries to her spine and many internal organs. Visiting her 3 weeks after the shooting and a week after her hospital discharge (Whitcomb, 2015), a reporter found her requiring round-the-clock care for her physical condition. The home where she lived with her mother was decorated with balloons, teddy bears, and greeting cards, but her mother had been unable to afford a proper hospital bed, wheelchair, or walker. Instead, they were making do with donated and garage-sale equipment (Saslow, 2015). Cheyeanne had been given a booklet called *"Creating a Safe Place to Recover*" and was eligible for a victim restitution payment of $7,200. Apart from one session with a Veterans Affairs psychologist, she had had little opportunity to talk about the horrific event and the emotional scars she suffered. She was hypervigilant and startled by unexpected noises, had fits of anger, and expressed the type of "survivor guilt" that is common after such an event: "I just lied there. I didn't save anybody" (Saslow, 2015).

Cheyeanne is the youngest of three children, the first in her family to attend college. Her parents are divorced and her mother, Bonnie, had to leave her job as a waitress to care for Cheyeanne full-time. Bonnie has faced many difficulties of her own, requiring multiple heart surgeries; at 52 she was on her fourth pacemaker. Her older children had problems with lawbreaking and substance addiction. Getting Cheyeanne out of the house for a change of scenery has been a major struggle. Though the Roseburg community has displayed banners with slogans such as "Roseburg Will Prevail," there has been little support for the needs of individual survivors recovering from their wounds, physical and emotional. Cheyeanne and Bonnie have been encouraged to "think positive," but such thoughts and phrases are of limited use (Saslow, 2015).

When we advocate for resilience, we believe that most of us can choose to fight back after a trauma and attempt to right ourselves. However, we must emphasize that some people lack access to support and resources that make it easier, or even possible, to do so. This does not mean that those with scarce resources should give up, but rather recognizes that they will have a more difficult road to travel. Understanding these limitations may allow us to be more patient with ourselves or with others who are striving to recover from trauma.

We sincerely hope that the words and deeds of the generous individuals in this book will be as inspirational to you as they have been to us, and that these individuals will serve as role models for you as you face the upcoming challenges of your life.

# References

Alvarez, L. (2008). Nearly a fifth of war veterans report mental disorders, a private study finds. *New York Times*, April 18. Accessed February 15, 2010 at www.nytimes.com/2008/04/18/us/18vets.html

American Academy of Pediatrics (2001). Children, adolescents, and television. *Pediatrics*, 107(2), 423–426.

American Academy of Pediatrics (2013). *Pediatric Clinical Practice Guidelines & Policies: A Compendium of Evidence-Based Research for Pediatric Practice*, 13th edn. Elk Grove Village, IL: American Academy of Pediatrics.

American Psychiatric Association (2013). *Diagnostic and Statistical Manual of Mental Disorders*, 4th edn. Arlington, VA: American Psychiatric Association.

American Psychological Association (2010). *The Road to Resilience*. Washington, DC: American Psychological Association. Accessed June 25, 2010 at www.apa.org/helpcenter/road-resilience.aspx

Amstadter, A. B., Myers, J. M. & Kendler, K. S. (2014). Psychiatric resilience: longitudinal twin study. *The British Journal of Psychiatry: The Journal of Mental Science*, 205(4), 275–280.

Bartone, P. T. (1999). Hardiness protects against war-related stress in Army Reserve forces. *Consulting Psychology Journal: Practice and Research*, 51(2), 72–82.

Bartone, P. T. (2007). Test–retest reliability of the Dispositional Resilience Scale-15, a brief hardiness scale. *Psychological Reports*, 101(1), 943–944.

Bonanno, G. A. (2004). Loss, trauma, and human resilience: Have we underestimated the human capacity to thrive after extremely aversive events? *American Psychologist*, 59, 20–28.

Bonanno, G. A. (2005). Resilience in the face of potential trauma. *Current Directions in Psychological Science*, 14, 135–138.

Bremner, J. D., Southwick, S. M., Johnson, D. R., Yehuda, R. & Charney, D. S. (1993). Childhood physical abuse in combat-related post-traumatic stress disorder in Vietnam veterans. *American Journal of Psychiatry*, 150, 235–239.

Bremner, J. D., Narayan, M., Staib, L. H. *et al.* (1999). Neural correlates of memories of childhood sexual abuse in women with and without posttraumatic stress disorder. *American Journal of Psychiatry*, 156, 1787–1795.

Brooker, K. (2002). Starting over. *Fortune*, January 21, 50–68.

Carver, C. S. (1998). Resilience and thriving. Issues, models, and linkages. *Journal of Social Issues*, 54, 245–266.

Centers for Disease Control and Prevention (2010) FastStats: Obesity and Overweight. Accessed February 24, 2010 at www.cdc.gov/nchs/fastats/overwt.htm

Centers for Disease Control and Prevention (2013). Adult participation in aerobic and muscle-strengthening physical activities – United States, 2011. *MMWR. Morbidity and Mortality Weekly Report*, 62(17) 326–30.

Charney, D. S., Deutch, A., Krystal, J. H., Southwick, S. M. & Davis, M. (1993). Psychobiological mechanisms of posttraumatic stress disorder. *Archives of General Psychiatry*, 50, 294–305.

Charney, D. S., Nagy, L. M., Bremner, J. D. *et al.* (1996). Neurobiological mechanisms of human anxiety. In B. S. Fogel, R. B. Schiffler & S. M. Rao (eds.) *Neuropsychiatry*, pp. 257–278. Baltimore, MD: Williams & Wilkins.

Choi, U. S., Sung, Y. W., Hong, S., Chung, J. Y. & Ogawa, S. (2015). Structural and functional plasticity specific to musical training with wind instruments. *Frontiers in Human Neuroscience*, 9, 597.

Chopra, D. & Tanzi, R. E. (2012). *Super Brain: Unleashing the Explosive Power of Your Mind to Maximize Health, Happiness and Spiritual Well-Being*. New York, NY: Random House.

Christeson, W., Taggart, A. D. & Messner-Zidell, S. (2009). *Ready, Willing, and Unable to Serve: 75 Percent of Young Adults Cannot Join the Military: Early Education Across America Is Needed to Ensure National Security.* Washington, DC: Mission: Readiness.

Christeson, W., Taggart, A. D., Messner-Zidell, S. & Mission: Readiness (U.S.) (2010). *Too Fat to Fight: Retired Military Leaders Want Junk Food Out of America's Schools: A Report by Mission: Readiness.* Washington, DC: Mission: Readiness.

Christeson, W., Kiernan, M., Cusick, J. *et al.* (2012). *Still Too Fat to Fight: A Follow-Up Report to Too Fat to Fight.* Washington, DC: Mission: Readiness.

Clark, B. (2006). A survivor's story. PBS Nova interview transcript. Accessed March 9, 2010 at www.pbs.org/wgbh/nova/wtc/above.html

Cohen, R. (2010). Op-Ed columnist: The Narcissus society. *New York Times,* February 22.

Connor, K. M. & Davidson, J. R. (2003). Development of a new resilience scale: The Connor–Davidson Resilience Scale (CD-RISC). *Depression and Anxiety,* 18, 76–82.

Coutu, D. L. (2002). How resilience works. *Harvard Business Review,* May, 46–55.

Cramer, S. C., Sur, M., Dobkin, B. H. *et al.* (2011). Harnessing neuroplasticity for clinical applications. *Brain,* 134(6), 1591–1601.

Dao, J. (2010). At War: Notes from the front lines: Presidential condolences and troop suicides. *New York Times,* February 1. Accessed February 15, 2010 at http://atwar .blogs.nytimes.com/2010/02/01/presidential-condolences-and-troop-suicides/

Dudley, K. J., Xiang Li, Kobor, M. S., Kippin, T. E. & Bredy, T. W. (2011). Epigenetic mechanisms mediating vulnerability and resilience to psychiatric disorders. *Neuroscience and Biobehavioral Reviews,* 35, 1544–1551.

Dwyer, J., Lipton, E., Flynn, K., Glanz, J. & Fessenden, F. (2002). 102 minutes: Fighting to live as the towers died. *New York Times,* May 26. Accessed October 13, 2017 at http://www.nytimes.com/2002/05/26/nyregion/fighting-to-live-as-the-towers-died.html

Easterbrook, G. (2003). *The Progress Paradox: How Life Gets Better While People Feel Worse.* New York, NY: Random House.

Elbert, T., Pantev, C., Wienbruch, C. & Rockstroh, B. (1995). Increased cortical representation of the fingers of the left hand in string players. *Science,* 270(5234), 305–307.

Feder, A., Nestler, E. J. & Charney, D. (2009). Psychobiology and molecular genetics of resilience. *Nature Reviews,* 10, 446–466.

Giller, E. (1999). What is psychological trauma? This article originated as a workshop presentation at the Annual Conference of the Maryland Mental Hygiene Administration, "*Passages to Prevention: Prevention across Life's Spectrum,*" May 1999. Accessed February 24, 2010 at www.sidran.org/sub.cfm? contentID=88&sectionid=4

Guarino, Col. Larry (1990). *A POW's Story: 2801 Days in Hanoi.* New York, NY: Random House.

Hasin, D. S., Stinson, F. S., Ogburn, E. & Grant, B. F. (2007). Prevalence, correlates, disability, and comorbidity of DSM-IV alcohol abuse and dependence in the United States: Results from the National Epidemiologic Survey on Alcohol and Related Conditions. *Archives of General Psychiatry*, 64(7), 830–842.

Healy, J. & Holson, L. M. (2015). Oregon gunman's father dismayed by lack of gun legislation. *New York Times*, October 3. Retrieved from www.nytimes.com/2015/ 10/04/us/death-of-gunman-in-oregon-college-shootings-is-ruled-suicide .html?_r=0

Hobfoll, S. E. (2001). The influence of culture, community, and the nested-self in the stress process: Advancing conservation of resources theory. *Applied Psychology: An International Review*, 50(3), 337–421.

Jacobsen, L. K., Southwick, S. M. & Kosten, T. R. (2001). Substance use disorders in patients with posttraumatic stress disorder: A review of the literature. *American Journal of Psychiatry*, 158, 1184–1190.

Johnson, D. C., Polusny, J. A., Erbes, C. *et al.* (2008). The response to stressful experiences scale (RSES). *Military Medicine*, 176(2) 161–169.

Kessler, R. C., Sonnega, A., Bromet, E., Hughes, M. & Nelson, C. B. (1995). Post-traumatic stress disorder in the National Comorbidity Survey. *Archives of General Psychiatry*, 52, 1048–1060.

Kobasa, S. C. (1979). Stressful life events, personality, and health: An inquiry into hardiness. *Journal of Personality and Social Psychology*, 37, 1–11.

Kobasa, S. C., Maddi, S. R. & Kahn, S. (1982). Hardiness and health: A prospective study. *Journal of Personality and Social Psychology*, 42, 168–177.

Kroft, S. (2001). Sandler O'Neill fights back. *CBS News*, October 4. Accessed December 4, 2009 at www.cbsnews.com/stories/2001/10/04/60minutes/ main313589.shtml

Kumar, J., Muntner, P., Kaskel, F. J., Hailpern, S. M. & Melamed, M. L. (2009). Prevalence and associations of 25-hydroxyvitamin D deficiency in US children: NHANES 2001–2004. *Pediatrics*, 124, e362. DOI:10.1542/peds.2009–0051.

Layne, C. M., Warren, J. S., Watson, P. J. & Shalev, A. Y. (2007). Risk, vulnerability, resistance, and resilience: Toward an integrative conceptualization of posttraumatic adaptation. In T. K. M. Friedman & P. Resick (eds.), *Handbook of PTSD: Science and Practice*, pp. 497–520. New York, NY: Guilford Press.

Liberzon, I., King, A. P., Ma, S. T. *et al.* (2014). Interaction of the *ADRB2* gene polymorphism with childhood trauma in predicting adult symptoms of posttraumatic stress disorder. *JAMA Psychiatry*, 71(10), 1174–1182.

Litz, B. T. (2005). Has resilience to severe trauma been underestimated? *American Psychologist*, 60, 262.

Lukas, E. S. (1984). *Meaningful Living: A Logotheraphy Guide to Health*. New York, NY: Grove Press.

Luthar, S. S. (2006). Resilience in development: A synthesis of research across five decades. In D. Cicchetti & D. J. Cohen (eds.), *Developmental Psychopathology*, Vol. 3: *Risk Disorder, and Adaptation*, 2nd edn, pp. 740–795. New York, NY: Wiley.

Luthar, S. S., Cicchetti, D. & Becker, B. (2000). The construct of resilience: A critical evaluation and guidelines for future work. *Child Development*, 71, 543–562.

Maddi, S. R. (2005). On hardiness and other pathways to resilience. *American Psychologist*, 60(3), 261–262.

Maguen, S., Lucenko, B. A., Reger, M. A. *et al.* (2010). The impact of reported direct and indirect killing on mental health symptoms in Iraq War veterans. *Journal of Traumatic Stress*, 23(1), 86–90.

Malik, M. L., Connor, K. M., Sutherland, S. M. *et al.* (1999). Quality of life and posttraumatic stress disorder: A pilot study assessing changes in sf-36 scores before and after treatment in a placebo-controlled trial of Fluoxetine. *Journal of Traumatic Stress*, 12(2), 387–393. DOI:10.1023/A:1024745030140

Masten, A. S. (2001). Ordinary magic: Resilience processes in development. *American Psychologist*, 56, 227–238.

McEwen, B. S. (2007). Physiology and neurobiology of stress and adaptation: Central role of the brain. *Physiological Reviews*, 87, 873–904.

McKay, M. J. (2002). '60 Minutes' looks at September 11. *CBS News*, September 5. Accessed September 2, 2010 at www.cbsnews. com/stories/2002/09/05/60min utes/main520965.shtml

Mehta, D., Gonik, M., Klengel, T. *et al.* (2011). Using polymorphisms in *FKBP5* to define biologically distinct subtypes of posttraumatic stress disorder: evidence from endocrine and gene expression studies. *Archives of General Psychiatry*, 68(9), 901–910.

Münte, T. F., Altenmüller, E. & Jäncke, L. (2002). The musician's brain as a model of neuroplasticity. *Nature Reviews Neuroscience*, 3(6), 473–478.

Nader, P. R. (2003). Frequency and intensity of activity of third-grade children in physical education. National Institute of Child Health and Human Development Study of Early Child Care and Youth Development Network. *Archives of Pediatric and Adolescent Medicine*, 157, 185–190. Accessed 2010 at http://aappolicy.aappublications.org/cgi/content/full/pediatrics;117/5/1834

National Center for PTSD, Department of Veterans Affairs (2009). How common is PTSD? Accessed January 2009 at www.ptsd.va.gov/

Nestler, E. J. (2012). Epigenetics: Stress makes its molecular mark. *Nature*, 490, 171–172.

Neumeister, A., Charney, D.S., Belfer, I. *et al.* (2005). Sympathoneural and adrenomedullary functional effects of alpha 2C-adrenoreceptor gene polymorphism in healthy humans. *Pharmacogenetics and Genomics*, 15, 143–149.

Nocera, J. (2006). After 5 years, his voice can still crack. *New York Times*, September 9.

Norrholm, S. D. & Ressler, K. J. (2009). Genetics of anxiety and trauma-related disorders. *Neuroscience*, 164(1), 272–287.

Norris, F. H. (1992). Epidemiology of trauma: Frequency and impact of different potentially traumatic events on different demographic groups. *Journal of Consulting and Climnical Psychology*, 60, 409–418.

Norris, F. H. & Sloane, L. B. (2007). The epidemiology of trauma and PTSD. In M. J. Friedman, T. M. Keane & P. A. Resick (eds.), *Handbook of PTSD*, pp. 78–98. New York, NY: Guilford Press.

Occupational Safety and Health Administration, U.S. Department of Labor (2002). *A Dangerous Worksite: The World Trade Center.* Washington, DC: author. Accessed March 12, 2010 at https://www.osha.gov/Publications/WTC/danger ous_worksite.html

Ogden, C. L., Carroll, M. D., Kit, B. K. & Flegal, K. M. (2014). Prevalence of childhood and adult obesity in the United States, 2011–2012. *Journal of the American Medical Association*, 311(8), 806–814.

Oishi, S. (2010). The psychology of residential mobility: Implications for the self, social relationships, and well-being. *Perspectives on Psychological Science*, 5(1), 5–21.

Ortiz, D. (2001). The survivor's perspective: Voices from the center. In E. Gerrity, T. M. Keane & F. Tuma (eds.), *The Mental Health Consequences of Torture*. New York, NY: Kluwer Academic/Plenum.

Philpott, T. (2002). *Glory Denied: The Saga of Vietnam Veteran Jim Thompson, America's Longest-Held Prisoner of War*. New York, NY: Plume Books.

Prince-Embury, S. (2008). The resiliency scales for children and adolescents, psychological symptoms, and clinical status in adolescents. *Canadian Journal of School Psychology*, 23(1), 41–56.

Rothbaum, B. O., Foa, E. B., Riggs, D. S., Murdock, T. & Walsh, W. (1992). A prospective examination of post-traumatic stress disorder in rape victims. *Journal of Traumatic Stress*, 5(3), 455–475.

Rüber, T., Lindenberg, R. & Schlaug, G. (2015). Differential adaptation of descending motor tracts in musicians. *Cerebral Cortex*, 25(6), 1490–1498.

Rutter, M. (1985). Resilience in the face of adversity: Protective factors and resistance to psychiatric disorder. *British Journal of Psychiatry*, 147, 598–611.

Saad, L. (2008). Few Americans meet exercise targets: Self-reported rates of physical exercise show little change since 2001. Gallup, Inc., January 1 (press release). Accessed February 24, 2010 at www.gallup.com/poll/103492/few-americans-meet-exercise-targets.aspx

Saslow, E. (2015). A survivor's life. *Washington Post*, December 5. Retrieved from www.washingtonpost.com/sf/national/2015/12/05/after-a-mass-shooting-a-sur vivors-life/

Simon, S. (2002). Jimmy Dunne gets back to business: Firm works to recover from unthinkable losses on Sept. 11. *National Public Radio*, September 7. Accessed December 4, 2009 at www.npr.org/news/specials/091102reflections/jimmy dunne/index.html

Singleton, O., Vangel, M., Lazar, S. W. *et al.* (2014). Change in brainstem gray matter concentration following a mindfulness-based intervention is correlated with improvement in psychological well-being. *Frontiers in Human Neuroscience*, 8, 33.

Skelton, K., Ressler, K. J., Norrholm, S. D., Jovanovic, T. & Bradley-Davino, B. (2011). PTSD and gene variants: New pathways and new thinking. *Neuropharmacology*, 62(2), 628–637.

Southwick, S. M., Vythilingam, M. & Charney, D. (2005). The psychobiology of depression and resilience to stress: Implications for prevention and treatment. *Annual Review of Clinical Psychology*, 1, 255–291.

Southwick, S. M., Gilmartin, R., McDonough, P. & Morrissey, P. (2006). Logotherapy as an adjunctive treatment for chronic combat-related PTSD: A meaning-based intervention. *American Journal of Psychotherapy*, 60(2), 161–174.

Southwick, S.M., Davis, L., Aikins, D. E. *et al.* (2007). Neurobiological alterations associated with PTSD. In M. J. Friedman, T. M. Keane & P. A. Resick (eds.), *Handbook of PTSD: Science and Practice*, pp. 166–189. New York, NY: Guilford Press.

Southwick, S. M., Ozbay, F., Charney, D. & McEwen, B. S. (2008). Adaptation to stress and psychobiological mechanisms of resilience. In B. J. Lukey & V. Tepe (eds.), *Biobehavioral Resilience to Stress*, pp. 91–115. Boca Raton, FL: CRC Press.

Southwick, S. M., Litz, B., Charney, D. S. & Friedman, M. J. (eds.) (2011). *Resilience and Mental Health: Challenges Across the Lifespan*. Cambridge: Cambridge University Press.

Southwick, S. M., Bonanno, G. A., Masten, A. S., Panter-Brick, C. & Yehuda, R. (2014). Resilience definitions, theory, and challenges: Interdisciplinary perspectives. *European Journal of Psychotraumatology*, 5(1), 25338.

Stahl, S. M. (2011). Psychotherapy as an epigenetic 'drug': psychiatric therapeutics target symptoms linked to malfunctioning brain circuits with psychotherapy as well as with drugs. *Journal of Clinical Pharmacy and Therapeutics*, 37(3), 249–253.

Stellman, J. M., Smith, R. P., Katz, C. L. *et al.* (2008). Enduring mental health morbidity and social function impairment in World Trade Center rescue, recovery, and cleanup workers: The psychological dimension of an environmental health disaster. *Environmental Health Perspectives*, 116(9), 1248–1253.

Twenge, J. M. & Campbell, W. K. (2009). *The Narcissism Epidemic: Living in the Age of Entitlement*. New York, NY: Free Press.

US Census Bureau, Population Division, Fertility & Family Statistics Branch (2006). America's Families and Living Arrangements: 2005. Accessed February 24, 2010 at www.census.gov/population/www/socdemo/hh-fam/cps2005.html

Vaillant, G. E. (2002). *Aging Well: Surprising Guideposts to a Happier Life from the Landmark Harvard Study of Adult Development*. New York, NY: Little, Brown & Co.

Watkins, L. E., Han, S., Harpaz-Rotem, I., Mota, N. P. *et al.* (2016). *FKBP5* polymorphisms, childhood abuse, and PTSD symptoms: Results from the National Health and Resilience in Veterans Study. *Psychoneuroendocrinology*, 69, 98–105. DOI:10.1016/j.psyneuen.2016.04.001

Wayne, L., with Deutsch, C. (2002). It isn't easy, but Sandler thrives. *New York Times*, September 10. Accessed January 22, 2010 at http://sandleroneillfamily.com/articles/nyt091002.htm

Whitcomb, D. (2015). Girl critically wounded in Oregon college massacre is released from hospital. *Reuters*, October 13. Retrieved from www.reuters.com/article/us-usa-shooting-oregon-idUSKCN0S72UM20151013

World Health Organization (2006). Report of a workshop on tracking health performance and humanitarian outcomes. Accessed November 22, 2009 at www.who.int/hac/events/

Zhang, T. Y., Labonte, B., Wen, X. L., Turecki, G. & Meaney, M. J. (2012). Epigenetic mechanisms for early environmental regulation of hippocampal glucocorticoid receptor gene expression in rodents and humans. *Neuropsychopharmacology Reviews*, 38(1), 111–123.

Zhou, Z., Zhu, G., Hariri, A. R. *et al.* (2008). Genetic variation in human NPY expression affects stress response and emotion. *Nature*, 452(7190), 997–1001.

# CHAPTER 2

# Optimism: Belief in a Brighter Future

Optimism ignites resilience, providing energy to power the other resilience factors. It facilitates an active and creative approach to coping with challenging situations.

How do we define optimism? Optimism is a future-oriented attitude, a confidence that things will turn out well. Optimists believe that good things will happen to them, and that with enough hard work, they will succeed. Pessimists, in contrast, see the future as dim. They believe that bad things will happen to them and doubt that they have the skills and stamina to achieve their goals. In other words, optimists and pessimists have very different expectations.

Can optimism be measured? Many researchers think so, and they attempt to measure it with tools such as the Life Orientation Test (the LOT), a questionnaire that includes statements such as "In uncertain times, I usually expect the best," and "I hardly ever expect things to go my way." Respondents rate each statement on a five-point scale ranging from "strongly disagree" to "strongly agree" (Scheier, Carver & Bridges, 1994).

Psychologists such as Shelley Taylor (1998) have identified two styles of optimism: dispositional optimism (also called trait optimism), which pervades the individual's outlook and tends to be stable from one situation to another; and situational optimism, in which the individual may feel hopeful and expect a favorable outcome in one situation but not in another. While some of the highly resilient people we interviewed for this book displayed trait optimism, for others optimism depended on the situation. Still, they managed to build on whatever small glimmers of optimistic thinking they could find under adverse circumstances.

Of the many people we interviewed, Deborah Gruen is perhaps the one who best exemplifies the spirit and power of dispositional optimism. Her life story suggests the ways in which optimism can contribute to resilience, not only for the individual, but also for those around her.

Deborah's difficulties began at birth. When Deborah was born in 1987, her father had just been appointed an assistant professor of neonatology at the Yale Medical School. Jeff Gruen was happily married to Susan Gruen and they had one healthy daughter, Michele. Jeff was enjoying success at work and had recently won a grant to fund his research; he was excited about the arrival of his second child. Several months earlier, Susan had been accepted to law school and was poised to embark on a new career of her own.

The Gruens knew that their new baby would be a girl, and they had already chosen the name Deborah. Susan Gruen was meticulous in the care of her unborn fetus: she ate well, exercised regularly, took no medication, and avoided alcohol and cigarettes. As a neonatologist, Jeff Gruen made certain that his wife received all of the finest in fetal testing.

When Susan went into labor, Jeff drove her to the hospital, where her obstetrician and the other medical staff found no reason to expect anything other than a normal delivery and a healthy infant. But when Deborah emerged into full view, Jeff was stunned. He recalls,

> She had a large lipoma (fatty tumor) at the base of her spine, about the size of a half grapefruit. She had normal anatomy, but she didn't have normal posture from the waist down, and she was somewhat flaccid. There was some movement of her legs – but not a lot. She moved her hips and toes and feet, but it wasn't normal movement. It was never normal movement. I couldn't believe it. Disbelief – and I would say emotional shock, if there is such a thing.

Susan, still bleeding from the delivery, began crying. "What's going on?" she pleaded. "I need to know. What's going on?"

A pediatric radiologist was summoned for a computed tomography scan, an ultrasound, and an MRI. This was state-of-the-art medicine at the time, and the Gruens were lucky to be at a university hospital, Yale New Haven Hospital. A few hours later they knew: their new baby had a lipomyelomeningocele, a fatty tumor at the base of the spinal cord. Her vertebrae were malformed, and some were impinging on the spinal cord itself.

> The radiologist was concerned about the spinal cord so he calls Duncan, the neurosurgeon. Duncan looks at the scans and says, "We need to operate right now. The longer these vertebrae impinge, the more function she will lose." So your kid has to have surgery, and she's not even 12 hours old. We were just devastated. I didn't know what to do, so I went to see my section chief, Ian. I was standing there with Ian, and I just fell apart, sobbing. Susan is upstairs crying and screaming. They are telling me to do an operation. I don't even know Duncan. I mean, I know him professionally. I don't know what to do. I just don't know what to do. I am crying uncontrollably. Finally, Ian just hugged me.

The surgery was successful: once the spinal canal was widened by removing the impinging vertebrae, Deborah's condition improved rapidly. Still, there was no assurance that she would ever walk. There was a real possibility that her condition would be degenerative, worsening year by year and putting her at risk for chronic problems such as impaired bladder and bowel functions. As a doctor, Jeff clearly understood that Deborah faced a long road ahead.

After two weeks in neonatal intensive care, Deborah came home. Because Deborah's spine was so unstable, she was fitted for a "clam shell." This was a cast made of molded plastic with Velcro hinges that extended from her neck to the top of her thighs. The device restricted the movement of her torso, back, and hips. When her parents removed Deborah from the clam shell for short periods in order to bathe her, they were instructed to support her so that her back would remain as straight as possible. They were told to remain vigilant and resist the natural instinct to cuddle her into a fetal position. Susan remembers walking on eggshells, constantly worrying that she might lift or bend Deborah the wrong way and damage her baby's spinal cord.

For the first few days, Deborah cried nonstop. Concerned that she was in pain, her parents took her back to the hospital. It turned out they'd put her clam shell on upside down.

Jeff and Susan were overwhelmed at times, feeling helpless to make things better for their baby and deeply fearful about her future. Would she be rejected from preschool because she needed a walker? Would her physical disability prevent her from participating in everyday childhood activities? How would she feel about being short? Deborah was born in the autumn, a time when the Gruens customarily go apple-picking. Shortly after Deborah's birth, Susan wondered whether her new daughter would ever be able to pick apples with them. Jeff replied, "Of course she will. If she can't walk, I'll carry her."

When the infant Deborah was formally named and blessed at the synagogue, the rabbi ended his prayer with the words, "And may we all dance at her wedding." Susan whispered to Jeff, "I hope so."

To her parents' relief, Deborah began to develop normally in many ways: feeding, swallowing, smiling, and occasionally moving her legs. Months later, she had another long but successful surgery to untether her spinal cord. Three weeks after this surgery, however, just as the family was beginning to settle into a routine, Susan Gruen noticed several drops of clear fluid at the base of Deborah's back. She immediately called her husband, who suspected a cerebral spinal fluid leak, a potentially life-threatening situation. Deborah was rushed to the emergency room and admitted for yet another surgery. "I was in the lab and I remember driving home, just screaming. I was on Interstate 95 and I was screaming," Jeff recalls.

> We worried about her every minute of every waking hour. We called each other two or three times per day. Susan would ask, "Do you think she will ever walk? Do you think she is going to be paralyzed?" I was really worried about her life in a chair. I was really worried about her kidneys and urinary infections; I was always worried about an

asymptomatic UTI [urinary tract infection] and how would we know. An asymptomatic UTI can lead to pyelonephritis [kidney infection] and eventually kidney failure. I was also worried that she would be incontinent or have to be cathed [catheterized]. I didn't really want her in a chair. I worried about having to pick her up for the rest of her life, and I worried that she would become dependent. I knew she would need multiple operations and there might be a mishap.

During the second and third hospitalizations, the Gruens received conflicting opinions about Deborah's need for a fourth surgery, a fusion of several thoraco-lumbar vertebrae that would further stabilize her spinal cord. She was only nine or ten months old, and some consultants believed she was too young for the procedure. They recommended postponing it for several years because she wasn't going to walk anyway, but others argued that the surgery should be done immediately. The Gruens agonized over the decision. Finally, they chose to have the surgery as soon as possible, even though the surgeon had never before performed this operation on a child as young as Deborah. Because HIV infections had become a major concern in blood banks, Jeff and Susan donated their own blood in case Deborah needed emergency transfusions. Eventually, at the age of five, Deborah required a fifth surgery.

With time, Deborah's condition stabilized. However, as expected, her physical growth and motor development were compromised.

She never crawled. She dragged herself across the floor. And then she used a walker . . . She had this little stand that the physical therapist made, like a box, and then literally strapped the kid into the stand. It locked her legs in, so she could start putting weight on her legs. It's a funny thing, the leg thing, because to us you don't really think about it, but to her using her legs requires active thought, even to this day.

Even though – or perhaps because – there were countless distressing and heartbreaking potential scenarios, the Gruens eventually learned not to fret about the future, but instead to help Deborah negotiate the present. Of course, negotiating the present wasn't always easy. They did their best to treat Deborah as they would any other child, just as they had treated Michele. But they also knew that Deborah was not like other children.

When Deborah was a preschooler, one of Susan's friends invited her to swim at the Ridgetop Club. Susan reluctantly agreed. She was apprehensive about how club members would respond to Deborah – who was able to walk only by using a pair of bright pink crutches – and how Deborah would respond to them. Would they stare at her, as happened so often in unfamiliar settings? Would the other kids welcome Deborah? Could she keep up with them? Susan recalls,

So she got into the pool and as her mother, I'm dying, because, oh my God, everyone is looking at her. What's going to happen? Well, nothing happened. She swam, she did great, she gets out of the pool just like everybody else. Probably one of the kids picked her up, hugged her and then it was on to the next little game.

Looking back, Jeff and Susan reflect on how overwhelming the first five years of Deborah's life were for them as parents. When they weren't working, they spent most of their "free" time trying to keep their heads above water, trying to solve each new unexpected problem, one day at a time. Their primary goal was to help Deborah live as normal a life as possible. Their experience highlights the fact that traumas are family events; they affect everyone in the household. While young Deborah coped with her disability, life was also a challenge for those who loved her and wanted to do everything possible to help her grow and thrive.

Despite predictions that Deborah would never walk, she did gradually learn to walk with two canes. And the invitation to the swim club turned out to be especially lucky: Deborah continued to swim, first for fun and then competitively. In 2004, at age 16, she traveled to Athens to compete in the Summer Paralympic Games, where she won the bronze medal in the 100-meter breast stroke. In 2005, this outgoing, gregarious, and popular young woman was invited to swim on a number of prestigious National Collegiate Athletic Association (NCAA) swim teams, including those at Yale, Princeton, and Brown. Having the highest academic average in her high school class and being valedictorian, Deborah was awarded early admission to Yale University, where she majored in economics and competed on the varsity Women's Swimming and Diving Team. Her speed at the 2008 Paralympics in Beijing earned her another bronze medal. By 2010, she had won medals in nearly a dozen international swimming competitions and set four world, pan-American, and American records in her class.

At age 18, she articulated her future ambition: "I am hoping to serve as a United States senator. I have my eye on Senator Joe Lieberman's job." In the ensuing years, she continued to show potential to make that dream come true: she graduated summa cum laude and Phi Beta Kappa from Yale and was accepted to Georgetown University's School of Law.

Emerging from such a rough beginning and living with such a severe lifelong disability, how has Deborah Gruen succeeded in so many areas of her life? The answer is complex and multi-faceted: her parents never gave up hope, provided unconditional love and support, treated Deborah like any able-bodied child, and expected others to do the same; her sister Michelle served as a role model who protected Deborah only when absolutely necessary, at the same time pushing her to face her fears and achieve her goals; her friends never excluded Deborah from their activities, even if it meant waiting for her; and Deborah was inherently very bright and born into a highly accomplished family that valued ideas, education, moral and ethical principles, hard work, and community service. But perhaps most important, Deborah was and remains an optimist. In fact, her sister has never heard Deborah complain about her disability. "She is just mentally tough. She walks around like you and me, like she has no problem. She has always been that way. I don't remember her ever having a problem with it."

# Blind Optimism Doesn't Work

Contrary to popular belief, optimism as a resilience trait does not mean blindly ignoring life's problems or viewing the world through "rose-colored glasses." In their book *The Resilience Factor*, Karen Reivich and Andrew Shatté (2003) refer to "realistic optimism." As do pessimists, realistic optimists pay close attention to negative information that is relevant to the problems they face. However, unlike pessimists, they do not remain focused on the negative. They tend to disengage rapidly from problems that appear to be unsolvable: they know when to cut their losses and turn their attention to solvable problems.

Diane Coutu (2002) discusses the importance of paying close attention to negative information in the context of business success:

> That's not to say that optimism doesn't have its place: In turning around a demoralized sales force, for instance, conjuring a sense of possibility can be a very powerful tool. But for bigger challenges, a cool, almost pessimistic, sense of reality is far more important... Facing reality, really facing it, is grueling work. Indeed, it can be unpleasant and emotionally wrenching. (Coutu, 2002, p. 48)

She goes on to observe that this flinty realism pays off when an organization needs to overcome a major challenge or bounce back from a disaster. Assessing obstacles realistically helps to surmount them.

Sandra Schneider, a psychologist at the University of South Florida, suggests that realistic optimism is qualitatively different from the blind variety: "A realistic outlook improves chances to negotiate the environment successfully, whereas an optimistic outlook places priority on feeling good. But are realistic and optimistic outlook necessarily in conflict?" Schneider points out that in many cases, optimism and realism don't conflict, but "there remain numerous 'optimistic biases' that do involve self-deception, or convincing oneself of desired beliefs without appropriate reality checks" (2001, p. 250).

Many other researchers have documented examples of unrealistic optimistic beliefs. Psychologist Tali Sharot of University College, London, and her colleagues at New York University found, for example, that "people expect to live longer and be healthier than average, they underestimate their likelihood of getting a divorce, and overestimate their prospects for success on the job market" (2007, p. 102). This kind of illusory superiority has been called the "Lake Wobegon effect" after the fictional town created by author Garrison Keillor, where "all the children are above average." Researchers have observed this effect in driving, among other behaviors; the popular book *Traffic: Why We Drive the Way We Do* includes a chapter titled "Why you're not as good a driver as you think you are." She writes, "... if we were to ask ourselves, 'How's my driving?' research has shown that the answer would probably be a big thumbs-up – regardless of one's actual driving record" (Vanderbilt, 2008, p. 60).

It is not hard to see how excessive or unrealistic optimism can be detrimental, or even dangerous. As noted by Justin Kruger and David Dunning of Cornell University (1999), it tends to lead to "an underestimation of risk, an overestimation of ability, and inadequate preparation." For an individual confronted with a major trauma like being shot down and taken prisoner, being blindly optimistic could easily be the last mistake he or she would ever make.

Former POW Admiral James Stockdale clearly recognized the dangers of blind or "rosy" optimism. He shared his misgivings about optimism in a speech addressed to the Class of 1983 at the West Point United States Military Academy:

> We pretty much knew each other's outlook and most guys thought it was really better for everybody to be an optimist. I wasn't naturally that way; I knew too much about the politics of Asia when I got shot down. I think there was a lot of damage done by optimists; other writers from other wars share that opinion. The problem is, some people believe what professional optimists are passing out and come unglued when their predictions don't work out. . . babbling optimists are the bane of existence to one under stress. (Stockdale, 1984)

Humanitarian Hellen Keller likely would have agreed. Although her life was a testament to optimism, Keller was no Pollyanna. She believed that her own brand of optimism was the product of years of deprivation and hardship.

Born in 1880 in a small town in Alabama, Helen Keller contracted a life-threatening infection when she was 19 months old. Doctors at the time called it "brain fever"; it is now believed to have been scarlet fever or meningitis. She nearly died. When the fever lifted and Helen began to recover, her family rejoiced, not yet knowing that the illness had forever "closed her eyes and ears" (Keller, 1903b).

The next five years were marked by "outbursts of passion," screaming, daily (and sometimes hourly) temper tantrums and fits of violent and uncontrollable behavior. In 1887, when Helen's parents had reached their limit and seriously considered institutionalizing their daughter, Anne Sullivan came into Keller's life and "the light of love shone on me that very hour." With unwavering patience, Sullivan persisted in the daunting task of teaching Helen to understand language and to communicate so that "the barren places between my mind and the minds of others blossomed like the rose" (Keller, 1903b).

If those around her had lacked hope, Keller might have lived her entire life in severe isolation. Without optimism, her parents would not have hired a teacher, and Anne Sullivan would not have weathered her student's tantrums and would not have tried again and again to cultivate those "barren places."

The barriers of blindness and deafness seemed insurmountable. But, eventually, Helen learned to associate words with objects, feelings, and concepts. Under Sullivan's creative tutelage, Helen learned to understand letters and words traced on her hand and then to read Braille. Her progress was so rapid and extraordinary that within a few years she became a "phenomenon," receiving widespread publicity and meeting with world dignitaries, including Alexander Graham Bell and President Grover Cleveland.

After four years of study at the Cambridge School for Young Ladies, Keller applied to Radcliffe College. Doing so unexpectedly tested her resilience: Keller was informed only a day or two before the entrance exam that the mathematical portion would be given in a style of Braille unfamiliar to her, so that she had to learn an entirely new set of symbols overnight. Nevertheless, she wrote,

> I do not blame anyone. The administrative board of Radcliffe did not realize how difficult they were making my examinations, nor did they understand the peculiar difficulties I had to surmount. But if they unintentionally placed obstacles in my way, I have the consolation of knowing that I overcame them all. (Keller, 1903b)

Radcliffe admitted her. There, Keller began to write about her life and her philosophy. In her essay "Optimism," she describes the superficiality and contingency of the type of happiness that people ordinarily seek, what she called "false optimism."

> Most people measure happiness in terms of physical pleasure and material possession. Could they win some visible goal which they have set on the horizon, how happy they would be! Lacking this gift or that circumstance, they would be miserable. If happiness is to be so measured, I who cannot hear or see have every reason to sit in a corner with folded hands and weep. (1903a, pp. 12–13)

And yet Keller saw herself as happy and optimistic, writing: "If I am happy in spite of my deprivations, if my happiness is so deep that it is a faith, so thoughtful that it becomes a philosophy of life, if, in short, I am an optimist, my testimony to the creed of optimism is worth hearing." Keller saw adversity as a prerequisite for real optimism.

> A man must understand evil and be acquainted with sorrow before he can write himself an optimist and expect others to believe that he has reason for the faith that is in him. I know what evil is... I can say with conviction that the struggle which evil necessitates is one of the greatest blessings. It makes us strong, patient, helpful men and women. It lets us into the soul of things and teaches us that although the world is full of suffering it is full also of the overcoming of it. My optimism then does not rest on the absence of evil, but on a glad belief in the preponderance of good and a willing effort always to cooperate with the good that it may prevail. I try to increase the power God has given me to see the best in everything and everyone, and make that Best a part of my life. (1903a, pp. 16, 17)

# How Does Optimism Increase Resilience?

Barbara Fredrickson, a psychologist from the University of North Carolina, has developed what she calls the broaden-and-build model of positive emotions (Fredrickson, 2001). She begins by differentiating the functions of negative and positive emotions and notes that negative emotions such as anger, fear, and disgust help us to survive by preparing us for danger. They do this by activating the sympathetic nervous system, which increases physiological arousal. This "fight–flight" reaction narrows our visual focus and tends to restrict our behaviors to those that are essential for attacking or fleeing.

Fredrickson observes that positive emotions, in contrast, have been shown to reduce physiological arousal and to broaden our visual focus, our thoughts, and our behavior. When people experience positive emotions and an accompanying broadening of attention and behavior, their thinking tends to become more creative, inclusive, flexible, and integrative. Experiments have shown that inducing a positive mood (for example, by showing participants a funny movie or reading them a funny story) increases people's scope of attention, their ability to solve problems actively, and their interest in socializing and in strenuous as well as leisurely activities (Isen, 1990; Phillips *et al.*, 2002; Fredrickson & Branigan, 2005; Catalino & Fredrickson, 2011). Thus, by broadening attention and action, positive emotions can contribute to our creativity, physical health, relationships with family and friends, our ability to acquire new knowledge, and our psychological resilience (Catalino, Algoe & Fredrickson, 2014).

This capacity to broaden attention and build resources can help people cope with stress. Those who frequently experience positive emotions generally have the ability to step back from the maelstrom and observe stressful situations from multiple perspectives. Three coping mechanisms related to broadened attention include: positive reappraisal of trying circumstances; goal-directed, problem-focused coping; and the infusion of meaning into ordinary events. We will briefly discuss these coping mechanisms now, and elaborate on them later in the book.

First, when optimists broaden their attention, they increase their capacity to positively reappraise situations that initially appear to be negative. The process of reframing allows them to approach hardship as a challenge and to find opportunity embedded in adversity. Optimists who are realistic do not deny the difficulties they face, but they do tend to look for a silver lining.

Deborah Gruen is expert at positive reappraisal. When she received her "early acceptance" letter from Yale, she was ecstatic. Her long hours of studying and grueling workouts in the pool had paid off. Gaining acceptance to a college like Yale is no small feat. In the midst of her excitement, as she read and re-read the admissions letter, Deborah noticed a website that posted profiles of the applicants who had accepted early admission to Yale. Reading about the other students, she began to feel intimidated by their level of accomplishment and worried that she wouldn't be able to measure up. But soon she reappraised the situation; she started to think about how interesting her new classmates were and how much fun it would be to get to know them.

A second characteristic of optimists is that they tend to cope with stress by actively employing strategies to solve problems. They gather information, acquire necessary skills, plan, set goals, make decisions, resolve conflicts, and seek social support. In a series of studies of individuals who were providing care to AIDS patients, researchers from the University of California at San Francisco found that positive emotion in caregivers was positively related to active problem-solving strategies, such as pursuing realistic and attainable caregiving goals. That is, the greater the optimism in the caregiver, the more he or she actively cared for patients (Folkman, 1997; Moskowitz *et al.*, 1996; Catalino, Algoe & Fredrickson, 2014). Similarly, findings from a University of Miami study of breast cancer patients suggest that optimistic patients who expect a positive outcome tend to embrace and actively pursue their treatment goals (Carver *et al.*, 1993).

In short, research has shown that optimism and positive expectations tend to promote active striving, while pessimism and negative expectations are associated with feelings of weakness and helplessness that may lead to unhelpful behaviors such as self-pity, resentment, denial, and avoidance of problems.

A third characteristic of optimists is that they are more likely than pessimists to report that their lives are meaningful. A large body of research supports this observation (Heintzelman & King, 2014). While it is widely believed that a sense of meaning and purpose enhances positive emotions and happiness, researchers have recently begun to ask whether it also works the other way – whether positive emotions and feelings of happiness can enhance one's belief that life has meaning. In a group of fascinating experiments, Laura King and colleagues (King & Hicks, 2009) from the University of Missouri examined the relationship between positive emotion, negative emotion, and meaning in life. Participants rated their sense of meaning and purpose in life and how much they experienced positive and negative emotions on a given day. The Purpose in Life scale evaluated the degree to which participants agreed or disagreed with statements such as "My personal existence is very purposeful and meaningful," and "I regard my ability to find meaning, purpose or a mission in life to be very great." The research team found that the greater the positive emotion a participant reported on a given day, the more he or she experienced life as meaningful on that day.

In a separate experiment (King *et al.*, 2006), the team demonstrated that a sense of meaning in life could be increased by inducing a positive mood. In the laboratory, each participant read one of three mood-inducing scripts on a computer screen. Participants in the positive mood-inducing group read a script about being hailed as a hero after reuniting a lost child with her parents. Those in the negative mood-inducing group read about running a yellow light, crashing into another car, and tragically killing a baby. The neutral script simply described a student's plans for the day. Results indicated that participants' judgments about meaning in life were enhanced only in the positive mood-induction group and not in the neutral or negative groups. We will have more to say about the relationship between meaning in life and resilience in Chapter 11.

The findings in these experiments, in conjunction with those from numerous other studies, are consistent with Fredrickson's broaden-and-build theory of positive emotions. In this theory, positive emotions broaden the scope of attention, expand and open the individual's mind to new types of information, enhance cognitive flexibility, and increase the capacity to form creative and meaningful connections among elements of an experience. As a result, the optimist may be more likely than the pessimist to see the "big picture" and to view daily experiences within a larger framework of meaning.

# Optimism Is Good for Your Physical and Mental Health

Optimism has widespread implications for physical and mental health. Numerous scientific studies have shown that optimists tend to be more satisfied with their lives, feel psychologically healthier, and display greater physical well-being than people who are not optimists (Carver & Scheier, 2014; Olson *et al.*, 2014; Serlachius *et al.*, 2015; Affleck & Tennen, 1996). For example, in a review of more than 90 studies on the topic, Carver and Scheier (2014) found that optimistic individuals, compared with pessimists, tend to have more successful careers and social relationships, be healthier, and be more engaged in the pursuit of their goals.

Optimism has been associated with better physical health in various populations, such as women with breast cancer (Carver *et al.*, 1993) and cardiac patients recovering from open heart surgery (Scheier *et al.*, 1989). In one study, heart transplant patients with positive expectations before surgery were found to be in better physical health after surgery than patients without positive expectations (Giltay *et al.*, 2006). Greater optimism has also been associated with less pain and fewer post-operative symptoms in patients undergoing coronary bypass surgery (Ronaldson *et al.*, 2014). And among patients who had experienced acute coronary syndrome (commonly referred to as heart attack and/or unstable angina), those who were assessed upon admission as optimistic were found to be in better physical health 12 months later, even after controlling for factors such as baseline health, age, ethnicity, social deprivation, and clinical risk factors (Ronaldson *et al.*, 2015). A meta-analysis review (Dubois *et al.*, 2015) of studies involving 100 or more cardiology patients found a significant association between positive psychological constructs and reduced rates of mortality and re-hospitalization that was independent of the severity of illness; and in a Women's Health Initiative study that followed 95,000 healthy women over the course of eight years, optimists were less likely than pessimists to develop coronary heart disease, or to die from any cause. Optimism has also been associated with better quality of life among patients with Parkinson's disease (Gison et al., 2015).

Several classic research investigations have also reported that optimists may live longer than pessimists. In a remarkable study involving 180 nuns from School Sisters of Notre Dame in Milwaukee, Deborah Danner and colleagues at the University of Kentucky examined the relationship between signs of good cheer and optimism at the time of initiation into the Sisterhood and subsequent length of life (Danner, Snowdon & Friesen, 2001). At the School Sisters of Notre Dame, it is customary for women to write a brief autobiographical sketch shortly before taking their vows of commitment to God and the Church. The researchers analyzed these autobiographical sketches, which the nuns had written decades earlier, by quantifying numerous variables within the sketches, such as degree of unhappiness, level of religious devotion, intellectual complexity of the sketch, and amount of positive emotion. Of all the variables, only positive emotion was related to longevity: 90 percent of nuns whose autobiographical sketches fell within the most cheerful quarter were still alive at age 85, compared with 34 percent of those in the least cheerful quarter; at age 94 the figures were 54 percent compared with 11 percent.

It is possible that optimism protects against some of the negative effects of stress. For example, in a study of Israeli civilians who were exposed to SCUD missile attacks during the Gulf War of 1991, optimists developed fewer stress-related psychological illnesses, such as PTSD and depression, and used fewer medical services than did pessimists (Zeidner & Hammer, 1992). Over the longer term, a 2015 study of former Vietnam prisoners of war found that "optimism was the strongest predictor of psychological health" and that it "provides long-term protective benefits" (Segovia et al., 2015).

It is even possible that optimists have increased immunity to infectious diseases. In a fascinating experiment conducted by Sheldon Cohen, professor of psychology at Carnegie Mellon University, study subjects were required to live in a hotel for one week where they ate only what they were served by the research staff, were not permitted to leave the hotel, and did not have close physical contact with other research participants. On the first day of the experiment, all participants were infected with a cold virus. Consistent with a large body of research showing that positive emotions are associated with better health than are negative emotions, fewer participants assessed as having higher positive emotions developed colds. Those who did had fewer runny noses, less sneezing and congestion, and less mucus (Cohen et al., 2003).

Further support for the relationship between optimism and immune function comes from a study by Susanne Segerstrom from the University of Kentucky and Sandra Sephton of the University of Louisville. They evaluated first-year law students at five different points in time for their academic optimism (i.e. expecting to do well in school), positive and negative emotional state, and cell-mediated immunity (i.e. immunity that protects against microbes, such as viruses). They found that changes in optimistic expectancies were accompanied by changes in immunity, and this association was partly explained by changes in positive emotions (Segerstrom & Sephton, 2010). More recently, Jennifer Stellar and colleagues (2015) found that greater dispositional optimism was associated with lower levels of markers of inflammation. If chronically elevated, inflammation has been linked with depression, cardio-vascular disease, and diabetes.

Although researchers do not fully understand the mechanisms by which positive emotions benefit physical health, it is likely that the immune system and hormones, such as cortisol and growth hormone are involved. It is also likely that optimists in general choose healthier lifestyles than do pessimists: they may adopt healthier eating patterns, exercise more, drink less alcohol, enjoy a more supportive social network and be less likely to abuse drugs.

# The Neuroscience of Optimism

Is there something special about the biology of people who are able to remain optimistic and hopeful in the face of extremely stressful life events? The answer is complex and only partly understood but it begins with genetics. As we noted in Chapter 1, twin studies are one of the most productive methods for studying the heritability of personality traits such as optimism. If personality were solely determined by genes, then identical twins should have identical personality traits, because their genes are identical. This should hold true whether they have been raised together or apart – that is, in different environments and by different caretakers. However, it doesn't hold true. Rather, the results of many twin studies strongly suggest that only 30 to 50 percent of most personality traits are genetically transmitted, including optimism. That means that the other 50 to 70 percent depends on environ-ment, including the efforts we make to reach our potential and maximize our positive experiences. With regard to optimism, no one gene stands out. Instead, it is likely that numerous genes and gene variants each contribute a small amount to the expression of optimism. For example, when researchers at the University of California–San Diego explored the heritability of opti-mism and resilience, they selected 65 genes and gene variants to be included in their analysis (Rana *et al.*, 2014).

Three brain regions that play a central role in optimism are: the prefrontal cortex; the amygdala; and reward systems including the anterior cingulate cortex (ACC), ventral-tegmental area, and the nucleus accumbens (Feder, Nestler & Charney, 2009). As described in Chapter 1, the prefrontal cortex serves as the brain's "executive center"; it is essential for guiding behavior, regulating emotions, and understanding the difference between potential rewards and punishments. It is also essential for imagining the future and setting goals – functions that relate directly to optimism. The prefrontal cortex enables us to engage in optimistic processes such as hoping for the best and imagining a bright future, anticipating and preparing to meet a challenge, and making plans to achieve and enjoy success.

The second brain area involved in optimism is the amygdala. Recall from Chapter 1 that the amygdala plays a role in triggering "raw emotions" such as fear or excitement. In this way, the amygdala plays a role in our ability to experience positive emotions. There is also evidence that the amygdala plays an important role in imaging future emotional events including positive events (Sharot, 2007).

Areas of the brain involved in reward circuitry – the ACC, ventral-tegmental area, and nucleus accumbens – also appear to play a central role in optimism. These areas are associated with the rewarding effects of social attachment, eating, sex, and other pleasurable stimuli. Reward circuitry is generally active when we are engaged in behaviors that we enjoy. On the other hand, acute stress tends to reduce activity in these circuits (Nestler & Carlezon, 2006). The neurotransmitter commonly associated with reward is dopamine. Alice Isen and her colleagues at Cornell University (Isen, 1990) have found that dopamine improves cognitive flexibility and perspective-taking. These researchers, and others, believe that the broadened perspective and flexible cognitive style that accompany positive emotions may be related to increased dopamine (Ashby, Isen & Turken, 1999; Isen, 1990).

In order to understand how the brain generates the positive bias that characterizes optimism, psychologist Tali Sharot (2007) and colleagues at New York University instructed subjects to imagine both positive (e.g., winning an award) and negative (e.g., ending a romantic relationship) future events while undergoing functional MRI (fMRI). When participants imagined a positive future event, activation of the amygdala and the ACC increased. The greatest activation of these regions occurred in participants with the highest scores on a measure of dispositional optimism, the LOT-R (Life Orientation Test-Revised).

In our own research with colleagues at the National Institutes of Mental Health (Vythilingham *et al.*, 2008), we investigated brain reward systems in highly resilient US Special Forces soldiers compared to healthy civilians. In one experiment, we collected fMRI data while study participants performed a task in which they were instructed to press a button quickly enough to either win money or avoid losing money. When the civilian control subjects "won" money (or anticipated doing so), activity in reward centers and the prefrontal cortex (top-down control) increased. When they "lost" money, activity in these areas decreased. But in the brains of Special Forces soldiers, we observed equal activation of the reward systems whether they "won" or "lost" money in the task. The fact that the soldiers showed no relative reduction in reward center activity when they "lost" money suggests that the brain reward system of resilient individuals may be relatively impervious to stress or adversity. Perhaps people who are resilient tend to have a dopamine reward system that is relatively resistant to dopamine depletion and that functions well even under highly stressful conditions (Charney, 2004).

Consistent with the above findings, Richard Davidson and colleagues have found that optimism is associated with high activity in the left prefrontal cortex with prolonged engagement of subcortical reward circuitry. Depression, on the other hand, has been associated with low prefrontal activity and inability to sustain reward circuitry activation. The ability to savor and sustain positive emotion is "critical to daily function well-being and to health" (Heller *et al.*, 2015, p. 10503).

While the ability to sustain and savor positive emotions is an essential component of optimism, the capacity to focus on and engage negative emotions also appears to be important. For example, in a study by our research team at the Icahn School of Medicine at Mount Sinai, we used fMRI to examine emotional responses to negative stimuli among three groups of women: 14 women who had been sexually assaulted and developed PTSD, 14 who had been sexually assaulted and had not developed PTSD, and 14 who had never been sexually assaulted (New *et al.*, 2009). Each subject was shown 60 emotionally negative pictures during the study. Immediately before viewing each negative picture, subjects were given one of three instructions: to "enhance," to "diminish," or to "maintain" their emotional response to that picture. Nontraumatized healthy controls were best able to decrease their emotional responses to negative pictures as measured by subjective ratings and degree of PFC activation. Unexpectedly, the trauma-exposed resilient group had greater PFC activation following the "enhance" instruction than did the trauma-exposed PTSD group. These findings suggest that the ability to focus effortfully on negative emotional responses and engage cognitive/linguistic areas of the brain in order to manage, diminish or extinguish the negative emotion may be an important component of resilience.

# How Optimists and Pessimists See the World

During the course of any day, each of us is exposed to a barrage of sensory information, an endless stream of sights, sounds and smells. Out of this morass of information, in order to survive, we need to selectively focus on those stimuli that are most relevant to our well-being. The brain does this by preferentially drawing our attention to situations that are negative or dangerous, and also to situations that are positive and can bring pleasure. That which brings pleasure, such as food and sex, keeps us alive and perpetuates our species, while what is dangerous, such as a snake or a stranger, may threaten our survival. Of these two biases, our attention to the negative is generally stronger than attention to the positive, particularly when the negative involves threat or danger. In this sense, fear rules; when fear competes with pleasure, it usually wins out. As noted by researcher Elaine Fox, director of the Affective Neuroscience Laboratory at the University of Essex, our natural attentiveness to danger and negative stimuli protects us, but also makes it more difficult for us to be optimistic (Fox, 2012). This is particularly challenging in a world where the local, national and international media intentionally focus on stories about war, global warming, crime, epidemics, terrorism, and other frightening events. Media editors know that readers and viewers are naturally drawn to the negative: bad news sells, and bad news goes viral.

Yet, while humans tend to focus more on negative and positive situations more than neutral ones, Fox (Fox, 2012; Fox *et al.*, 2015) has found that individuals vary considerably in attention bias. For example, compared to optimists, people who are chronically anxious or pessimistic have a tendency to focus on potentially negative or threatening stimuli and to avoid focusing on potentially positive situations. They are captivated by bad news, tend to view ambiguous situations as threatening, constantly keep an eye out for possible threats and dangers, and vividly picture what might go wrong in any particular situation. On the other hand, while nonanxious or optimistic people notice and pay attention to relevant negative information, they are drawn toward pleasant or positive stimuli, and easily imagine what can go right.

## How Optimists and Pessimists Interpret Events

By carefully analyzing thought patterns and spoken words, psychologists like Martin Seligman have found that pessimists and optimists employ very different explanatory styles (ways of explaining events to themselves and others). When bad things happen to pessimists, they tend to believe that the negative consequences will last forever (permanence) and will intrude into many areas of their lives (universality). They commonly describe the event using words such as "always" or "never." Optimists, on the other hand, tend to respond to adverse events by viewing the consequences as temporary and limited in scope. They are more likely to use words such as "sometimes" or "lately." In addition, optimistic people tend to have an internal locus of control (Guarnera & Williams, 1987) – the belief that they can influence events in their lives.

For example, a pessimist whose romantic relationship falls apart might conclude that he will fail in all future romances (permanence), that his nonromantic relationships are also doomed (universality), and that he inherently lacks some quality or skill needed to form lasting relationships (external locus of control). When pessimists face a stressful situation, they tend to exaggerate their appraisal of threat, blame or criticize themselves, underestimate their capacities, and over-generalize the nature and extent of the problem.

In contrast, an optimist whose romance fizzles may conclude that he and his partner were not well suited for each other, that he has learned from the experience – making it more likely that his next romantic relationship will work out – and that he possesses the necessary qualities and skills to succeed in present and future relationships, both romantic and platonic. When threatened or challenged, optimists tend to contain their appraisal of threat, create positive appraisals about themselves, and focus on their strengths.

Pessimists and optimists tend to employ opposite explanatory styles in good times, too. In response to good events, pessimists often view their gains as temporary and specific to the particular event itself. Optimists, on the other hand, generally anticipate longstanding and widespread benefits.

# Four Ways to Become More Optimistic

What about those of us who are not born optimists? If we did not inherit "optimism genes," is it still possible to become more optimistic? Fortunately, for most of us the answer is yes. Based on a large body of scientific evidence, we suggest four ways to increase optimism.

1. Focus attention on the positive things around us.
2. Intentionally think positive thoughts and do not dwell on negative thoughts.
3. Reframe the negative and interpret events in a more positive light.
4. Behave and take action in ways that build positive feelings.

If we habitually focus our attention on the negative, think negative thoughts, interpret events negatively, constantly complain, worry, and act as if we are miserable, we will tend to see the world as a dark and threatening place. But if we pay attention to both the positive and the negative, ignore irrelevant negative information, let go of the negative that we cannot change, interpret information in a more positive light, and take action to solve problems that are solvable, then we will tend to see the world as exciting, challenging, and hopeful. Using these four methods to become more optimistic is basically a matter of building habits that enhance optimism.

# Focus on the Positive

First, we can learn to change our attention bias and shift our focus of attention, so that instead of habitually noticing the negative and threatening, we build the habit of also noticing the positive and hopeful stimuli in our environment. In her book, *Rainy Brain, Sunny Brain* (2012), Elaine Fox describes brain imaging research showing that people who are anxious and pessimistic have an unconscious habit of paying attention to negative stimuli, while optimistic people unconsciously pay attention to positive stimuli. If a habitually pessimistic person can learn to shift attention to positive stimuli, this new habit will help the person to build optimism.

One technique to achieve this shift is called cognitive bias modification (CBM) (Fox, 2013). CBM uses computer programs to change automatic negative biases at a preconscious level. The computer screen displays negative, unpleasant pictures (e.g., a snarling dog or a scowling person) and positive, pleasing images (e.g., a playful puppy or a smiling person) along with a target that directs the viewer's attention. Typically, the individual practices on the computer or mobile device for 15 to 20 minutes daily for anywhere from two days to two weeks. By repetitively, over hundreds of trials, directing the subject's attention to positive rather than neutral or negative images on their screen, CBM gradually shifts the individual's automatic negative attention bias to a more positive one (Beard, 2011; Fox, 2013).

Another technique, which requires no software, is to bring some of the unconscious negative attentional bias to consciousness. Each of us can make a conscious effort to be aware of the stimuli around us and to focus on the stimuli that are pleasing and positive.

# Cultivate Positive Thoughts

A second technique for increasing optimism is to train ourselves to think or insert positive thoughts and to avoid dwelling on negative ones. Each time we think a positive thought, we make a new memory trace in our brain and build a mental habit of positive thinking. Further, we can strengthen the benefits of thinking a positive thought by savoring it: holding the thought in the forefront of our attention for 5, 10, or even 20 seconds (Hanson, 2009). Research using fMRI has shown that brain areas associated with resilience are activated when positive memories are savored (Speer, Bhanji & Delgado, 2014).

Veteran Lew Meyer used positive thinking after he was captured in Vietnam during the 1968 Tet Offensive and held as a POW for four and a half years. Optimism did not come naturally for Meyer, but by accessing memories of his life at home with his wife, he trained himself to become a positive thinker.

> We had this book in our house. My wife Gail read it and re-read it and quoted things and pushed me and pushed me. I started reading it. Then I ended up occasionally skimming through it and looking for a certain chapter... I started re-reading it [in my memory] in solitary.

The book was *The Power of Positive Thinking* by the Protestant minister Norman Vincent Peale. The book has sold over five million copies since its publication in 1952 and has helped countless people learn to practice optimism.

While Peale believed that having faith in God and drawing strength from the divine were largely responsible for personal power and resilience, he also believed that our emotions and feelings are largely determined by our thoughts. He believed that when we think negative thoughts, we are likely to feel anxious, worried, angry, and sad; but if we think positive thoughts, we will tend to feel happy, energized, and peaceful. It is also possible that when we feel depressed or anxious we tend to think negative thoughts and that when we are happy we tend to think positive thoughts.

In either case, Peale's practical recommendations include visualizing yourself as happy and successful, and avoiding building up obstacles in your imagination. Peale also recommended cultivating friendships with hopeful people. Optimism and pessimism can both be "contagious," so it is often beneficial to intentionally surround ourselves with people who are positive, confident, and encouraging.

Deborah Gruen may be a good example of the kind of optimist with whom we would like to associate. A former neighbor and babysitter recalls visiting Deborah in Boston Children's Hospital after she had undergone painful surgery.

> We were waiting in her room, and I remember that everyone was quiet, depressed and sad. No one was talking. Yet, as soon as Deborah was brought in, the entire room lit up. She was lying in a cart of some sort because she couldn't be in the sitting position, and she was so bandaged and fragile-looking. But once she started talking, you totally forgot that she had just had a serious surgery. It was amazing.

As Deborah's mother observed, "Deborah doesn't let other people get her down. She stays really positive. She is an uplifting person. I don't see how you can spend time with her and not get energized."

# Interpret Events Positively

A third technique to enhance positive emotions and optimism focuses on changing our explanatory style, the way in which we interpret experiences in our life. We can learn to confront and often refute negative thoughts that are unrealistic or exaggerated. In fact, this practice is fundamental to cognitive behavioral therapies, which we will discuss in detail later in the book.

Many people make destructive statements about themselves (e.g. "How stupid can I be?" or "I blew it again.") during trying times and setbacks, but psychologists Martin Seligman, Lisa Aspinwall, Albert Ellis, and others have observed that optimists are highly skilled at refuting or in some cases ignoring these negative statements. Optimists often employ a number of strategies and techniques that are taught in cognitive behavioral therapy. These techniques teach the learner to recognize automatic negative thoughts and then dispute those thoughts so that new, more positive patterns of thinking can replace the old ones. In essence, cognitive behavioral therapy teaches people how to change their habitual automatic explanatory style (Aspinwall & Staudinger, 2002).

An optimistic coping style can involve not only increasing positive thoughts and refuting negative ones, but also affirming the coexistence of both. In their research on positive and negative emotions, David Spiegel and colleagues from Stanford University (Speigel & Classen, 2000) have found that women with metastatic breast cancer benefit from a group therapy technique he has called "supportive-expressive therapy." This therapy requires the capacity to co-activate positive and negative emotions and then tolerate and withstand the resulting unpleasant tension. Squarely confronting, engaging, and grappling with the negative, as well as the positive, may facilitate the process of "working through" and possibly resolving or even transcending a major life stressor. Spiegel has observed that patients who actively use these techniques survive longer and experience better quality of life in the form of lower rates of anxiety and depression, and less physical pain. His work supports the views of James Stockdale and Helen Keller who describe the power of realistic optimism that focuses on the positive without denying the negative.

In practical terms, we offer the following self-help tips for building a more positive explanatory style:

## When Something Bad Happens

- Remember that these difficulties won't last forever. Take one day at a time. Where now there may only be pain, over time good things will return.
- Keep the adverse event or situation within its limits; don't let it pervade other areas of your life.

- Think of strengths and resources you can use to help deal with the problem.
- Notice what is good, for example, acts of kindness by those who recognize your struggle.

## And When Something Good Happens

- Give yourself credit for whatever part you played in making it happen.
- Allow yourself to feel grateful for whatever part you *didn't* play in it – the efforts or generosity of others, or just simple good luck.
- Get the most out of it: think of ways to expand the scope and duration of the positive event or situation.

In his book, *Authentic Happiness*, Martin Seligman discusses the importance of making a conscious choice to build a more positive explanatory style; he recommends responding to negative thoughts "as if they were uttered by an external person whose mission is to make your life miserable" (2002, p. 181). Sometimes it is helpful to ask yourself specific questions in order to refute negative beliefs. These may include:

- What is the evidence for this negative belief?
- Is there a less destructive way to look at this belief?
- What are the implications of this belief?
- Am I catastrophizing or exaggerating the potential negative impact of the situation?
- Am I over-generalizing, falsely assuming that this particular situation has broad implications?
- How useful is my pessimistic approach to the problem at hand?

## Behave in Positive Ways

Finally, a fourth way to enhance positive emotions and to decrease negative emotions relies on changing behavior rather than attention or thoughts. *Behavioral activation* is a therapeutic intervention that has been used to successfully treated depression. It is based on the idea that behaviors affect mood and that depression is often fueled by too much reinforcement for depressive behaviors (e.g., avoidance and withdrawal, crying, repetitively talking about sadness, staying in bed) and not enough reinforcement for healthy nondepressed behaviors (e.g., exercise, socializing, pursuing and accomplishing goals). Thus, the therapy typically involves increasing positive behaviors and reducing negative behaviors. Psychologists often refer to these, respectively, as activation behaviors (those that accomplish goals and increase mastery) and avoidance behaviors (those that keep the person "stuck" in a negative place).

Behavioral activation essentially works from the outside in: first it changes behaviors, which then, in turn, change moods or emotions. As noted by research psychologist Christopher Martell, behavioral activation encourages the patient to "act according to a goal rather than a feeling" (Addis, Jacobson & Martell, 2001, p. 116). Thus, behavioral activation seeks to reduce negative emotions and increase positive emotions by systematically increasing behaviors that are known to be related to the positive emotions in a particular patient (Sudak, Majeed & Youngman, 2014).

This behavioral approach accords with the advice offered more than a century ago by the pioneering American psychologist William James to "act as if"; if we act as if everything is all right, our behavior will make us feel more like things are indeed all right. As James wrote,

> Action seems to follow feeling, but really action and feeling go together; and by regulating the action, which is under the more direct control of the will, we can indirectly regulate the feeling, which is not... Thus the sovereign voluntary path to cheerfulness, if our spontaneous cheerfulness be lost, is to sit up cheerfully, to look round cheerfully, and to act and speak as if cheerfulness were already there... So to feel brave, act as if we were brave, use all our will to that end, and a courage-fit will very likely replace the fit of fear. (Richardson, 2012, p. 131)

Based on behavioral activation research, we can recommend the following, either on one's own or in conjunction with a therapist.

- Activity monitoring: Keep a written record of your daily activities (both activation behaviors and avoidance behaviors) and how these activities make you feel. Over time, this record will likely show a pattern of association between activation behaviors and increased positive feelings.
- Assessment of goals and values: Verbalize or write down your values and goals, which may then serve as motivators that help you to sustain activation behaviors.
- Activity scheduling: Use a daily planner to set aside time for activities that are consistent with your values and goals, and that you find increase your positive mood.

Not all of the above techniques will be effective for everyone, but we hope readers will find at least some of them to be helpful.

# Conclusions About Optimism

The determinants of optimism are numerous and include genetic, developmental, neurobiological, cognitive, and social factors among others. Accordingly, there are many potential ways to enhance realistic optimism and positive emotions, such as focusing attention on the positive things around us, cultivating positive thoughts, refuting negative thoughts that are unrealistic or exaggerated, increasing positive and negative behaviors, spending time with optimistic and supportive people, engaging in meaningful and altruistic pursuits, and in some cases psychotherapy and/ or prescribed medication to boost mood.

A note of caution is in order. As we discussed in Chapter 1, individuals who suffer pronounced alterations in mood, such as those with major depression, should seek help from a qualified professional who can assess and treat the mood disorder. Therapy for actual mood disorders often combines counseling and medication, such as antidepressants. Specific recommendations for diagnosis and treatment of depression are beyond the scope of this book. However, we hope readers will benefit from this discussion of optimism.

Is realistic optimism an important component of resilience? Yes. In fact, during an interview with a Special Forces instructor we asked, "Do Special Forces soldiers tend to be pessimistic or optimistic?"

"Definitely optimistic," the instructor replied. "We can't afford to have a really negative pessimist on one of our teams because pessimism is infectious and brings everybody down... All it takes is one guy getting excited and negative about something we can handle that causes other people to doubt the situation or the leadership. . . If one of our guys is too pessimistic, we try our best to work with him, but if he can't get it right, then we remove him from the team. It's pretty simple really. If you want to be on one of our teams and you don't have optimism, then you better figure out how to get it."

# References

Addis, M. E., Jacobson, N. S. & Martell, C. R. (2001). *Depression in Context: Strategies for Guided Action*. New York, NY: W. W. Norton.

Affleck, G. & Tennen, H. (1996). Construing benefits from adversity: adaptational significance and dispositional underpinnings. *Journal of Personality*, 64, 899–922.

Ashby, F. G., Isen, A. M. & Turken, A. U. (1999). A neuropsychological theory of positive affect and its influence on cognition. *Psychological Review*, 106, 529–550.

Aspinwall, L. G. & Staudinger, U. M. (eds.) (2002). *A Psychology of Human Strengths: Fundamental Questions and Future Directions for a Positive Psychology*. Washington, DC: American Psychological Association.

Beard, C. (2011). Cognitive bias modification for anxiety: Current evidence and future directions. *Expert Review of Neurotherapeutics*, 11(2): 299–311. DOI:10.1586/ern.10.194

Carver, C. S., Pozo, C., Harris, S. D. *et al.* (1993). How coping mediates the effect of optimism on distress: A study of women with early stage breast cancer. *Journal of Personality and Social Psychology*, 65, 375–390.

Carver, C. S. & Scheier, M. F. (2014). Dispositional optimism. *Trends in Cognitive Science*, 18(6), 293–299.

Caspi, A., Sugden, K., Moffitt, T. E. *et al.* (2003). Influence of life stress on depression: Moderation by polymorphism in the 5-HTT gene. *Science*, 301, 386–389.

Caspi, A., McClay, J., Moffitt, T. *et al.* (2002). Role of genotype in the cycle of violence in maltreated children. *Science*, 297, 851–855.

Catalino, L. I. & Fredrickson, B. L. (2011). A Tuesday in the life of a flourisher: The role of positive emotional reactivity in optimal mental health. *Emotion*, 11(4), 938–950.

Catalino, L. I, Algoe, S. B. & Fredrickson, B. L. (2014). Prioritizing positivity: An effective approach to pursuing happiness? *Emotion*, 14(6), 1155–1161.

Chang, E. C., Maydeu-Olivares, A. & D'Zurilla, T. J. (1997). Optimism and pessimism as partially independent constructs: Relations to positive and negative affectivity and psychological well-being. *Personality and Individual Differences*, 23, 433–440.

Charney, D. S. (2004). Psychobiological mechanisms of resilience and vulnerability: Implications for successful adaptation to extreme stress. *American Journal of Psychiatry*, 161, 195–216.

Cohen, S., Doyle, W. J., Turner, R. B. *et al.* (2003). Emotional style and susceptibility to the common cold. *Psychosomatic Medicine*, 65, 652–657.

Coutu, D. (2002). How resilience works. *Harvard Business Review*, May, 46–55.

Danner, D. D., Snowdon, D. A. & Friesen, W. V. (2001). Positive emotions in early life and longevity: Findings from the nun study. *Journal of Personality and Social Psychology*, 80(5), 804–813.

DuBois, C. M., Vesga Lopez, O., Beale, E. E. *et al.* (2015). Relationship between positive psychological constructs and health outcomes in patients with cardiovascular disease: A systematic review. *International Journal of Cardiology*, 195, 265–280.

Feder, A., Nestler, E. J. & Charney, D. (2009). Psychobiology and molecular genetics of resilience. *Nature Reviews*, 10, 446–466.

Folkman, S. (1997). Positive psychological states and coping with severe stress. *Social Science & Medicine*, 45(8), 1207–1221.

Fox, E. (2012). *Rainy Brain, Sunny Brain.* New York, NY: Basic Books.

Fox, E. (2013). The essence of optimism. *Scientific American Mind*, Jan/Feb: 22–27.

Fox, E., Dutton, K., Yates, A., Georgious, G. A. & Mouchlianitis, E. (2015). Attentional control and suppressing negative thought intrusions in pathological worry. *Clinical Psychological Science*, 3(4), 593–606.

Fredrickson, B. L. (2001). The role of positive emotions in positive psychology: The broaden-and-build theory of positive emotions. *American Psychologist*, 56(3), 218–226.

Fredrickson, B. & Branigan, C. (2005). Positive emotions broaden the scope of attention and thought-action repertoires. *Cognition & Emotion*, 19(3), 313–332.

Giltay, E. J., Kamphuis, M. H., Kalmijn, S., Zitman, F. G. & Kromhout, D. (2006). Dispositional optimism and the risk of cardiovascular death: The Zutphen Elderly Study. *Archives of Internal Medicine*, 166, 431–436.

Gison, A., Rizza, F., Bonassi, S., Donati, V. & Giaquinto, S. (2015). Effects of dispositional optimism on quality of life, emotional distress and disability in Parkinson's disease outpatients under rehabilitation. *Functional Neurology*, 30(2), 105–111.

Goldman, S. L., Kraemer, D. T. & Salovey, P. (1996). Beliefs about mood moderate the relationship to illness and symptom reporting. *Journal of Psychosomatic Research*, 41, 115–128.

Guarnera, S. & Williams, R. L. (1987). Optimism and locus of control for health and affiliation among elderly adults. *Journal of Gerontology*, 42(6), 594–595.

Hanson, R. (2009). Taking in the good. *Greater Good Magazine*, November 1, University of California, Berkeley: Greater Good Science Center.

Heintzelman, S. J. & King, L. A. (2014). Life is pretty meaningful. *The American Psychologist*, 69(6), 561–574.

Heller, A. S., Johnstone, T., Shackman, A. J. *et al.* (2009). Reduced capacity to sustain positive emotion in major depression reflects diminished maintenance of fronto-striatal brain activation. *Proceedings of the National Academy of Sciences, USA*, 106(52), 224445–224450.

Heller, A. S., Fox, A. S., Wing, E. K. *et al.* (2015). The neurodynamics of affect in the laboratory predicts persistence of real-world emotional responses. *The Journal of Neuroscience*, 35(29), 10503–10509.

Isen, A. M. (1990). The influence of positive and negative affect on cognitive organization: Some implications for development. In N. L. Stein, B. Leventhal & T. Trabasso (eds.) *Psychological and Biological Approaches to Emotion*, pp. 75–94. Hillsdale, NJ: Lawrence Erlbaum Associates.

Johnstone, T., van Reekum, C. M., Urry, H. L., Kalin, N. H. & Davidson, R. J. (2007). Failure to regulate: counterproductive recruitment of top-down prefrontal-subcortical circuitry in major depression. *Journal of Neuroscience*, 27(33), 8877–8884.

Kaufman, J., Yang, B. Z., Douglas-Palumberi, H. *et al.* (2006). Brain-derived neurotrophic factor-5-HTTLPR gene interactions and environmental modifiers of depression in children. *Biological Psychiatry*, 59, 673–680.

Keller, H. (1903a). *Optimism: An Essay*. New York, NY: Thomas Y. Crowell.

Keller, H. (1903b). *The Story of My Life*. New York, NY: Doubleday.

King, L. A. & Hicks, J. A. (2009). The detection and construction of meaning in life events. *Journal of Positive Psychology*, 4, 317–330.

King, L. A., Hicks, J. A., Krull, J. & Del Gaiso, A. K. (2006). Positive affect and the experience of meaning in life. *Journal of Personality and Social Psychology*, 90, 179–196.

Kruger, J. & Dunning, D. (1999). Unskilled and unaware of it: How difficulties in recognizing one's own incompetence lead to inflated self-assessments. *Journal of Personality and Social Psychology*, 77, 1121–1134.

Lilienfeld, S. O., Watts, A. L. & Smith, S. F. (2015). Successful psychopathy: A scientific status report. *Current Directions in Psychological Science*, 24(4), 298–303.

Moskowitz, J. T., Folkman, S., Collette, L. & Vittinghoff, E. (1996). Coping and mood during AIDS-related caregiving and bereavement. *Annals of Behavioral Medicine*, 18(1), 49–57.

Munafo, M. R., Brown, S. M. & Hariri, A. R. (2008). Serotonin transporter (5-HTTLPR) genotype and amygdala activation: A meta-analysis. *Biological Psychiatry*, 63, 852–857.

Murphy, S. E., Clare O'Donoghue, M., Drazich, E. H. *et al.* (2015). Imagining a brighter future: The effect of positive imagery training on mood, prospective mental imagery and emotional bias in older adults. *Psychiatry Res.*, 230(1), 36–43. DOI:10.1016/j.psychres.2015.07.059

Nestler, E. J. & Carlezon, W. A. (2006). The mesolimbic dopamine reward circuit in depression. *Biological Psychiatry*, 59, 1151–1159.

New, A. S., Fan, J., Murrough, J. W. *et al.* (2009). A functional magnetic resonance imaging study of deliberate emotion regulation in resilience and posttraumatic stress disorder. *Biological Psychiatry*, 66(7), 656–664.

Olson, E. A., Fanning, J. T., Awick, E. A., Chung, H. D. & McAuley, E. (2014). Differential trajectories of well-being in older adult women: The role of optimism. *Applied Psychology: Health and Well-Being*, 6(3), 362–380.

Peale, N. V. (1952). *The Power of Positive Thinking*. Englewood Cliffs, NJ: Prentice-Hall.

Phillips, L. H., Bull, R., Adams, E. & Fraser, L. (2002). Positive mood and executive function: Evidence from Stroop and fluency tasks. *Emotion*, 2, 12–22.

Poulin, M. J., Brown, S. L., Dillard, A. J. & Smith, D. M. (2013). Giving to others and the association between stress and mortality. *American Journal of Public Health*, 103(9), 1649–1655.

Rana, B. K., Darst, B. F., Bloss, C. *et al.* (2014). Candidate SNP associations of optimism and resilience in older adults: Exploratory study of 935 community-dwelling adults. *American Journal of Geriatric Psychiatry*, 22(10), 997–1006.

Reivich, K. & Shatté, A. (2003). *The Resilience Factor: Seven Keys to Finding Your Inner Strength and Overcoming Life's Hurdles*. New York, NY: Broadway Books.

Richardson, R. D., ed. (2012). *The Heart of William James*. Cambridge, MA: Harvard University Press.

Ronaldson, A., Molloy, G. J., Wikman, A. *et al.* (2015). Optimism and recovery after acute coronary syndrome: a clinical cohort study. *Psychosomatic Medicine*, 77(3), 311–318.

Ronaldson, A., Poole, L., Kidd, T. *et al.* (2014). Optimism measured pre-operatively is associated with reduced pain intensity and physical symptom reporting after coronary artery bypass graft surgery. *Journal of Psychosomatic Research*, 77(4), 278–282.

Saslow, E. (2015). A survivor's life. *Washington Post*, December 5. Retrieved from http://www.washingtonpost.com/sf/national/2015/12/05/after-a-mass-shooting-a-survivors-life/

Scheier, M. F., Carver, C. S. & Bridges, M. W. (1994). Distinguishing optimism from neuroticism (and trait anxiety, self-mastery, and self-esteem): A reevaluation of the Life Orientation Test. *Journal of Personality and Social Psychology*, 67(6), 1063–1078.

Scheier, M. F., Matthews, K. A., Owens, J. F. *et al.* (1989). Dispositional optimism and recovery from coronary artery bypass surgery: The beneficial effects of physical and psychological well-being. *Journal of Personality and Social Psychology*, 57, 1024–1040.

Schneider, S. L. (2001). In search of realistic optimism: Meaning, knowledge, and warm fuzziness. *American Psychologist*, 56(3), 250–263.

Segerstrom, S. C. & Sephton, S. E. (2010). Optimistic expectancies and cell-mediated immunity: The role of positive affect. *Psychological Science*, 21(3), 448–455.

Segovia, F., Moore, J. L., Linnville, S. E. & Hoyt, R. E. (2015). Optimism predicts positive health in repatriated prisoners of war. *Psychological Trauma*, 7(3), 222–228.

Seligman, M. E. P. (1998). *Learned Optimism: How to Change Your Mind and Your Life*. New York, NY: Free Press.

Seligman, M. E. P. (2002). *Authentic Happiness: Using the New Positive Psychology to Realize Your Potential for Lasting Fulfillment*. New York, NY: Free Press.

Serlachius, A., Pulkki-Raback, L., Elovainio, M. *et al.* (2015). Is dispositional optimism or dispositional pessimism predictive of ideal cardiovascular health? The Young Finns Study. *Psychology and Health*, 30(10), 1221–1239.

Sharot, T., Riccardi, A. M., Raio, C. M. & Phelps, E. A. (2007). Neural mechanisms mediating optimism bias. *Nature*, 450 (October 24), 102–115.

Skelton, K., Ressler, K. J., Norrholm, S. D., Jovanovic, T. & Bradley-Davino, B. (2011). PTSD and gene variants: New pathways and new thinking. *Neuropharmacology* 62(2), 628–637.

Speer, M. E., Bhanji, J. P. & Delgado, M. R. (2014). Savoring the past: Positive memories evoke value representations in the striatum. *Neuron*, 84, 847–856.

Spiegel, D. & Classen, C. (2000). *Group Therapy for Cancer Patients: A Research-Based Handbook of Psychosocial Care*. New York, NY: Basic Books.

Stellar, J. E., John-Henderson, N., Anderson, C. L. *et al.* (2015). Positive affect and markers of inflammation: Discrete positive emotions predict lower levels of inflammatory cytokines. *Emotion*, 15(2), 129–133.

Stockdale, J. B. (1984). *A Vietnam Experience*. Stanford, CA: Hoover Institution.

Sudak, Donna M., Majeed, M. H., Youngman, B. (2014) Behavioral activation: A strategy to enhance treatment response. *Journal of Psychiatric Practice*, 20(4), 269–275.

Taylor, S. E. (1998). Optimism/pessimism. Summary prepared by Shelley Taylor in collaboration with the Psychosocial Working Group. University of California at

San Francisco. MacArthur Research Network on SES & Health. Accessed July 8, 2009 at www.macses.ucsf.edu/research/psychosocial/optimism.php

Tindle, H. A., Chang, Y. F., Kuller, L. H. *et al.* (2009). Optimism, cynical hostility, and incident coronary heart disease and mortality in the Women's Health Initiative. *Circulation*, 120(8), 656–662.

Tsai, J., El-Gabalawy, R., Sledge, W. H., Southwick, S. M. & Pietrzak, R. H. (2015). Post-traumatic growth among veterans in the USA: results from the National Health and Resilience in Veterans Study. *Psychological Medicine*, 45(1), 165–179. DOI:10.1017/S0033291714001202

Tsai, J., Mota, N. P., Southwick, S. M. & Pietrzak, R. H. (2016). What doesn't kill you makes you stronger: A national study of U.S. military veterans. *J Affect Disord*, 189, 269–271. DOI:10.1016/j.jad.2015.08.076

Twenge, J. M. & Campbell, W. K. (2009). *The Narcissism Epidemic: Living in The Age Of Entitlement* (1st Free Press hardcover edn). New York, NY: Free Press.

Twenge, J. M., Miller, J. D. & Campbell, W. K. (2014). The narcissism epidemic: commentary on modernity and narcissistic personality disorder. *Personality Disorders*, 5(2), 227–229. DOI:10.1037/per0000008

Vanderbilt, T. (2008). *Traffic: Why We Drive the Way We Do (And What It Says About Us)*. New York, NY: Alfred A. Knopf.

Vythilingam, M., Nelson, E. E., Scaramozza, M. *et al.* (2008). Reward circuitry in resilience to severe trauma: An fMRI investigation of resilient special forces soldiers. *Psychiatry Research: Neuroimaging*, 172(1), 75–77.

Whitcomb, D. (2015). Girl critically wounded in Oregon college massacre is released from hospital. *Reuters*, October 13. Retrieved from http://www.reuters.com/article/us-usa-shooting-oregon-idUSKCN0S72UM20151013

Widom, C. S. (1977). A methodology for studying noninstitutionalized psychopaths. *Journal of Consulting and Clinical Psychology*, 45, 674–683.

Zanon, M., Novembre, G., Zangrando, N., Chittaro, L. & Silani, G. (2014). Brain activity and prosocial behavior in a simulated life-threatening situation. *Neuroimage*, 98, 134–146. DOI:10.1016/j.neuroimage.2014.04.053

Zeidner, M. & Hammer, A. L. (1992). Coping with missile attack: resources, strategies, and outcomes. *Journal of Personality*, 60, 709–746.

# CHAPTER 3

# Facing Fear: An Adaptive Response

Fear is ubiquitous. No one escapes its grip. Fear even strikes individuals who are widely admired for their courage. South African dissident Nelson Mandela reported that during his years of imprisonment and struggle against oppression, "I learned that courage was not the absence of fear, but the triumph over it. I felt fear myself more times than I can remember, but I hid it behind a mask of boldness. The brave man is not he who does not feel afraid, but he who conquers that fear" (1995, p. 622).

For some people, fear is constricting and even paralyzing, while for others it is energizing and serves as a catalyst for growth. Whether we allow it to diminish us or enlist it as an ally, fear has an enormous impact on how we conduct our lives. To become more resilient, sooner or later we will need to face our fears. In this chapter, we will discuss the importance of fear, its neurobiological underpinnings, and ways to manage and even take advantage of it.

## The Science of Fear

We begin this chapter with science because it will deepen your understanding of the survivor stories that follow. When we encounter something that frightens us, we react with the urge either to defend ourselves or to run away. This "fight-or-flight" response was first described by Harvard physiologist Walter Cannon in the early twentieth century. Cannon observed that, without any conscious effort on our part, our body mobilizes us to fight or to flee. Fear does us a great favor: it prepares us to react to danger.

The fight–flight response is mediated, in part, by a group of chemicals called catecholamines (which include epinephrine, norepinephrine, and dopamine). The nervous system releases these chemicals in response to perceived danger. Catecholamines shut down blood flow to the digestive system, which slows during dangerous situations, and instead shunt blood to the heart and skeletal muscles, which are needed for fighting or fleeing. Our reflexes sharpen and blood flow to capillaries decreases. This reduces bleeding if we are wounded.

In the brain, the catecholamine, norepinephrine, stimulates multiple brain regions, including the amygdala. It helps us to orient toward potentially dangerous stimuli, and then zero in on the most threatening stimulus in our immediate environment, such as a weapon or an attacker's fist. Increased levels of norepinephrine in the amygdala also enhance encoding and consolidation of memory, which makes memories that occur during dangerous situations especially strong and sometimes unforgettable.

To demonstrate the importance of norepinephrine in the formation of memories of arousing and traumatic events, Larry Cahill and James McGaugh at the University of California, Irvine, studied a group of college students and showed them a series of photographic slides. Some of the slides were neutral in content while others showed a traumatic event (a young child being hit by a car) (Cahill *et al.*, 1994). One week later, the college students came back for "surprise" memory testing. The students remembered the traumatic slides better than the neutral ones. Why? The researchers hypothesized that traumatic slides stimulated arousal, and an increase in norepinephrine in the amygdala, and that this norepinephrine enhanced memory consolidation.

To test this hypothesis, McGaugh and Cahill conducted a second experiment (McGaugh, 2000). They divided students into two groups and gave the first group a drug called Propranolol, which blocks norepinephrine. Propranolol is commonly used to treat high blood pressure. They gave the second group of students a placebo sugar pill. Both groups then viewed the same series of neutral and traumatic slides. As in the first study, the participants returned a week later for surprise memory testing. As predicted, the placebo group remembered the slides showing trauma better than the neutral slides, presumably because viewing the traumatic slides caused an increase in arousal and norepinephrine, which in turn caused an increase in memory consolidation. The Propranolol group, however, remembered the traumatic slides no better than the neutral slides – apparently because the drug had blocked the action of the norepinephrine which had been released upon viewing the images of trauma.

In light of these studies, we ourselves decided to evaluate further the effects of norepinephrine on memory (Southwick *et al.*, 2002), but we took a different approach: rather than blocking norepinephrine while subjects viewed this same series of slides, we increased norepinephrine shortly after the subjects had finished viewing them. We gave half of the volunteers a medication that briefly increases the body's release of its own norepinephrine. The others received a placebo pill. As expected, subjects with the greatest increases in norepinephrine remembered both neutral and traumatic slides better than did subjects with less robust increases in norepinephrine. Taken together, these and many other studies provide support for the finding that people remember emotionally arousing events better than emotionally neutral events, and that norepinephrine plays an important role in strengthening memory for these emotionally arousing events. Thinking back on your own life, out of the countless experiences that you have had, which ones do you remember the best? You remember experiences you had when you were emotionally aroused and your norepinephrine was elevated, that is, when you were happy, sad, angry or afraid.

# Fear Conditioning

Not only do people tend to remember emotionally arousing and traumatic events better than emotionally neutral events, but they also tend to remember the context in which arousing events occur (LeDoux, 1996, 2002, 2016). The brain's limbic system links the fear that accompanies a traumatic event to sights, sounds, odors, time of day, weather conditions, and other ordinarily neutral stimuli that are present during the frightening event. These contextual stimuli can then become fear-conditioned cues that are capable of triggering fear by themselves because of their previous association with danger. These contextual stimuli/cues now serve as predictors of potential current or future danger. Because the linking of fear with contextual stimuli occurs in the limbic system, we may not be consciously aware that these contextual stimuli can trigger a fear response on their own (LeDoux, 1996, 2016).

For example, imagine that you are walking through a park near your home, a place where you have frequently taken pleasant and relaxing walks. This time, however, someone runs up behind you, holds a knife to your throat, grabs your wallet, shoves you to the ground, kicks you, and runs away. The park that you once enjoyed now becomes a fear-conditioned stimulus. From now on, each time you walk near the park, its newly formed association with danger makes you feel anxious. In fact, you may become afraid of all parks, not just this one.

This process, known as classical conditioning, is familiar to those who know the story of Russian physiologist Ivan Pavlov and his dogs. Seeking to study digestion in dogs, Pavlov measured their saliva flow when they were fed meat powder. He began to notice that the dogs salivated even before being fed, as soon as they heard the sound of the researcher's footsteps approaching their cages. The dogs had come to associate the sound of footsteps with meat powder so that the footsteps themselves caused the dogs to salivate. Classical conditioning works similarly in humans: we have a response (in this case a negative response, fear) when we are exposed to formerly neutral stimuli (such as the sights, smells, and sounds of a park) that have been paired with a traumatic event (being attacked).

A friend of ours, John, was mystified by a personal experience that involved fear conditioning. One spring, John noticed that every time he walked outdoors into his garden, he immediately began to feel both afraid and nauseated. When he walked back into the house, the fear and nausea rapidly dissipated. This sequence lasted for a few weeks, and then one day it just stopped; walking into the garden no longer bothered him. John remained baffled until one evening, months later, he suddenly identified the trigger for his fear and nausea: the song of a particular type of migrating bird that passed through his town for several weeks each spring. But why would birdsong trigger anxiety and such an unpleasant reaction? Because a year earlier, John had been diagnosed with cancer and was receiving chemotherapy. Naturally, he was frightened by the cancer and the chance that he might not survive, and like many patients, he suffered from nausea as a side effect of the chemotherapy. Each time he came home from a treatment, he sat in the garden hoping to ease his anxiety and recover from his nausea. At that time of the year, the migrating birds were singing in his garden. At a purely unconscious level, John's limbic system formed an association between the birdsong and his feelings of fear and nausea.

Returning to the example of the assault in the park, suppose you were attacked on a hot and humid day. In the days, weeks, months and even years after the attack, you might find yourself unaccountably feeling anxious every time the weather is hot and humid. In our own research, we have observed this phenomenon in veterans who had narrowly escaped death during combat. Years later, they, too, may feel afraid when the weather resembles the weather on the day that they risked death, yet they cannot explain why they feel afraid. Anniversary reactions can operate in a similar way. Survivors may feel anxious on the anniversary of a traumatic event without consciously associating their current anxiety with the original trauma. Instead, they may search for something in their current life that might explain their anxiety.

Why does the brain have a mechanism to strengthen memory for dangers and the conditions under which the dangers occur? The answer is survival. An organism that remembers a past danger (through enhanced consolidation) can recognize a similar current or future danger and respond accordingly. Similarly, the organism that remembers the context or stimuli that were associated with a past danger (through fear conditioning) will react to similar stimuli as if the danger were present again. In other words, the neutral stimuli that have been transformed into fear-conditioned stimuli now serve as predictors of potential danger. And, of course, the animal or person that can predict danger is likely to survive and pass on its genes.

Formation of memory for dangerous events and for associated fear-conditioned stimuli occurs quickly and tends to be very durable. In fact, these memories may last a lifetime. Joseph LeDoux, a pioneer in the neurobiology of fear, puts it this way:

> If an animal is lucky enough to survive one dangerous encounter, its brain should store as much about the experience as possible, and this learning should not decay over time, since a predator will always be a predator. In modern life, we sometimes suffer from the exquisite operation of this system, since it is difficult to get rid of this kind of conditioning once it is no longer applicable to our lives, and we become conditioned to fear things that are in fact harmless. Evolution's wisdom sometimes comes at a cost. (2002, p. 124)

# Can We Prevent or Undo Fear Conditioning?

Once we live through a terrifying experience, does that mean that we will be haunted by fear-conditioned memories of the experience for the rest of our lives? Fortunately, no. The story of Al DeAngelis' skydiving trip provides an example of how "getting back on the horse" right away can alter memory consolidation.

On Memorial Day, in 1989, 26-year-old DeAngelis and several friends drove to a small airport in northwestern New Jersey for an afternoon of skydiving. None of them had ever been skydiving before, so to prepare for "static-line jumping" (parachuting without a partner), they had each trained for four to six hours to learn how to leap out of a plane, deploy a parachute, and land without injury.

When they arrived at the airport, they were surprised at the condition of their airplane. The exterior was patched together, and although it was built to carry eight to ten passengers, the interior had no seats. As Al put it, "It was no Cessna." However, nobody had promised them a luxury plane, so they began to joke and laugh about the V.I.P. accommodations as they assembled their gear. They boarded the plane along with the pilot and a jump master, sat on the floor, and waited for takeoff. However, despite numerous attempts, the engine failed to turn over. Finally, the pilot called air traffic control for help. "So they bring a truck to jump-start the plane... It was a big joke," Al recalls. "'Oh my God, they're going to jump-start our plane. I just can't wait to get out.' We were kidding around." Eventually, the engine started, and the plane took off, but before it reached cruising altitude, an enormous explosion shook the plane. Within seconds, Al and his friends were covered with oil, and the cabin had filled with smoke.

> I couldn't even see the guy next to me or in front of me. As soon as this happened, the pilot screamed "Mayday!" He was trying to get control of the plane, but I guess the

> motor wasn't operating properly and it threw a rod; it actually blew a part of the motor out along with the hydraulics and electronics... The jump master was totally panicked, screaming and running back and forth – that's why I remember it so vividly, because I thought, of all the people in the plane, he is the one who is supposed to be the calmest.

When the smoke inside the cabin briefly cleared, Al could see the jump master opening the side door of the plane. Al remembers thinking, "I'm either going to burn to death or get thrown out of the plane." Somehow, in spite of the chaos and blinding smoke, the pilot, who had spent years flying large jets for a major airline, successfully landed the burning plane in a rural field. After what seemed like an eternity, the plane finally came to a stop and everyone, including the pilot, jumped out and raced away from the wreckage.

> As soon as we got away from the plane, we didn't really say anything to each other; we were just standing around; we were scared... The pilot had a pack of cigarettes – I guess he is a smoker, and I have never even had a cigarette in my life. I took one of his cigarettes. I smoked that thing probably in two breaths, I was so nervous. The pilot was so scared he couldn't light his cigarette, he was shaking so much. We all had bumps and bruises, but nobody was seriously hurt.

A police helicopter soon landed on the site, and fire trucks and ambulances arrived. After Al and his co-workers were medically evaluated by emergency medical technicians, they were offered an ambulance ride to the nearest hospital. But each of them refused; all they wanted was a ride back to the airport so they could get their cars and drive home.

> As we were driving back to the airport, I started getting really nervous, and I got nervous to the point where I started to shake a little bit. So we got to the airport, and I told my friends, "I am going up on the next flight." I said, "If I don't go up on this next plane, I am never going to get in an airplane again, let alone skydive again." They thought I was crazy.

When Al told the sky-diving company that he wanted to go up again in the next available plane, they were amazed but they agreed.

> When they began to put the parachute on me, I started to shake so much that my knees – like in a cartoon or in a movie – were quivering to the point where I couldn't stand. So I sat down on a table and they strapped the chute on me while my knees were shaking. I was trying not to. I did not want them to see it; I was wearing a jumpsuit, but I was shaking... Then they gave us a few minutes, and I kind of got myself together so that I could stand up.
>
> As I was walking towards this airplane, which, again, looked a little shady, the new pilot jokingly said, "I heard you guys were in a crash. I don't think we'll get in another one." You know, kidding around, trying to ease my mind... So I got on the plane, and as we started to taxi and take off, I am telling you, I could not wait to get out of that plane. I never felt so motivated in my life. I just wanted to get to the door and jump out. And sure enough, I did it, and when I landed, it was probably the greatest feeling that I have had in my entire life. I did it and got it out of the way.

Al DeAngelis went on to a successful career as a forensic detective in Monmouth County, New Jersey, where he has routinely faced danger and fear. He has worked in uniform and under cover, on narcotics squads and SWAT (Special Weapons And Tactics) teams. As a young man, he learned one of the most important lessons in facing fear: when you're bucked off a horse – or a plane – get back on as soon as possible.

Why was Al DeAngelis able to return from his terrifying outing feeling good? Research shows that new memories remain unstable or malleable for a short period of time immediately after the event. During this unstable period, memories are being encoded and consolidated into long-term storage through a mechanism that involves the synthesis of proteins. In rats, this malleable period of memory consolidation may last no longer than an hour or two. In humans, the period appears to be longer. If we intervene during this window of time, when the new memory is "unstable," it may be possible to alter consolidation of the memory.

Our colleague, Roger Pitman at Harvard Medical School, conducted an experiment addressing this theory, extending the research by James McGaugh that we described earlier. In 2002, Pitman intervened with accident victims who came into an emergency room. Beginning within six hours after the trauma, these patients took either a placebo or the drug Propranolol for 10 days. Recall that Propranolol is known to block the increase of norepinephrine that naturally occurs during and soon after a traumatic event. Pitman and his colleagues hypothesized that taking Propranolol shortly after the trauma would interfere with consolidation, making the memory less emotionally arousing and upsetting in the future.

At an assessment three months later, the Propranolol-treated patients showed no difference in level of PTSD symptoms compared to patients who received a placebo; however, they did have significantly reduced physiological reactions (heart rate, skin conductance) upon listening to a recorded account of their own traumatic experience. These findings are encouraging for possible medical interventions in the future aimed at decreasing the potency of traumatic memories. However, it is important to note that studies using medication to decrease the intensity of traumatic memories are in their infancy; currently there are no medications approved by the Food and Drug Administration to specifically alter emotionally arousing and fear-related memories.

As we saw in the story of Al DeAngelis, encoding and consolidation can be altered immediately after an event without medication. But what happens if you don't get back on the plane right away? Is it too late months or even years later? The answer appears to be no. Until recently it was believed that a memory remains essentially unchanged once it has been consolidated into long-term storage. However, newer research suggests that every time a memory is retrieved, it once again becomes fragile and unstable for a brief period of time until it is consolidated again.

The process is called reconsolidation. This unstable period provides another window of time during which the memory may be disrupted or updated and transformed. In other words, each time a memory is recalled, it can be weakened, strengthened, or otherwise modified during reconsolidation. Research in animals and more recently in humans holds promise for both pharmacological (e.g., Propranolol) and behavioral (e.g., extinction training) interventions aimed at modifying fearful memories, not only shortly after a trauma, but also later, even years later, when fearful memories are retrieved and re-consolidated (Hartley & Phelps, 2010; Brunet *et al.*, 2008; Schiller *et al.*, 2010; Quirk *et al.*, 2010; Lee, Nader & Schiller, 2017). Researchers have also suggested that the process of reconsolidation plays an important role in psychotherapy (Lane *et al.*, 2015). When a patient recalls and re-evaluates a past experience with the guidance of a psychotherapist, the new reconsolidated memory is different and – one hopes – more positive and adaptive. Ideally, the new memory then serves as a "corrective experience," leading to a more positive emotional response when the memory is again recalled (Alberini & Ledoux, 2013).

# The Neuroscience of Extinction

The process of overcoming a learned fear is called extinction (LeDoux, 1996, 2002, 2016; Clem & Schiller, 2016). It involves the brain structures that we discussed earlier (the amygdala, prefrontal cortex (PFC), and hippocampus). To extinguish a fear-conditioned memory, a person must be exposed to the fear-inducing stimulus in a safe environment, and this exposure needs to last long enough for the brain to form a new memory. This new memory conveys that the fear-conditioned stimulus is no longer dangerous in the present environment. Brain imaging findings suggest that extinction may involve a strengthening of the capacity of the PFC to inhibit amygdala-based fear responses (Phelps *et al.*, 2004).

Several approaches to treating anxiety have been shown to be effective in promoting extinction. In essence, these therapies encourage the patient to confront fear and anxiety head-on. To understand why such treatments are effective for disorders, such as PTSD and phobias, it is important to note that avoidance is a hallmark of anxiety disorders. Although it is natural for trauma survivors to avoid situations that remind them of the original trauma and therefore make them anxious, avoiding such situations prevents them from updating or transforming their fear-based learning and memories. This is why many successful psychotherapies involve some form of confrontation with the fear.

One of these therapies, known as flooding or direct exposure therapy, requires prolonged exposure to the memory of the traumatic event. In her book *Stress and Trauma*, Patricia Resick (2001) describes the therapy as consisting of "extended exposure to moderate or strong fear-producing cues. In addition to confronting fear cues in imagination, flooding also involves confrontation with the conditioned fear cues *in vivo*" (p. 153). In the imagination component, patients are asked to recount the traumatic experience with eyes closed and in as much detail as possible, describing sights, sounds, smells, and sensations, as well as what they were thinking and feeling. These sessions are recorded, and the client then listens to the recording repeatedly on subsequent days. In the in-vivo component, clients "gradually confront safe situations that evoke moderate levels of anxiety and then follow up with confrontations of more fearful situations" (p. 153).

Just as we saw earlier with the use of Propranolol to reduce the consolidation of fear-conditioned memories, researchers are also developing pharmacological methods designed to facilitate extinction of traumatic memories. Because extinction involves new learning, and the protein molecule known as the NMDA receptor is critical to learning, Barbara Rothbaum and colleagues at Emory University experimented with giving the NMDA receptor partial agonist D-cycloserine (DCS) with exposure therapy. DCS is a drug that activates the NMDA receptor, which then enhances learning of the new memory. Rothbaum's team hypothesized that the combination of exposure therapy and DCS would speed up the process of extinction, and their findings supported this hypothesis: patients taking DCS showed significantly faster improvement than did subjects taking a placebo. Other more recent published studies on the efficacy of combining DCS with exposure therapy have not been as positive as Rothbaum's (Mataix-Cols *et al.*, 2017). However, the prospect of augmenting extinction-based therapies, like prolonged exposure, with medications that affect learning is promising.

A related treatment approach is eye-movement desensitization and reprocessing therapy. In this therapy, the patient is asked to remember the trauma in detail while visually tracking the therapist's finger as it moves back and forth (Resick, 2001). It was initially proposed that lateral eye movements would facilitate the mental processing of the trauma. However, studies by Roger Pitman and others suggest that exposure is the key therapeutic element and that the eye movement component may not be crucial.

Cognitive processing therapy (CPT) also involves confronting fear. It uses the Socratic method of teaching, in which the teacher poses questions and the student, by answering them, learns new ways of understanding. CPT focuses on emotions such as anger, humiliation, shame, guilt, and sadness, which trauma survivors often experience in addition to fear and anxiety. It is not uncommon for trauma victims to believe, for example, that they could have done something to prevent the traumatic event or acted more heroically to minimize harm, even if in reality such actions would have been impossible. They tend to blame themselves and to imagine that others blame them as well. For example, a crime victim may have unrealistic beliefs such as,

"I shouldn't have gone to the ATM that night." A therapist using CPT asks questions aimed at helping the patient to arrive at the more realistic conclusion that he or she could not have predicted that a robber would choose that particular ATM on that particular evening, and that the fault lies with the thief, not with the victim.

Another related technique involves helping trauma survivors understand when and why various fear-conditioned stimuli make them feel anxious and afraid in their current life. For example, as mentioned earlier, a trauma survivor may feel anxious at the same time every year but not understand why. By becoming aware that the brain unconsciously associates this time of year with a traumatic event that occurred during the same season or on the same day of the year in the past, the survivor is better able to anticipate current and future "anniversary reactions." In addition, the survivor is better able to interpret and understand the origin of emotions that previously may have been confusing and overwhelming. Our friend John's experience with birdsong provides a good example. Once he became consciously aware of the connection between birdsong, nausea, and anxiety, he was better able to understand and anticipate this yearly reaction. John believes that this understanding has provided him with an increased sense of control because now when the birds return, he can remind himself, "This anxiety that I am feeling now is not related to anything that is happening to me in the present but instead to the circumstances of the past when I was worried about my cancer." Similarly, therapy can bring to consciousness other cues associated with a trauma – certain sights, sounds, odors, weather conditions. Emerging laboratory evidence has shown that becoming consciously aware of an unconscious fear-conditioned association may help to inhibit or reduce feelings of fear related to the conditioned cue (Jovanovic & Norrholm, 2011). It may be that with conscious awareness one can appraise the current situation as no longer dangerous, and this process is likely to facilitate prefrontal cortical inhibition of the amygdala.

However, you do not necessarily have to undergo therapy to transform or extinguish a fearful memory. The experience of our good friend Janine Solejar provides a relevant example. Solejar coped with longstanding fear when she literally got back on a horse after a long hiatus. She recalls:

> I was 14 and we had just gotten a horse for Christmas named Macy. One Sunday my sister brought Macy out in our driveway so the whole family could take turns riding. I had taken riding lessons for a few years, and had been told horses can tell if you're scared, but I always said I wasn't afraid of horses at all. I felt very confident as the older sister, so I decided to ride down the street instead of just staying in the yard.
>
> Apparently Macy saw this as a chance to escape – or maybe she was having a fear response of her own? Anyway, she took off at a trot, then a canter, and then a full-out

gallop. I tried to pull the reins and yell "Whoa!" as I'd been taught, but it didn't work with Macy. She just kept running faster and faster. A car went by and spooked her even more. At that point I was totally panicked. Neighbors who saw it happen said the reins were flapping loose and I was yelling, "Oh, no! Oh, no!" Finally, after what seemed like forever, Macy lunged in a mud puddle and I fell off. Landing on the pavement felt like a great relief to me. A man who had been working in his yard ran over and asked if I was all right. I started reciting my name and address, like an automated recording.

That night we were watching TV and *Bonanza* came on. Someone jumped on a horse and started galloping away, and I started shrieking and put my hands over my eyes and had to get up and run out of the room, I had such an overwhelming feeling of panic seeing that man on the galloping horse. Of course, I knew in my head that he was an actor and it was all just staged for TV, but at the gut level that didn't matter. I was sure he was going to fall off, and I didn't want to have to watch. I was afraid of all horses after that.

Although Janine's traumatic experience lasted only a few minutes and did not result in any permanent injury, she continued to fear horses and reminders of horses for several years. However, like Al DeAngelis, Janine Solejar found a way to confront her fear without medical intervention, but she did not seek it out, and it did not happen until several years after the mishap.

When I was 17, I was visiting some friends, Ruth and Barbara, who had a horse named Danny that they assured me had always been very gentle and was now quite old and didn't even have any teeth anymore. They encouraged me to try riding again, saying they would lead Danny around by the reins. I was shaking so badly I had trouble mounting, and then I think I just sat there kind of frozen while Ruth and Barbara walked Danny around their garden for about 10 minutes. I was still pretty shaky when I got off, but after that I was OK around horses. I was even able to enjoy riding again. To this day, more than 40 years later, I still feel fear when I relive the memory of the runaway, but it doesn't paralyze me anymore.

Janine formed a new memory of riding a horse, a memory in which being on the horse was safe. This new memory then successfully competed with the fearful memory of her earlier, frightening experience. In fact, decades later, after many years of being out of touch with horses, Janine rode a horse again and the horse bucked. However, "My training kicked in. I automatically kept my weight on the stirrups and held my seat. When the horse stopped bucking, I was shaken but not too scared to continue the ride."

# Feeling Fear Is Only Human

Although in this chapter we emphasize the value of surmounting one's fears, at this juncture we do want to acknowledge that fear is inevitable; at times, everyone feels afraid.

Journalist Sebastian Junger came to understand overwhelming fear while embedded with US troops in Afghanistan. He is the author of books such as *War, A Death in Belmont*, and *The Perfect Storm*, and co-director of *Restrepo*, a documentary film about the Afghan war. He is known for his hands-on coverage of military combat, high-risk civilian occupations, and other life-threatening situations. Although Junger seems relatively comfortable with high-stress situations, he nevertheless admits to moments of sheer terror, such as the time that he and a colleague, an Iranian-born photojournalist, were pinned down in a foxhole in Afghanistan as Taliban missiles pelted the surrounding hillside.

> There was nothing exciting about it, nothing even abstractly interesting. It was purely, exclusively bad... No matter how small the odds were, the idea that I could go straight from life to nonexistence was almost unbearable... Bravery – the usual alternative to fear – also held no appeal, because bravery could get you killed. It had become very simple: It was their war, their problem, and I didn't want any part of it. I just wanted off the hill. (2001, pp. 207–208)

Eventually Junger and the photographer got their wish to get "off the hill." It came in the form of an order to abandon their position and run for their lives. As they ran, Junger recalls,

> Mainly there was the sound of my breathing: a deep, desperate rasp that ruled out any chance of hearing the rockets come in... Ten minutes later it was over: we sat behind the next ridge and watched Taliban rockets continue to pound the hill, each one raising a little puff of smoke, followed by a muffled explosion. From that distance they didn't look like much; they almost looked like the kind of explosions you could imagine yourself acting bravely in. (2001, p. 208)

## Don't Let Fear Hang Around for Too Long

As Junger notes, his experience of intense fear was fleeting. But what happens to a person when fear persists for a long time? Imagine yourself as a soldier in combat, exposed to one danger after another, day after day, for months, or even years. Or suppose you are a woman in an abusive marriage. Because of your situation, you live with fear day in and day out. In such circumstances, chronic stress and fear can wear you down mentally and physically. As the Canadian endocrinologist Hans Selye described some 50 years ago, repeated exposure to such threats will eventually lead to exhaustion. Chronic fear is counter-productive.

When fear, stress, or hypervigilance continue unabated for a long time, the effects can be serious. In a patient information article entitled "Stress and your health," eminent neuroscientists Bruce McEwen and Robert Sapolsky (2006) describe the symptoms that can arise from chronic stress:

- stomach upsets and diarrhea,
- overeating,
- weakening of the immune system,
- insomnia,
- decreased interest in physical activity,
- decreased sex drive,
- anxiety and depression.

Through its tendency to increase blood pressure, heart rate, cholesterol and triglycerides, blood sugar, and appetite, chronic stress can even lead to an increased risk of heart disease.

Recent evidence (Arnsten, 2009, 2015; Sapolsky, 2017) suggests that prolonged stress can damage the PFC and the hippocampus. Damage to either of these brain areas can make it more difficult to shut off the fear response, and leaves the person feeling anxious and afraid much of the time. Thus, while fear can benefit us in the short run, unabated fear can harm us.

# Practical Applications: Learning to Face Fear

Learning to face fear is essential for resilience. Tim Cooper, Gordon Smith, and Mark Hickey, instructors in the Special Forces SERE School, believe that we can all learn to face our fears by using a number of tested techniques. Some of these techniques focus on thinking, while others focus on behaviors. Even if you have no plans to join the military, these techniques will be useful when facing your own fears or perhaps recovering from a traumatic experience.

# View Fear as a Guide

For Sergeants Cooper, Smith, and Hickey, to master fear one must first accept it, even welcome it. Rather than appraising fear as something to avoid, these men have trained soldiers to view fear as normal, as a guide and even as an opportunity to grow. When afraid, they focus on their goal or mission,

> Fear is normal. You try to tell the student that throughout life, you'll experience fear in some form or fashion; but the difference between that and panic is control. You let your fear guide you. You respect it. I mean, I got bit by a snake, a copperhead. OK, not a smart move, but I'm not going to panic because that's just going to make the symptoms worse.

In his 2007 book, *In Extremis Leadership: Leading as if Your Life Depended on It*, Col. Thomas Kolditz, head of the Department of Behavioral Sciences and Leadership at the United States Military Academy at West Point, points out that fear is largely a chemical reaction. It is a natural bodily process; it does not signify weakness. From a neuroscience perspective, under normal nonstressful conditions, moderate levels of catecholamines, such as norepinephrine, enhance functioning of the PFC. However, when brain catecholamine levels rise too high, they tend to take the PFC "off-line," meaning that the PFC no longer adequately inhibits the amygdala. At that point, the fight–flight response predominates and the individual may panic and become impulsive.

Cooper intuitively understands the difference between fear and panic.

> You can control fear. I can almost even use it for my benefit. But with panic, I can't control it. And if I let fear get so big that it turns into panic, then that's when it immobilizes me, keeps me from doing what I need to do.

When Cooper notes that he can almost use fear for benefit, he is pointing out that moderate levels of fear (and moderate levels of catecholamines) may actually sharpen focus and decision-making. And when he cautions against letting fear "get so big that it turns into panic," he means that panic (excessively high levels of catecholamines) can greatly compromise prefrontal cortical functioning and rational decision-making. During combat, soldiers sometimes refer to this compromised cognitive state as "the fog of war," which means stress-related loss of mental clarity and rational decision-making.

# View Fear as an Opportunity

In addition to viewing fear as a helpful warning and guide, medic and SF instructor Mark Hickey believes that fear is good because it keeps him on his toes and serves as a platform for developing courage, self-esteem, and a sense of mastery. When Hickey experiences fear, he often thinks, "I'm scared, but I can learn from this," or "This is a test that's going to make me stronger." During dangerous missions or training exercises, he feels "apprehension and excitement mixed with fear," and as he puts it,

> I think that fear is good because it keeps you sharp. They say when you don't become afraid at all, that's when mistakes start happening, when you take things for granted. When you still have that little bit of fear, you recheck your equipment. You make sure things are as they should be.

Indeed, a certain amount of fear is adaptive.

# Focus on the Goal or Mission

Many of us who are facing fear waste precious time and resources by focusing too much on potential negative and catastrophic scenarios and by fretting about the unknown. Instead, SF instructors teach soldiers to concentrate on goals and on the mission of the group, even when they are grappling with fear.

Cooper recommends that soldiers ask themselves,

> What are my goals? What is my mission? What is the mission of my group? In order to meet my goals and accomplish my mission, I know that I must make a choice: either back down and fail, or face this fear and forge ahead. It's that simple.

When Cooper advises a frightened trainee who is about to make his first night parachute jump from 20,000 feet, he tells the trainee to concentrate on his or her own personal goals and remember that he or she is part of a team with a shared mission:

> Look, I need you out there right now. You need to be helping me, I need you involved in this. Don't worry about it, dude, I'm afraid too. This is an unnatural act for humans; otherwise we'd all be flying to work, we'd all be flying home. Bottom line is: I understand your nervousness... But you have to think, there's a bigger task, there's a bigger goal and it's bigger than you and it's bigger than me. We have to go out and get a job done. And I need you as a part of this, so, come on – let's you and I go ahead and knock this out.

The SF instructors we interviewed also recommend a number of behaviors that they have found helpful in dealing with fear. These include acquiring as much information as possible about what is feared, learning and practicing the skills necessary to face the fear, developing a plan and a back-up plan, confronting fear in the company of a friend or colleague or spiritual presence whenever possible, and taking a calculated leap of faith.

# Acquire Information About What Is Feared

The former Navy pilot and Vietnam POW Al Carpenter understands the importance of recognizing and learning about what is feared.

> A big part of true fear is the fear of the unknown, when you don't know what's gonna happen to you. You can't anticipate, but you think it's gonna be horrible. But most of the scenarios that we, as combat pilots, might face, we have already learned about from other people [instructors and colleagues], from our own experiences, or whatever. So we were prepared.

In the military, fighter pilots or SF team members are required to complete many hours of didactic classroom work that addresses a wide array of topics. These didactics are necessary for optimal performance during complex, challenging, and often dangerous missions. The goal is to expose soldiers to as many potential mission scenarios as possible so that they will not be surprised or overwhelmed by the unknown. The military believes that knowledge is power. To master fear successfully, first learn as much as possible about what is feared.

# Learn and Practice the Skills Necessary to Master the Fear

Once we acquire sufficient information about what is feared, we can learn and practice the skills needed to master the fear. Whenever possible, those skills should be practiced repetitively until they become automatic or second nature. This is what psychologists call achieving automaticity.

West Point instructor Col. Thomas Kolditz advises us to focus on our breath:

> Of all the autonomic responses to the adrenalin rush – including heart rate, respiration, skin conductivity, and muscle tension – the one that we can best control consciously is respiration. Deep, controlled breathing is largely incompatible with the other elements of the fear response. Physical relaxation can get you to the point where mental relaxation, and therefore outward focus, can be re-established and maintained. (2007, p. 122)

When we asked former POW pilots about how they felt while ejecting from fighter jets that had burst into flames while traveling at hundreds of miles per hour, many did not remember feeling a great deal of fear at the actual time of the ejection. We learned that they had so fully achieved automaticity that they did not report feeling afraid. Instead, they remember responding almost "automatically" to a checklist of skills they had mastered during countless hours of training, where they had practiced mock ejection scenarios so many times that an actual real-life ejection required little thought. Lt. Al Carpenter describes his ejection over North Vietnam:

> It was the back end of the aircraft that was ablaze. I really needed to take care of myself, get out of there... So I started climbing very rapidly. I was at full power, still on fire. My intention was to climb to about 9,000 feet, shut the engine down purposely, hope that the fire would go out, and try to get a re-light and possibly I could get back to the ship.
>
> Well, that was a pretty optimistic approach. But it was the only game in town at that point. On my way to 9,000 feet, passing about 5,500 feet, the airplane lurched... I lost my oxygen. I lost all my electrical power. I deployed my emergency generator and I got electrical power back and then I lost it again, and then basically all I had were pressure instruments. Nothing else was working. The control stick went full forward and right. My right rudder pedal slammed full forward. The plane lurched sideways and started to roll right. What had happened really is that the tail burned off, and it started to turn and

that caused me to start a slow rudder roll. Well, I was headed up and I was climbing at a pretty good rate... The aircraft continued to roll all the way to inverted.

And there's something about most aviators, we just really don't want to eject inverted, 'cause you have visions of becoming a lawn dart. I had already stowed all the stuff, with my kneeboard, my flashlight, and anything that might hurt me on the way out. I waited for the airplane to become upright. I looked down at the airspeed just before I punched out: it was at 550 knots and climbing very rapidly. I'd already ejected a couple of months before that, in August, back at the ship at 200 knots, and that was a nice, calm deliberate ejection. No problem.

But this one was just incredibly violent. Incredibly violent. When the canopy went off, the noise outside was just incredible. It was like lying on train tracks with a freight train going over you... And as the seat fired and I went up the rails, I could feel this knife edge come down across me, which was the air blast on my body. You know how fast these things are happening. And still the mind becomes so acutely aware, you just compress everything and get it in slow-motion.

Then your training kicks in and you determine what you're going to do next. Well, I was now floating in the chute. I opened my eyes to assess the situation and my first reaction was, I lost my vision. It was totally black. I knew that my eyes were open, but I had absolutely no vision whatsoever. And in the race that your mind goes through trying to make sense out of all of this, I first thought, well, maybe my optic nerves have been severed. How would that happen? Who knows? And then the next thought was, well, maybe I've lost my face 'cause the pain was so incredible all over, I had no idea what might be damaged.

So I thought, well, I have to survive so we'll just go on. And the first thing you do after you eject from a jet like that is reach up and get rid of your oxygen mask. So I reached up with both hands but felt incredible pain in one shoulder. Finally, I hit something that was very hard and smooth and felt like it was wet.

Yup. I've wiped off my face. But for some reason, I went around to the side, I guess to see if I still had ears or something, and here's my oxygen mask. Boy, that was a good feeling. I grabbed the ear piece of my helmet, and I pulled it around and, bingo, I could see. It was like the Wizard of Oz, you know, everything becomes Technicolor for Dorothy. But that was one of the best feelings of my life. So then I knew why I couldn't see. My eyes had been encased in the helmet ear piece.

For most people, such a situation would evoke paralyzing fear, but not for Carpenter. When asked if he felt afraid or terrified, he replied,

Not really, I was just taking care of business... Now, I know that sounds like an oversimplification, but it's the absolute truth... You don't get fearful. You get tense. You tighten up. And all your senses are alert and you're aware that you need to do your best job. And it's not that you're not afraid, but you're not overcome with fear. We had trained a great deal... you just do it. How conscious are you driving down the road of every movement that you make? You're not, because that's training through experience. It's that kind of a thing.

# Face Fear with Friends or Colleagues

Most people find it easier to face fear in the company of other people, particularly those whom they know and trust. (We will discuss this concept of social support in greater depth in Chapter 6.) Confronting fear with others tends to help in various ways. It may increase our ability to make a realistic appraisal of the feared situation. It may also reduce physiological stress responses, such as elevated heart rate and blood pressure, hyperventilation, and stomach "butterflies." With supportive friends or colleagues by their side, people tend to feel more confident and are better able to cope with problems by finding constructive solutions rather than by avoidance. It is much easier to jump out of a plane, rappel down the face of a cliff, go to the hospital for a cancer biopsy, attend a divorce hearing, begin the first day of college, or risk arrest while demonstrating against political injustice when you are doing it with a colleague, friend, or loved one.

# Face Fear with Spiritual Support

Religious or spiritual support can also provide the perspective and strength needed to face one's fears. (We will discuss the power of spirituality further in Chapter 5.) For General Hugh Shelton, fear is no match for God.

If you're getting ready to do something really dangerous, like jump out of an airplane at 30,000 feet in the middle of the night, having a strong faith in God is very important. When the bullets are flying, if you're scared to death that you are going to die because you're worried about what comes after life on this Earth, I think that takes away from your confidence. I was always confident that God was by my side: He was there when I went out of the airplane; He was there when the bullets were flying. It bothered my wife that I was never afraid of dying. Do I want to die? No, but I wasn't worried about it. I was worried about the people on the left and right and the people I was entrusted to care for, but not about myself.

Elizabeth, a social worker who was kidnapped, raped, and thrown off a bridge, also uses spiritual insight to fight fear. She has mastered this technique.

I see fear as energy. I try to come into the body and feel where it is lodged, and breathe into it and allow it to flow. If it is not moving, I turn to my spiritual practices, which include chanting, meditation, body movement and yoga, to help the stuck energy move. Once it is moving, the essential self underneath – the inner spirit – is more accessible and the fear has no more power over me. Making the decision to turn and face my fear rather than repress or run from it is half the battle. I believe we all have the capacity to do this; however, we need to know that we have the choice.

Elizabeth's approach resembles the Buddhist practice of mindfulness in which emotions and fear are faced head on. Mindfulness involves observing one's thoughts and emotions without judging them. In his book *Mindfulness in Plain English*, the Buddhist monk Bhante H. Gunaratana (2002) notes that mindfulness and meditation require attention to reality and resemble Elizabeth's practice of going toward the fear. Gunaratana writes:

> Meditation is running straight into reality. It does not insulate you from the pain of life but rather allows you to delve so deeply into life and all its aspects that you pierce the pain barrier and go beyond suffering...
>
> In order to observe our fear, we must accept the fact that we are afraid. We can't examine our own depression without accepting it fully. The same is true for irritation and agitation, frustration and all those other uncomfortable emotional states. You can't examine something fully if you are busy rejecting its existence. (pp. 25, 139)

To deal with fear, Gunaratana writes,

> Observe the fear exactly as it is. Don't cling to it. Just watch it rising and growing. Study its effect. See how it makes you feel and how it affects your body. When you find yourself in the grip of horror fantasies, simply observe those mindfully. Watch the pictures as pictures. See memories as memories. Observe the emotional reactions that come along and know them for what they are. Don't try to repress the memories or the feelings or the fantasies. Just step out of the way and let the whole mess bubble up and flow past. It can't hurt you. It is just a memory. It is only a fantasy. It is nothing but fear. (p. 108)

Thich Nhat Hanh, a well-known Buddhist monk who was nominated for the Nobel Peace Prize in 1970 for his role in the Vietnam War Paris Peace Talks, recognizes that all of us are afraid. "Fear is always there within us: the fear of getting old, the fear of getting sick, the fear of dying, the fear of being abandoned by our loved ones. It is very human to be fearful and to worry about it" (Hanh, 2003, p. 148).

However, he also understands that hiding from fear is not the answer.

> If you try to run away, instead of confronting or embracing your ill-being, you will not look deeply into its nature and will never have the chance to see a way out. That is why you should hold your suffering tenderly and closely, looking directly into it, to discover its true nature and find a way out. (Hanh, 2000, p. 84)
>
> The Buddha advised us to invite these fears to the upper level of our consciousness, recognize them and smile at them. To do so was the daily practice for monks and nuns in the time of the Buddha, as it is for monks and nuns now. Every time your fear is invited up, every time you recognize it and smile at it, your fear will lose some of its strength. When it returns to the depth of your consciousness, it returns as a smaller seed. That is why the practice should be done every day, especially when you are feeling mentally and physically strong. (Hanh, 2003, p. 148)

# Get Someone or an Organization to Push You

But facing fear is never easy, even with the help of friends or colleagues. As a result, organizations that specialize in overcoming fear, such as the military, have developed a host of methods to "coax" or "encourage" their members. Tim Cooper says that Special Forces training is designed to overcome fear.

> Just about every course will have something that bothers somebody at some time. And they'll try to push you through that. They'll be screaming, yelling in your face . . . calling you all types of names and talking about your mom . . . basically trying to physically push you over the wall, without touching you. They don't give you any space to retreat. It's all designed to get you to force yourself past the fear. Then once you go through it, they'll congratulate you and pat you on the back and tell you, "Good boy." And once you go over the edge and you're doing fine, you look back and say, "You know, it wasn't a problem."

Special Forces instructor Mark Hickey has a similar approach: "I can say from my own experience that after you do one thing and conquer it, the next thing is a little bit easier, whereas if you let the first one knock you out, it's going to be even harder to try to overcome the next one."

Just as the military designs its training to strengthen members and foster growth by pushing its members beyond their current level of comfort, numerous civilian organizations do the same. Examples include Outward Bound wilderness expeditions, police and fire academy training, high school and college athletic teams, and challenging educational programs (e.g., law school, intensive foreign language training).

Fear is ubiquitous. No one escapes its grip. But what is the best way to deal with it? The bottom line: the best way around fear is through it. To conquer fear, one must face fear. That is what resilient people do.

# References

Alberini, C. M. & Ledoux, J. E. (2013). Memory reconsolidation. *Current Biology*, 23(17), R746–750.

Arnsten, A. F. T. (2009). Stress signaling pathways that impair prefrontal cortex structure and function. *Nature*, 10, 410–422.

Arnsten, A. F. (2015). Stress weakens prefrontal networks: molecular insults to higher cognition. *Nature Neuroscience*, 18(10), 1376–85.

Brunet, A., Orr, S. P., Tremblay, J. *et al.* (2008). Effect of post-retrieval propranolol on psychophysiologic responding during subsequent scriptdriven traumatic imagery in posttraumatic stress disorder. *Journal of Psychiatric Research*, 42(6), 503–506.

Cahill, L., Prins, B., Weber, M. & McGaugh, J. L. (1994). β-Adrenergic activation and memory for emotional events. *Nature*, 371, 702–704.

Clem, R. L. & Schiller, D. (2016). New learning and unlearning: strangers or accomplices in threat memory attenuation? *Trends in Neurosciences*, 39(5), 340–351.

Gunaratana, B. H. (2002). *Mindfulness in Plain English*, expanded and updated edition. Somerville, MA: Wisdom Publications.

Hanh, T. N. (2000). *The Path of Emancipation: Talks from a 21-Day Mindfulness Retreat*. Berkeley, CA: Parallax Press.

Hanh, T. N. (2003). *No Death, No Fear: Comforting Wisdom for Life*. New York, NY: Riverhead Trade.

Hartley, C. A. & Phelps, E. A. (2010). Changing fear: The neurocircuitry of emotion regulation. *Neuropsychopharmacology*, 35(1), 136–146.

Jovanovic, T. & Norrholm, S. D. (2011). Neural mechanisms of impaired fear inhibition in posttraumatic stress disorder. *Frontiers in Behavioral Neuroscience*, 5, 1–8.

Junger, S. (2001). The lion in winter. In *Fire*. New York, NY: W. W. Norton.

Kolditz, T. A. (2007). *In Extremis Leadership: Leading as If Your Life Depended on It*. Hoboken, NJ: John Wiley & Sons.

Lane, R. D., Ryan, L., Nadel, L. & Greenberg, L. (2015). Memory reconsolidation, emotional arousal, and the process of change in psychotherapy: New insights from brain science. *Behavioral & Brain Sciences*, 38, e1.

Lang, S., Kroll, A., Lipinski, S. J. *et al.* (2009). Context conditioning and extinction in humans: Differential contribution of the hippocampus, amygdala and prefrontal cortex. *European Journal of Neuroscience*, 29(4), 823–832.

LeDoux, J. E. (1996). *The Emotional Brain*. New York, NY: Simon & Schuster

LeDoux, J. E. (2002). *Synaptic Self: How Our Brains Become Who We Are*. New York, NY: Viking.

LeDoux, J. (2016). *Anxious: Using the Brain to Understand and Treat Fear and Anxiety*. New York, NY: Penguin Books.

Lee, J. L. C., Nader, K. & Schiller, D. (2017). An update on memory reconsolidation updating. *Trends in Cognitive Sciences*, 21(7), 531–545.

Mandela, N. (1995). *The Long Walk to Freedom*. New York, NY: Back Bay Books.

Mataix-Cols, D., Fernandez de la Cruz, L., Monzani, B. *et al.* (2017). D-cycloserine augmentation of exposure-based cognitive therapy for anxiety, obsessive-compulsive, and posttraumatic stress disorders: a systematic review and meta-analysis of individual participant data. *JAMA Psychiatry*, 74(5), 501–510.

McEwen, B. & Sapolsky, R. (2006). Stress and your health. *Journal of Clinical Endocrinology & Metabolism*, 91(2), e2.

McGaugh, J. L. (2000). Memory: A century of consolidation. *Science*, 287, 248–251.

Phelps, E. A., Delgado, M. R., Nearing, K. I. & LeDoux, J. E. (2004). Extinction learning in humans: Role of the amygdala and vmPFC. *Neuron*, 43, 897–905.

Quirk, G. J., Pare, D., Richardson, R. *et al.* (2010). Erasing fear memories with extinction training. *Journal of Neuroscience*, 30(45), 14993–14997.

Resick, P. A. (2001). *Stress and Trauma*. Hove: Psychology Press Ltd.

Sapolsky, R. M. (2017). *BEHAVE: The Biology of Humans at Our Best and Worst*. New York, NY: Penguin Books.

Schiller, D., Monfils, M.-H., Ledoux, J. E. *et al.* (2010). Preventing the return of fear in humans using reconsolidation update mechanisms. *Nature*, 463(7277), 49–53.

Southwick, S. M., Davis, M., Horner, B. *et al.* (2002). Relationship of enhanced norepinephrine activity during memory consolidation to enhanced long-term memory in humans. *American Journal of Psychiatry*, 159, 1420–1422.

CHAPTER 4

# Moral Compass, Ethics, and Altruism: Doing What Is Right

In an age of moral relativism, situational ethics, and social Darwinism, it may seem irrelevant to talk about "moral compass." Some believe that over the past century, psychology, with its focus on the unconscious, has transformed what once were moral judgments into nonjudgmental assessments of behavior, sometimes to the point where individuals are now absolved of responsibility for the choices they make. However, concerns about the loss of moral responsibility are not new. Throughout history, social critics have decried the decay in moral values, especially among members of the young generation.

Is the moral climate in today's society really worse than that of our parents' or grandparents'? Perhaps. In her book *A Better Man*, author Kelly H. Johnson argues that "in addition to the perennial trials of peer pressure, hormones and popularity, young men must now grapple with a media-saturated culture that places enormous emphasis on physical appeal, material wealth and celebrity status" (Johnson, 2009). Power, money, sex, and violence are glorified while values such as courage, integrity, and kindness are often ignored. Former US Secretary of Education William Bennett made headlines by publishing books entitled *The Book of Virtues* and *Moral Compass* because they stood out as some of the only contemporary resources for parents, educators, and others wishing to instill moral values in today's youth.

In our interviews, we found that many resilient individuals possessed a keen sense of right and wrong that strengthened them during periods of extreme stress and afterward, as they adjusted to life following trauma. Another pillar of their value system was altruism – selflessness, concern for the welfare of others, and giving to others with no expectation of benefit to the self.

Yet people in today's world often speak of "compassion fatigue": we are overwhelmed by all the dreadful events and conditions in the world that we may feel powerless to make a difference. As Daryl Cameron and Keith Payne (2011) found in their research, we are more likely to respond altruistically when we focus on a more narrowly defined problem or an individual case. For years beginning in 2012, the worldwide media reported on millions of refugees fleeing government upheaval and violence in Syria and other countries in the region, yet there was little response from donors. Aid organizations found themselves unable to cope with the scope of the problem. Then, in August 2015, a photograph went viral of a dead toddler who washed up on a beach after his family attempted to make a sea crossing to Turkey (CBS/AP, 2015). The heartbreaking image inspired many people around the world to donate to the refugee cause to an extent not previously seen.

Morality and ethics are complex topics; they have been debated and expounded upon over the centuries by many esteemed philosophers and religious leaders. We are certainly not proposing to compete with such authorities. However, we have found that many resilient individuals articulate a core set of moral principles and strive to adhere to them. In this chapter, we argue that actively identifying your core values, assessing the degree to which you are living by these values, and challenging yourself to adopt a higher standard can strengthen character and build resilience.

# Epictetus at the Hanoi Hilton

James Bond Stockdale, the independent candidate for Vice President of the United States in 1992, was a highly decorated veteran; he received two Distinguished Flying Crosses, three Distinguished Service Medals, two Purple Hearts, and the Congressional Medal of Honor. He also served as president of the Naval War College, was a senior fellow of the Hoover Institute, and was the holder of eight honorary degrees. Midway through his naval career, in the spring of 1960, Stockdale received orders to enroll in a master's degree program in International Relations at Stanford University. There he took a philosophy course called "The Nature of Good and Evil" with readings that included works by Plato, Aristotle, Socrates, Koestler, and Dostoevsky. Stockdale's professor was a military veteran himself, and on the last day of the course he gave Stockdale a gift: a copy of *Enchiridion*, a manual for the combat officer written in AD 50 by the Greek philosopher Epictetus. The professor explained to Stockdale, "I think you might find this useful."

Epictetus, the son of a Roman slave, was sold into slavery himself at age 15. According to legend, after being chained, beaten, and crippled for life, he was sold to a man who would later murder the Roman emperor. Over the next 10 years, Epictetus served as an apprentice to the best Stoic teacher in the empire and eventually gained his freedom, becoming a highly respected and well-known philosopher.

Stockdale was puzzled by the parting gift. He wondered how the teachings of a classical Stoic philosopher could apply to his life as a fighter pilot. But trusting in the wisdom of his professor, he kept the copy of *Enchiridion* by his bedside at each of his duty stations, on every ship he sailed. He read and reread it, studying it and trying to live according to its messages about the importance of discipline; self-control; endurance and perseverance; virtue and moral character; courage; toughness tempered by compassion; attempts to be the very best; and dignity in the face of deprivation and suffering. However, Stockdale did not fully appreciate its value until day his plane was shot down over Vietnam.

Parachuting from his crippled fighter jet, Stockdale struck the ground with enough force to fracture a bone in his back and severely damage his leg. Still, even though he would not be able to stand on his injured leg for years, he drew strength and inspiration from the words of Epictetus: "Lameness is an impediment to the body but not to the will." According to Epictetus, one can never be the victim of another – only the "victim" of himself.

> When I ejected from that airplane in 1965, I left my world of technology and entered into the world of Epictetus. I was alone and crippled; self-reliance was the basis for daily life. The system of values I carried with me into this realm was to be tested by my captors. The payoff was my self-respect. I would keep it or it would be torn from me and used as leverage against my senses of purpose and stability. (Stockdale, 1984, p. 4)

For the first four years as a prisoner, Stockdale lived in solitary confinement because the North Vietnamese knew that he was a commanding officer and they wanted to prevent him from giving orders to the other prisoners in the Hanoi Hilton. Stockdale was rarely isolated, however, because his cell shared walls with other American POWs, and they communicated using the Tap Code, a system in which prisoners tapped messages to one another on prison walls.

As the senior ranking officer at the Hanoi Hilton, Stockdale knew that it was his duty to retain command over his fellow POWs and to provide them with leadership, direction, inspiration, and military orders. At first, he turned for guidance to the Military Code of Conduct, which states that the American chain of command will remain in effect for those who are captured or imprisoned; that captured soldiers will divulge only name, rank, serial number, and date of birth; that they will resist by all means available; and that they will make every effort to escape.

Some POWs supported adherence to a strict interpretation of the Code of Conduct, advocating death before giving up classified information. Stockdale did so as well until he was forced to face reality. In the fall of 1965, the North Vietnamese began to use torture during their interrogations of American prisoners. In late October of that year, Stockdale received detailed descriptions of North Vietnamese brutality from Lt. Rod Knutson, the first fellow POW to be tortured in North Vietnam.

Like Stockdale, Knutson had strong beliefs about moral behavior, but instead of Epictetus, he cited his father as a key source of those beliefs.

I grew up in Billings, Montana. In third grade a friend of mine and I stole mail from a neighbor's mailbox and threw it into a fish pond. We didn't know there was a check inside one of the envelopes. Later that day, my father confronted me. He picked me up under my armpits, set me on the kitchen counter, and planted his big old palms on either side of my hips. He got his nose about six inches from my face and said, "I'm going to stop right here and look you in the eye and see if you can earn my trust and confidence. And if you tell me the truth, it will be different than if I just punish you. I want you to tell me what you did with Mrs. Chase's mail and what you did with her check."

So after a long wait during which he didn't blink or move, I finally said, "Yeah, I took it and I tore it up and we threw it in the fish pond." He looked at me for a minute, and then, after putting his arms around me, thanked me for telling the truth. Then, he jerked me off the counter and marched me across the street to Mrs. Chase. I had to apologize and volunteer to clean her fish pond for the next five years.

Anyway, while I was in prison, a Vietnamese interrogator would be right there, nose to nose with me, asking me questions, saying I had to answer. And my old dad was standing right there, too...

By the time they got me to Hanoi, to the Hoa Lo Prison, I was in pretty bad shape, pretty beat up. I couldn't get out of the truck when they untied me. They pulled me out, just threw me like a sack of beans on the pavement, and then picked me up and dragged me inside and put me in an interrogation room. When I wouldn't answer any questions beyond name, rank, serial number, and date of birth, a guard stationed behind me took a rifle butt and smacked it into the side of my head. I was knocked off my chair, and I went sprawling across the floor. After the interrogation, they put me in a cell about the size of a table. On either side was a concrete pallet about 18 inches wide. At the foot of the concrete pallet, there was a set of leg stocks built into the concrete, two little shallow cut-out areas and a steel bar that swung over the top and locked.

The cell was filthy. I can't even describe how filthy it was. It had a toilet bucket that was rusted, full of feces and urine and flies. A rat was in the cell, trying to carry off a crust of bread. I called outside my cell door to see if there were any other POWs, and a guard came and smashed me in the face – I wasn't allowed to make any noise.

The next morning, a guard came to the cell with eleven questions on a sheet of paper. He jammed the pen in my hand and pointed to the paper. I just shook my head at him and said, "No, I'm not going to do that." He roughed me up and handed me the paper again. This time I said, "You want me to sign this? You want me to sign this? OK, I'll sign it!" I rammed the pen through the paper and tossed it aside. That sounds very John Wayne, but it led to a torture session that lasted five days.

They beat me with fists and a club, until my backside was just hamburger. Blood was splattering everywhere. They tied my arms behind my back, which is one of their favorite torture tricks. They use thin line and tie it into your muscle, cutting off all circulation to your lower arms. Your hands puff up like a rubber glove that's been blown into a balloon. They never let me up to go to the bathroom, so I was lying in my own bodily fluids. When they did finally let me up, well, I couldn't get the flight suit off, and

I couldn't stand up or sit down. A thick scab, which had previously been my rear end, had attached itself to my flight suit, and everything was welded together.

Knutson withstood nearly 16 consecutive days of brutal torture, but ultimately he felt profound despair over having told the North Vietnamese more than the "basic four": name, rank, serial number, and date of birth. Although Knutson fabricated facts about his family and background, he nevertheless felt devastated and guilt-ridden over having "broken."

When some prisoners heard that Knutson had "broken," they thought he was weak. Stockdale, however, understood that Knutson's torture signaled a frightening change in how the North Vietnamese were to treat American POWs and he also recognized that other prisoners did not really understand the horrific nature of Knutson's ordeal.

Now, Stockdale faced a major dilemma that was to preoccupy him for the remainder of his prison term. The Military Code of Conduct was clear, and as a Navy officer, Stockdale was bound by military law to uphold the Code and to order his men to obey it. But after hearing about Knutson's torture, Stockdale knew that the Code would be impossible to follow; every POW, no matter how tough or determined, had his breaking point and under torture would eventually provide more information than the "basic four." As the senior ranking officer, what guidelines should he provide his fellow POWs? How should he advise them to deal with torture? Stockdale turned to Epictetus and Stoicism.

Stoic philosophy is largely focused on personal control, reducing vulnerability, and living by a set of time-honored standards that promote dignity, even under the harshest of conditions. At the core of personal control is the ability to differentiate that which is within your control from that which is beyond it. Stockdale put it this way:

> . . .a Stoic always keeps separate files in his mind for (A) those things that are "up to him" and (B) those things that are "not up to him." Another way of saying it is (A) those things that are "within his power" and (B) those things that are "beyond his power." Still another way of saying it is (A) those things that are within the grasp of "his Will, his Free Will" and (B) those things that are beyond it. . . In short, what the Stoics say is "Work with what you have control of and you'll have your hands full." (Stockdale, 1995, p. 190)

For Stockdale, "station in life" generally belongs in category B because often we have little or no control over it. One moment, Stockdale recalls, he was "on top," the admired commander of more than 1000 men and more than 100 pilots, "confident" and "self-satisfied," a man who thought he had "found every key to success," but within minutes of being shot down he became "an object of contempt" and a "criminal" in the eyes of the North Vietnamese. In a matter of minutes, your station in life "can be changed from that of a dignified and competent gentleman of culture to that of a panic-stricken, sobbing, self-loathing wreck. . ." (Stockdale, 1995, p. 228).

Stockdale knew this firsthand, because, he, too, had been tortured. As a senior officer and vocal resister, Stockdale was regularly singled out for interrogations. Over the course of his four years in solitary, Stockdale was brutally interrogated on 15 occasions, and at times he was forced to provide information. He recounts in his book *In Love and War* (Stockdale & Stockdale, 1990) that after one extended round of torture, he became so depressed that he attempted suicide by cutting his wrists with a shard of broken glass.

His own experience with torture taught Stockdale to avoid creating unrealistic expectations and standards that could never be met. When prisoners fell short of their own expectations, Stockdale offered support, compassion, and forgiveness. Even when a POW resisted admirably and provided only information that was useless or of little value, he typically felt ashamed, believing that he had betrayed himself, his fellow prisoners, and his country. For example, Admiral Robert Shumaker remembers the first time he divulged any information to the North Vietnamese. After relentless torture, Shumaker could hold out no longer.

> My first experience [with divulging information] was just crushing – tears and sobbing. Not so much from the physical abuse, but from the realization that you hadn't lived up to your own expectations and the military's expectations of you. And I guess somewhere along the line you learn to become street smart and you learn to lie and you remember your lies and it's just kind of a departure from the American and George Washington dream of always telling the truth. (Stockdale, 1995, p. 187)

Stockdale knew that the suffering arising from starvation, harsh living conditions and physical pain paled in comparison with the agony of shame. He wrote that "a shoulder broken, a bone in my back broken, a leg broken twice were peanuts by comparison . . . Shame is heavy, a heavier burden than any physical wounds . . . the thing that brings down a man is not pain but shame" (Stockdale, 1995, p. 199).

In terms of the categories A (what is up to you) and B (what is not up to you), Stockdale recognized that the torture endured by Rod Knutson, Bob Shumaker, and so many others belonged in category B, because it was not up to them, not within their power, and not within the grasp of their free will. However, according to Stoic philosophy, each man did bear responsibility for those things that were within his power and the grasp of his free will. In her book *Stoic Warriors: The Ancient Philosophy Behind the Military Mind*, Nancy Sherman, a professor at Georgetown University and the inaugural holder of the Distinguished Chair in Ethics at the United States Naval Academy, discusses this Stoic imperative and its perspective on how to respond to forces that willpower cannot control:

> We are to continue to meet challenges, take risks and stretch the limits of our mastery. We are to continue to strive to the best of our efforts to achieve our ends. We are to push our agency to the limit. In this case, the message is one of empowerment. But at

the same time, we are to cultivate greater strength and equanimity in the face of what we can't change. We must learn where our mastery begins, but also where it ends.

(Sherman, 2005, p. 3)

Stockdale thought deeply about how to advise his fellow prisoners. Debates over how to interpret the Code and how to deal with torture became a regular and at times heated topic on those occasions when prisoners were able to communicate with one another. With Epictetus as his guide, Stockdale carefully weighed opposing viewpoints and gradually developed a set of rules that incorporated many of the basic values of Stoicism. Stockdale knew that "a structured set of values supporting a basic tenet of self-respect was fundamental to the performance of these men," and his goal was to make certain that the men "returned home with their heads held high" (Stockdale, 1984, p. 4).

His rules formed the acronym BACK US: B stood for bowing. Prisoners should never voluntarily bow in public. Refusing to do so would show the world that American prisoners had not been defeated, and if prisoners were visibly forced to bow by the North Vietnamese, any observer would see that US prisoners were being mistreated according to the Geneva Conventions. A = air. Stay off the air, refuse radio interviews and tape-recorded messages or confessions. C = crime. Never use the word "crime" and never admit to having committed a crime against the North Vietnamese people. K = don't kiss 'em goodbye when the time finally comes to be released. Never give the impression that the North Vietnamese were civilized in their treatment of prisoners and never show gratitude to the North Vietnamese, even if they granted prisoners early release for medical reasons. US = Unity over self.

Although the BACK US code incorporated specific rules, those rules took into account the reality of prison life. This is what Stockdale expected – that his men would resist to the best of their physical and moral capacity, would endure torture before divulging information, would tell their fellow prisoners how they had been tortured and what information they had given, and would make their torturers "begin all over again the next day." No one was to accept special favors from the North Vietnamese, and no one was to accept early release unless all prisoners were released at the same time. Fellow POW Steve Long described the implementation of the BACK US code:

> You had to be real careful in accepting things. They'd offer you a bath and you were very prone to accepting the bath but you learned that you shouldn't do that unless everybody gets a bath. Most of us were offered early release. The Vietnamese would tell us, if you give us information, then maybe we'll release you early. You'll go home in maybe thirty days. Well, our rules were no one accepts early release. Nobody goes home until we all go home.

South African leader Nelson Mandela provides a parallel example in his autobiography, *The Long Walk to Freedom*. In 1976, the South African Minister of

Prisons, Jimmy Kruger, paid Mandela a visit on the infamous Robben Island, where Mandela had served 12 years of a life sentence on charges of sabotage and conspiracy. As Mandela describes it,

> He came armed with a specific offer... If I recognized the legitimacy of the Transkei government [one of the so-called Bantustan homelands for black South Africans] and was willing to move there, my sentence would be dramatically reduced. I listened respectfully until he had finished. First, I said, I wholly rejected the Bantustan policy, and would do nothing to support it, and second, I was from Johannesburg, and it was to Johannesburg that I would return. Kruger remonstrated with me, but to no avail. A month later he returned with the same proposal, and again I turned him down. It was an offer only a turncoat could accept. (Mandela, 1995, pp. 481–483)

# The 9/11 Terrorist Attacks as a Moral Imperative

Recall from Chapter 1 the story of Jimmy Dunne, the only surviving managing partner at the investment firm Sandler O'Neill & Partners. As Dunne and his colleagues rebuilt the firm, they were motivated by their belief that they were morally obliged to bring the firm back from the brink of destruction. University of Pennsylvania researcher Steven F. Freeman and colleagues who studied Sandler O'Neil's resurrection wrote, "The firm, once an instrument, as one owner described it, 'for feeding the mouths of families,' became a moral enterprise: to honor the dead, care for both the family members of the deceased as well as the living, and deny the terrorists a victory... Moral purpose was a motivational factor in and of itself, spurring on the efforts of the partners and employees, as well as customers, suppliers, volunteers and other sources of external help" (Freeman, Hirschhorn & Maltz, 2004, p. 73). The workers were "selling not just for themselves but for their dead colleagues... any commissions generated by a client of a deceased Sandler employee would go to that employee's estate" (Brooker, 2002, pp. 60–61).

Outsiders displayed a spirit of cooperation unusual in the traditionally cutthroat Wall Street culture. Other investment firms donated office space and computers, and referred business to Sandler O'Neill. Overall, "a newly found moral purpose invigorated an entire community..." and the recovery effort became a "'virtuous circle' in which effort, opportunity, hope, and motivation created an upward spiral of confidence and performance" (Freeman, Hirschhorn & Maltz, 2004, pp. 72, 73).

Sandler O'Neill was by no means the only firm that felt this way. Many throughout Wall Street and the entire New York City business community believed that recovering and thriving would send a powerful message to the terrorists. The "virtuous circle" extended throughout the New York metropolitan region, inspiring businesses of all kinds to "show their stuff," recover from the economic losses of 9/11, and possibly even go on to achieve greater success than they had enjoyed before the attacks.

# One Person's Morality May Be Another Person's Evil

While most of the world's religions and cultures uphold a core set of moral principles having to do with truth, respect for human life, and treating others as we would like to be treated, people of good conscience can disagree on what is, and is not, moral and ethical. Diane Coutu makes this point with regard to organizations in her *Harvard Business Review* article, citing the values promoted among employees of businesses such as the Philip Morris tobacco company. "Companies can hold ethically questionable values and still be very resilient," she writes. "Philip Morris has very strong values, although we might not agree with them – for instance, the value of 'adult choice.' But there's no doubt that Philip Morris executives believe strongly in its values, and the strength of their beliefs sets the company apart from most of the other tobacco companies" (Coutu, 2002, p. 52).

As another example, someone who opposes war might nevertheless admire the resilience and moral courage of the many military veterans we describe in this book. The pacifist Joan Baez has written eloquently about the Vietnam War and the complex dynamics of living out one's nonviolent beliefs while honoring the sacrifices of POWs and other veterans. Her name is anathema in some military circles, and she has been lampooned in the *Doonesbury* comic strip as "Joanie Phoanie." Baez has used her talents to support nonviolent movements to protest wars, and to advocate for desegregation, and worker's rights. She was instrumental in establishing the US chapter of Amnesty International and has advocated for gay rights, environmental causes, and abolition of the death penalty.

After several years of outspoken opposition to the Vietnam draft – for which she had twice been arrested – Baez was asked in 1972 to join ex-Brigadier General Telford Taylor, Episcopal priest Michael Allen, and antiwar activist veteran Barry Romo on a visit to Hanoi. This trip was arranged by a peace group called The Liaison Committee. Its purpose was to deliver Christmas mail to American POWs and to express a spirit of friendship between the people of the United States and the people of North Vietnam.

This visit by Americans behind enemy lines was considered relatively safe because there had been no combat activity in North Vietnam for many months. On the third night of their two-week visit, however, the delegation was taken by surprise when their hotel lost electricity, sirens sounded, and guests were ushered into a bomb shelter beneath the building. They remained for days. As they later learned, this was the beginning of the 11-day Operation

Linebacker II, more commonly known as the "Christmas bombing" – the largest heavy bomber strikes launched by the US Air Force since the end of World War II. Baez later described the destruction she witnessed when she was allowed to leave the hotel.

> There was a man weeping to himself, and a surviving family moving about their small area like zombies. Everywhere were headbands of white cloth, the symbol of mourning for a relative... I saw a woman sitting on a small heap of rubble, pounding her fists on her thighs and crying with a despair that was ferocious. She would go from a wail to a moan to almost a growl, then sob wretchedly from her island of misery... Here was a shoe, here a half-buried little sweater, a piece of broken dish jammed into the earth, a book lying open, its damp pages stuck together... On the other side of a thirty-foot abyss I saw [another] woman bending low to the ground singing a strange little song as she hobbled back and forth over an area of ten or twelve feet of ground... [I asked the interpreter] what she was singing... Oh, heaven and earth. Such depths of sadness cannot exist. I crumpled to the ground and covered my face and sobbed. That woman's boy lay somewhere under her feet packed into an instantaneous grave of mud, and she, like a wounded old cat, could only tread back and forth over the place she'd last seen him, moaning her futile song. "Where are you now, my son?" (Baez, 1987/2009, pp. 217–218),

The experience served as an inspiration for Baez's 1973 album entitled *Where Are You Now, My Son?* Yet Baez was not one to follow the "leftist party line" as some might have expected; by 1979 she was speaking out in opposition to the Communist regime that then governed all of Vietnam. This put her at odds with many former compatriots in the antiwar movement. Decades later, Baez wrote of an encounter with four Vietnam veterans who were picketing one of her concerts.

> Their signs were uncomplimentary at best... but that is not the point. They have stories to tell that have not been heard: stories of real bravery, of deep sorrow, violence, killing, and death. We who have not experienced what they have can never understand their dilemma, and have no right to stand between them and the honor, respect, and compassion they deserve.
>
> I, of course, opposed the Vietnam War. I oppose all wars. I do not expect most people to understand that fact, certainly not the four soldiers who stood in front of me with signs reading "Joan Baez, Soldiers don't kill babies, liberals do" and "Joan Baez gave comfort & aid to our enemy in Vietnam & encouraged them to kill Americans!" However, the anger and disrespect they have mistakenly placed upon me is far less compromising than that which was placed upon them when they returned from the jungles of Vietnam. (Baez, 2009)

After she approached the veterans and had a conversation with them, Baez writes,

We each had unique reactions to this bizarre confrontation, which dared to become genuine communication. Mine was one of sorrow at their unresolved struggle, their rage, and the amount of time they'd spent trying to get their lives back. At their request I autographed their signs (on the back). I also dedicated a song to them during our concert that evening. Even though they continued to picket for a brief while, I felt I had made four new friends and come closer to mutual understanding. (Baez, 2009)

Resilience isn't reserved just for nice people like Baez and the soldiers she admired. Sadly, there are countless examples of highly resilient individuals throughout history who have used their resilience in self-serving, destructive ways. For example, Scott Lilienfeld and his colleagues at Emory University (Lilienfeld, Watts & Smith, 2015) write that psychopaths – defined as "charming, guiltless social predator[s]" (p. 301) – often achieve a high degree of success in their careers and/or personal lives. Psychopaths have also been described as "charming, aggressive, carefree people who are impulsively irresponsible but are good at handling people and looking out for number one" (Widom, 1977, p. 675), and as having "an uncaring nature, antisocial and aggressive behavior, and deficient prosocial emotions such as empathy, guilt, and remorse" (Marsh *et al.*, 2014, p. 15036). Lilienfeld and colleagues propose that seemingly admirable traits such as flinty determination and stoicism can make psychopaths impervious to the social consequences of their selfish, antisocial actions; they may be well aware that they have hurt others, but they don't care.

# Morality Requires Courage

To our knowledge, Admiral James Stockdale and Joan Baez never met. We can only imagine that they would have disagreed about war and a host of other topics. However, we can also imagine that they would have seen eye-to-eye on the importance of living by and standing by one's most deeply held values. The moral values that Stockdale treasured and relied on to bolster his resilience reiterate those values that have been admired over the centuries by nearly every world culture. However, they are not easily acquired because they all require courage. Taking his guidance from Plato and Aristotle, Stockdale defined courage as "endurance of the soul" (Stockdale, 1995, p. 16). It is "the measure of a man's ability to handle fear," (Stockdale, 1978, p. 2) and it must "be exercised in the presence of fear" (Stockdale, 1984, p. 56). Without fear, there can be no courage. Stockdale understood this, and while he respected the physical courage of soldiers who march into battle or pilots who land on aircraft carriers in stormy seas, he was most impressed by what many philosophers have called "moral courage."

Rushworth M. Kidder, who directs the Institute of Global Ethics, defines moral courage as "standing up for values... the willingness to take a tough stand for right in the face of danger... the courage to do the right thing... the quality of mind and spirit that enables one to face up to ethical challenges firmly and confidently without flinching or retreating" (Kidder, 2006, p. 72). Moral courage serves as the backbone for all of the great virtues. In fact, the eighteenth-century English diarist Samuel Johnson described it as "the greatest of all virtues; because, unless a man has that virtue, he has no security for preserving any other" (Boswell, 1791/2008). Former POW and former Presidential candidate John McCain asserts, "without courage all virtue is fragile: admired, sought, professed, but held cheaply and surrendered without a fight" (McCain, 2004, pp. 38–39).

Kidder suggests that moral courage requires three steps (p. 42). First, we must believe in and commit to a core set of moral values and principles. Second, we must recognize that by standing up for these principles we are likely to face danger. The danger may take many forms: physical injury, loss, rejection, shame, or disappointment. Third, to be morally courageous we must be willing to endure these consequences.

In Stockdale's mind, Rod Knutson easily met Kidder's criteria for moral courage, even though he "broke" and gave the North Vietnamese more than the "basic four" pieces of information. Knutson confronted fear and behaved honorably by taking as much punishment as possible and ultimately disclosing only fictional information. In retrospect, Knutson proved to be one of the toughest, most defiant and resilient of all the Hanoi Hilton prisoners.

# Altruism and Its Flip Side

On January 2, 2007, a 50-year-old Navy veteran and construction worker named Wesley Autrey had to take all three of Kidder's steps in a matter of seconds. He and his two daughters were waiting for a train in New York's 137th Street subway station, when a man standing near them on the platform collapsed and fell onto the train tracks. As passengers on the platform watched in horror, the headlights of an approaching train became visible in the tunnel. Making a split-second decision, Autrey jumped onto the tracks and lay on top of the victim, who was writhing in an apparent seizure. Telling him to lie still, Autrey pressed himself and the victim down between the tracks. Although the train's engineer slammed on the brakes, five cars passed over the men before the train screeched to a halt. Miraculously, although Autrey's coat was torn by the passing train, neither man was seriously injured. Autrey told the *New York Times*, "I don't feel like I did something spectacular; I just saw someone who needed help. I did what I felt was right" (Buckley, 2007).

Angela Diaz, mentioned in Chapter 1, exhibited altruism of another type. While Autrey made a split-second decision to risk his life, Diaz, who is Professor of Pediatrics and Adolescent Medicine, at the Icahn School of Medicine at Mount Sinai, made the deliberate decision to donate a kidney to the husband of a longtime friend and colleague. Initially, Diaz was not a suitable donor because she had a family history of diabetes and borderline blood tests, but she altered her lifestyle to bring her levels within the range of acceptability. She began to exercise regularly and modified her diet (*A Gift Between Friends*, 2012). A month later, her blood values had improved and she was cleared for surgery: the surgery was a success. Soon after returning home from the hospital, Diaz began to train for the New York City Marathon. Since 2010 she and other "Run for Teens" team members have competed annually in the New York City Marathon – raising tens of thousands of dollars for the Mount Sinai Adolescent Health Center.

What type of person donates a kidney to a friend? A closer look at the life of Angela Diaz helps to answer that question.

Angela was born in the Dominican Republic to a single mother who was extremely poor and who had not attended school because she had to work since childhood. Her mother loves Angela deeply. In order to support Angela, her mother moved to Santo Domingo for a job. Angela was left with her grand-mother, but at age nine months she was burned severely and thereafter rejoined her mother, was looked after by her mother's cousin and "the neighborhood" because her mother had such long working hours. When she was four years old, Angela slipped while carrying a jar of oil and lacerated her abdomen requiring emergency surgery. It was during her hospital stay that she first remembers wanting to become a doctor.

When Angela was eight, her mother moved to the United States but was unable to bring her children. Angela was taken in by her biological father, who had his own family, but her two maternal biological siblings moved in with their maternal grandmother. This was a painful time for Angela because she felt "very attached" to her mother and her mother's family; it was almost as if they had "disappeared." Sad and lonely, she spent most of her free time sitting quietly by herself in a small room that was attached to the back of the house. She remembers counting ants and playing with them as they scurried about the room.

Angela endured numerous hardships over the next four years including physical and emotional abuse, a civil war during which her house was ransacked, and a profound sense of isolation. When she was 12 her father helped obtain a visa that allowed her to visit the United States. Angela was overjoyed to be with her mother, but when the visa expired she couldn't bear to go back to the Dominican Republic, so she overstayed her visit and became an undocumented alien. Soon she was informed that in order to be eligible to get a green card to reside permanently in the United States she would need to live in the Dominican Republic for at least one year.

At age 14, Angela returned to the United States to live in West Harlem with her mother, grandmother, three maternal siblings, and her stepfather, as well as four aunts and an uncle who were about her age. Knowing very little English, she was placed in a classroom for immigrant children who spoke a variety of languages. She and her classmates were frequently bullied and sometimes beaten up because they were "different." Nevertheless, Angela enjoyed school and attended Brandeis High School, starting in tenth grade. While in high school she held three jobs to help the family financially; she tutored other students in math, science, and Spanish, washed dishes in a luncheonette, and helped out in a beauty salon on Saturdays.

During her final year of high school, Angela slipped into a deep depression, stayed home from school, and rarely left her room. But teachers and students from her school kept calling to ask how they could help, and Angela finally visited the Mount Sinai Adolescent Health Center. She had access to the Health Center because her school, knowing that she dreamed of becoming a doctor, had enrolled her in a program for inner-city youth who were interested in pursuing a career in healthcare. At the Health Center, Angela received compassionate and successful treatment for her depression. Having lived in poverty with no health insurance, this was the first time that she had access to comprehensive healthcare.

After graduating from high school, Angela enrolled in New York's City College. She attended sometimes during the day and sometimes at night depending on the type of job she had. At times during the day she worked in the same factory as her mother and stepfather, and at night she attended college classes. In the fall of her senior year, she decided to apply to Columbia Medical School because it was in her neighborhood.

One day, she walked into the admissions office and said "I want to be a doctor. What do I need to do to apply to your school?"

The admissions officer replied, "You need to take the required courses: biology, chemistry, physics, and so forth."

"I've already taken those," she said. "Can I apply?"

So the admissions officer gave her an application. Angela asked to borrow a pen and then sat down and filled out the forms. After an hour or so, she returned the completed application. The admissions officer asked, "What's this?"

Angela had no idea that most students spend weeks or months filling out their medical school applications. The admissions officer waived the application fee of 15 dollars because Angela didn't have any money with her.

Angela was accepted to the prestigious Columbia Medical School – the only school to which she applied. Just prior to starting the first year, Angela married and soon became pregnant. In fact, during medical school she was pregnant most of the time, with multiple miscarriages and she graduated from medical school nine months pregnant.

After medical school, Angela entered residency in pediatrics at Mount Sinai. She recalls feeling "very, very happy" as she took care of children and learned from senior mentors. During residency she was told that she had a gift for working with teenagers and residency was followed by a fellowship in adolescent medicine. Angela got pregnant during residency and delivered her second child during the fellowship. Upon completion of the adolescent medicine fellowship she was offered a staff position at the Mount Sinai Adolescent Health Center. Four years later, Angela was promoted to Director of the Center, a position that she has held for over 25 years.

The Mount Sinai Adolescent Health Center treats over 10,000 patients, ages 10–24, and their children if they have any. Many of the patients face a myriad of challenges: extreme poverty, racism, poor schooling, sexual and physical abuse, sex trafficking, rejection, and generally being ignored by society. To help these young people the Center employs over 100 staff members from 15 different disciplines.

Dr. Diaz finds great joy in working with adolescents because they are "real... raw... creative... authentic" and because they "don't have as many layers of socialization as adults." She and her staff "love these kids" and help them in any way possible: medically, psychologically, and socially.

"When kids come to the Center they come to a place where they are welcomed, respected, not judged, encouraged and loved," she said. "We cater to poor kids without insurance and see any young person who needs our services. They don't need an appointment. They can just walk in, even if they've never been seen in the Center. The staff is here to love, nurture, and develop these kids."

For Dr. Diaz the goal of the Health Center is to provide the basic fabric that we all need as humans: warmth; connectedness; the sense that we belong somewhere; the feeling that we matter.

"Little by little we help kids build themselves up," she said. "We help them find their voice. Everyone needs to find their voice. I think every kid's life gets a little better when they come here. Some kids' lives get transformed like mine was by the program."

Dr. Diaz believes that she would be living a very different life without the help she received at the Mount Sinai Adolescent Health Clinic. As she put it, "I was a high school dropout. I had so many issues. I was depressed and needed to heal from all the trauma. The staff just kept working with me. They never gave up on me. Without their intervention, I might never have gone back to school. They saved me. They gave me a chance."

And now, that is exactly what Dr. Diaz and the staff are doing every day: giving kids a chance. The Health Center staff understand that every child, no matter how ill or traumatized, possesses an inner reservoir of hope, strength and resilience – what psychologist Ann Masten calls "ordinary magic." For the staff, the goal is to provide the environment, resources and loving care that will help kids access that magic.

While growing up, Angela faced many of the same challenges that the kids at the Health Center face. This made her an expert: an expert in what it feels like to live in extreme poverty; to be abused and neglected; to feel hopeless and depressed. What has Angela done with her expertise? She has used it to lead, develop and dramatically expand the very same Health Center that saved her life.

Heroic acts like those of Autrey and Diaz, where one individual makes a sacrifice or takes a risk to benefit another, are examples of altruism. Social science research has shown that altruism is associated with resilience, positive mental health, and well-being in people with and without mental disorders. During World War II, a phenomenon known as "required helpfulness" was first described in citizens who cared for the immediate needs of others after aerial bombardments. Those who performed personally satisfying tasks that others viewed as socially necessary developed fewer trauma-related mood and anxiety symptoms than expected. Further, in a 1979 study, Stanley Rachman found that altruistic individuals with pre-air-raid psychological syndromes reported a decrease in their symptoms after bombardments. Carolyn Schwartz and Meir Sendor (1999) reported similar findings among individuals with multiple sclerosis; in this case, those who were trained to provide an empathic ear to fellow patients with multiple sclerosis experienced significant improvement in well-being. More recently, Michael Poulin and colleagues (Poulin *et al.*, 2013) interviewed more than 800 individuals about stressful events they had experienced in the past year, and also asked them how much tangible assistance they had provided to friends or family. The researchers then followed the participants for five years to see which of them died during that time. After adjusting for age, baseline health and functioning, and key psychosocial variables, they found that stressful events did not predict mortality risk among individuals who had helped others in the past year, but stress did predict mortality among those who had not.

In 2003, a team of University of Massachusetts researchers led by Carolyn Schwartz reported that altruism, or what some call social interest, was associated with better life adjustment, better marital adjustment, and less hopelessness and depression. Both giving and receiving help from others predicted better mental health, although giving help to others was a stronger predictor. Further, the researchers found that social interest moderated life stress and predicted physical health status. They theorized that the association between social interest, better mental health, and reduced stress may be related to a shift in attention from the self to others, enhanced self-confidence and self-acceptance, a reframing of one's own disease experience, and greater perceived meaning in life.

Altruism also appears to foster resilience among children who have survived highly stressful environments. In a longitudinal study of physically abused Israeli children, Hanita Zimrin and colleagues (1986) found that those children who adapted well over time were more likely to assume responsibility for someone else, like a sibling or a pet, than were those who fared poorly. Similarly, in Emmy Werner's classic study of children living in poverty on the Hawaiian island of Kauai, children who helped others in a meaningful way (e.g., by assisting a family member, a neighbor, or some other community member) were most likely to lead successful lives as adults (Werner & Smith, 1992).

We might say that altruism has a flip side: narcissism. Narcissistic individuals see themselves as the center of things, and constantly believe that they deserve more attention, understanding, and assistance than others. In his book *The Road to Character*, David Brooks cites a survey by the Gallup Organization that "asked high school seniors if they considered themselves to be a very important person" (p. 6). In 1950, 12 percent said yes. Two generations later, in 2005, an astounding 80 percent said yes (Brooks, 2006). Similarly, in a book titled *The Narcissism Epidemic*, Jean Twenge and colleagues (Quenqua, 2013; Twenge & Campbell, 2009; Twenge, Miller & Campbell, 2014) reported similarly, that today's young people score 30 percent higher on a test called the Narcissistic Personality Inventory (Raskin & Terry, 1988) than their peers did 20 years ago.

# The Neuroscience of Altruism and Other Moral Behavior

For centuries, scholars studying ethics and morality were mostly philosophers and religious thinkers. Recently, however, psychologists, anthropologists, and neuroscientists have begun to investigate the potential role of evolution and brain function in shaping and maintaining moral standards and societal values.

A large body of scientific evidence from infant research, ethology (the study of animal behavior), and experimental psychology suggests that altruism has had an important influence on behavior throughout human history, and that it represents a complex interplay of environmental and genetic influences. For example, among native South American forager-horticulturists, those individuals who produce and share more food than average are rewarded when they face hardship (e.g. an illness or an accident) by receiving larger quantities of food from a larger number of people than those who produce and share below-average amounts of food. Yakov Shapiro (1994) proposes that this practice, which has been called "reciprocal altruism," has many benefits and rewards, including enhanced reputation and power, more mating opportunities, and privileged access to resources when the community faces catastrophic stress.

Author Michael Shermer similarly argues for "the evolutionary origins of moral sentiments." He writes, "As a species of social primates, we have evolved a deep sense of right and wrong to reward reciprocity and cooperation and to attenuate selfishness and free riding" (Shermer, 2011).

Although we might think that selfish behavior reaps rewards and altruistic behavior requires sacrifice, brain imaging studies have shown that altruism has its own actions in the brain's reward centers. When people give to a charity or a cause they consider worthy, the nucleus accumbens lights up, releasing dopamine. This helps to explain the "helper's high" phenomenon described by Allan Luks (1988, 1991). In a survey of 3,000 people who volunteer in various capacities, those who engage in helping said they find it "like a drug" that elicits a pleasurable physical sensation, inner warmth, an energy spike, lower levels of pain, and greater well-being (Svoboda, 2013). Another study showed that when subjects decided to give to charity, levels of the hormone oxytocin rose. Oxytocin is associated with trust and caregiving, and promotes social bonding (Moll, 2014). And, when Paul Zak and colleagues (2007) administered oxytocin to subjects, the subjects were 80 percent more generous than control subjects who received a placebo sugar pill.

We do not yet know how the brain processes moral thinking and decision-making. In an emerging field called neuroethics, neuroscientists are trying to sort this out. A number of questions lie at the heart of this new science. Are moral and ethical values hard-wired into our brain? What regions of the brain play a role in moral and ethical decision-making, and are any of these areas also associated with resilience? Has morality, or some aspect of morality, been passed down through our DNA because it improves chances for survival? Can counseling, training, or medications enhance moral thinking and ethical behavior? If they can, would enhanced morality increase hardiness under stress?

To study social cooperation and altruism, some researchers are scanning the brains of research participants while they play specially designed games. An often-used game for this research is the Prisoner's Dilemma. It presents a scenario in which two players, isolated from each other, must each decide whether to betray the other player in exchange for a greater or lesser penalty. This research has found that mutual cooperation consistently activates brain regions (e.g., the dopamine nucleus accumbens system) that are known to be involved in the processing of reward. Thus, it appears that mutual cooperation, but not selfish behavior, tends to activate dopamine reward systems, which may leave the individual feeling good and wanting to repeat similar cooperative behaviors. Perhaps, through natural selection, this activation of reward systems has reinforced cooperation and group cohesion, which has helped human beings to survive.

This possibility is supported by twin studies that demonstrate strong heritability of prosocial behaviors such as cooperativeness, empathy, and altruism (Rushton, 2004). A recent genetic study compared the behavior of 101 healthy volunteers with and without a specific variation (polymorphism) of a gene (the catechol-$o$-methyl-transferase gene) that affects dopamine activity. After earning money in two challenging computer games, subjects were invited to donate money to a poor child from a developing country. Those with the specific gene variant donated twice as much as those without this polymorphism (Reuter *et al.*, 2010). While this finding is intriguing, it is important to note that many genes influence complex constructs and behaviors such as altruism.

In studies on personal values, researchers have also found that thinking about and affirming one's values can diminish perceptions of threat, reduce defensive responses to threatening information, and decrease rumination after failure. Focusing on personal values has even been found to buffer physiological and psychological stress responses during a challenging laboratory test. In a study involving college students, J. David Creswell and colleagues at the University of California (2005) found that those who reflected on and affirmed their own most important personal values immediately prior to a stressful laboratory test had significantly lower responses of the stress hormone cortisol compared to students who reflected on and affirmed values that were not personally important to them.

In a 2001 fMRI study, Joshua Greene and colleagues used a classic test of moral reasoning, the "runaway trolley" dilemma,[1] to examine which of two brain regions become activated when subjects wrestled with a moral dilemma. They compared activity in regions dedicated to reasoning (i.e., prefrontal cortex) with activity in regions involved in processing emotion (i.e., limbic system). This dilemma involved two different scenarios. In the first, research participants were asked to imagine themselves watching a runaway trolley travel down a track toward five strangers who would be killed if the trolley were to strike them. The participant was able to flip a switch that diverted the trolley onto another track, where one person (also a stranger) was standing. If the switch were flipped, one person would be killed instead of five. Most participants said that it was morally right to flip the switch. However, in the second scenario, the participant was asked to imagine that he or she was standing on a footbridge next to a stranger and that five people were trapped below in the path of an oncoming runaway trolley. Pushing the stranger onto the track was the only way to save the other five people. Even though the end result of the two scenarios would have been the same if the subject intervened (i.e., one person would die and five would survive), most participants said they would refuse to push the stranger into the path of the trolley.

---

[1] Dilemma originally designed by Philippa Foote and Judith Jarvis Thomson (Greene *et al.*, 2001).

Compared with the first decision, whether or not to flip the switch, the second decision, whether or not to actively kill someone, involved far more emotional processing and significantly greater blood flow in limbic brain regions. The same areas of the brain that become activated during grief or fear became activated during the decision to deliberately kill the one stranger even though it meant saving the lives of five other people. This study suggested that when emotional areas of the brain become activated, emotion may win out over logic and reasoning.

More recently, Marco Zanon and colleagues (Zanon *et al.*, 2014) presented participants with a virtual reality dilemma in which they could either escape from a burning building without stopping, or risk their own safety by stopping to rescue an injured person. Prosocial behavior– saving the other person – was predicted by differential activity in connectivity in two particular brain networks. Interestingly, it was weaker activity in one network paired with stronger activity in another that predicted choice to stop and help the injured person. Specifically, those who stopped to help had weaker activity in the anterior insula and anterior mid-cingulate cortex (known collectively as the salience network), which assesses the importance of a situation. This weaker activation of the salience network was associated with lower anxiety and lower assessment of the risk to oneself. At the same time, the rescuers had stronger activity in the medial prefrontal cortex, an executive area associated with accomplishing tasks.

Abigail Marsh and colleagues (Marsh *et al.*, 2014) assessed brain imaging profiles of individuals exhibiting prosocial behavior of a more extreme variety: people who, like Angela Diaz, had voluntarily donated a kidney. In this study, subjects had donated their kidney to an anonymous stranger. The researchers used structural and fMRI to compare brain patterns of "extraordinary altruists" with those of normal controls. They found that amygdala volume was larger and its responsiveness to fearful facial expressions was greater among altruists than controls. Interestingly, this pattern is opposite to patterns reported in psychopathic individuals – those on the opposite end of the "caring continuum" – who have been shown to have reduced volume in the amygdala and reduced responsiveness to fear-relevant stimuli.

## Sometimes There Are No Good Choices

It is important to realize that moral choices often involve dilemmas, some even more wrenching than the one posed by the hypothetical runaway trolley. In real life, trauma survivors are sometimes faced with far worse situations. Sometimes there is no "right" or "better" choice. Sister Dianna Ortiz describes the intolerable decision forced on a torture survivor she interviewed:

A father remembers not only his own horror and humiliation but also that of his teenage daughter and 9-year-old son, all of whom were detained by the military. "I was given another choice; I rape my daughter or the guard does it. . . I could not violate my own daughter. . . I lowered my eyes in shame. . . One guard held my face up, forcing me to watch this horrible scene. . . When they were through, they forced me to do what they had done to her. . . What kind of men are they? What kind of a father am I?" (Ortiz, 2001, p. 18)

Like the Vietnam POWs who "broke" under torture, and like many other trauma victims, a father who has survived such a horrific experience will understandably be haunted by memories and questions of "What else could I have done?" even when there were no viable alternatives. It is important to acknowledge that in some situations there may be no optimal "moral" choices.

# Training for Moral Compass

Is morality (or moral courage) innate, or can it be learned? This is a question that scholars have struggled with for centuries. While some doubt that morality and the courage to live by one's values can be taught, others believe that it can. Gus Lee, a former corporate whistleblower and later US Senate ethics investigator, writes in his book *Courage: The Backbone of Leadership* that "courage is not something with which we are born. . . Courage is a learned quality, an acquirable set of skills, a practiced competence. It's like boxing, except it's easier, it smells better, and it causes fewer nosebleeds" (Lee, 2007, p. 4).

In a more scholarly context, Helen Weng and colleagues (2013) conducted an experiment to see whether compassion and altruistic behavior could be increased through training. Trainees practiced 30 minutes a day for two weeks to cultivate feelings of compassion for loved ones, strangers, difficult people, and themselves; a control group practiced reinterpreting stressful personal events. Participants then played a game in which they could choose to make a monetary sacrifice to help a "victim" from whom money had been unfairly confiscated. Participants who had gone through the two weeks of compassion training were more altruistic and generous than were control participants. All participants also underwent fMRI studies, which showed that compassion training (but not reinterpretation training) was associated with neural activity in brain regions related to social cognition, emotion regulation, and reward processing. In sum, compassion training increased altruistic behavior mediated by alterations in neural activity and connectivity.

As an ordinary person, if I want to develop my moral courage, where do I begin? In his book *Moral Courage*, Rushworth Kidder outlines a three-step process (Kidder, 2006). First, I must perform a candid self-assessment. We all have core values and beliefs. What are mine? Which are the most important to me? Am I living by these principles and values? If not, where am I falling short? Am I motivated to change? Do I have the courage to do so?

Second, Kidder recommends that I discuss these questions with highly principled people whose ethics I admire. These discussions can help me to recognize and analyze the numerous situations in life where my actions have moral implications, and to honestly evaluate the risks inherent in defending my values.

Third, I act according to my values. I need to remain vigilant, because it is easy to make compromises and take short cuts. By repeatedly doing what I know to be right, and by taking a stand, particularly in challenging situations, I solidify my moral compass, and I grow stronger. As Aristotle wrote in his *Nicomachean Ethics*, "We become just by doing just acts, temperate by doing temperate acts, brave by doing brave acts."

But where should we begin? John McCain (2004) states it simply: "Do the duty before me." That is, there is no need to search for situations that require moral courage: these situations often present themselves to us in our daily life. In her book, *What Makes a Hero?* (2013), Elizabeth Svoboda points out that small acts of altruism on a daily basis will build a habit of helping others and prepare us to act heroically if a crisis occurs. In addition, we can practice heroism by imagining situations in which we would need to act. Stanford University's Heroic Imagination Project challenges students to surmount their own moral weaknesses through such imagination exercises.

What about our children? How do we teach them moral courage? One effective approach is the Giraffe Project, whose motto is "Moving people to stick their necks out for the common good." This project has developed a Heroes Program in which students in kindergarten to 12th grade listen to or read stories, stories about heroes tell similar stories about heroes in their own community and, finally, "become the story" by identifying a need in their community and working to address it though a service-learning project (Whang, 2010). As of 2007, the program had recorded the stories of more than 900 "Giraffes" and reached more than 30,000 students in the United States and abroad (through Giraffe Service Club International). YMCA camp director Matt Langdon devised a program of "Everyday Hero" workshops for children with a curriculum of spotlighting real-life heroes, performing daily small acts of "heroism," and articulating the moral lessons derived. In one school that tracked the results of participation in this program, disciplinary visits to the principal's office dropped by over 40 percent (Svoboda, 2013).

Adherence to our own moral compass is inextricably linked to resilience. We can become more faithful to our moral compass by taking an inventory of our most closely held beliefs and values, by learning from the writings and examples of ethical women and men, by discussing our beliefs with people whose values we respect, and then by practicing our values, particularly during times of adversity. Step by step, we can build our moral courage. When we most need to do the right thing, we will be ready.

# References

*A Gift Between Friends* (2012). *Mount Sinai Science & Medicine,* Fall 2012, Icahn School of Medicine at Mount Sinai. Retrieved at https://issuu.com/mountsinai/docs/mssm_fall2012_lowres

Aristotle (n.d.). *Nicomachaen Ethics* (W. D. Ross, Trans.). In D. C. Stevenson's The Internet Classics Archive. Retrieved from http://classics.mit.edu//Aristotle/nicomachaen.html

Baez, J. (1987/2009). *And a Voice to Sing With: A Memoir.* New York, NY: Simon & Schuster.

Baez, J. (2009). Joan's Corner: Notes from Joan. Idaho Falls. Blog post, updated 08/14/09. Accessed March 29, 2010 at www.joanbaez.com/joanscorner.html

Boswell, J. (1791/2008). *The Life of Samuel Johnson, LL.D.* London: Penguin Books.

Brooker, K. (2002). Starting over. *Fortune,* January 21, 50–68.

Brooks, D. (2016). *The Road to Character.* London: Penguin Books.

Buckley, C. (2007). Man is rescued by stranger on subway tracks. *New York Times* (January 3). Accessed September 3, 2010 at www.nytimes.com/2007/01/03/nyregion/03life.html

Cameron, C. D. & Payne, B. K. (2011). Escaping affect: how motivated emotion regulation creates insensitivity to mass suffering. *Journal of Personality & Social Psychology,* 100(1), 1–15.

CBS/AP (2015). Father of drowned Syrian tot makes heartfelt plea. December 23. Retrieved from www.cbsnews.com/news/father-of-drowned-syrian-tot-makes-heartfelt-plea

Coutu, D. (2002). How resilience works. *Harvard Business Review,* May, 46–55.

Creswell, J. D., Welch, W. T., Taylor, S. E. *et al.* (2005). Affirmation of personal values buffers neuroendocrine and psychological stress responses. *Psychological Science,* 16, 846–851.

Freeman, S. F., Hirschhorn, L. & Maltz, M. (2004). The power of moral purpose: Sandler O'Neill & Partners in the aftermath of September 11th, 2001. *Organization Development Journal,* Winter, pp. 69–81.

Greene, J. D., Sommerville, R. B., Nystrom, L. E., Darley, J. M. & Cohen, J. D. (2001). An fMRI investigation of emotional engagement in moral judgment. *Science,* 293(5537), 2105–2108.

Johnson, K. H. (2009). *A Better Man: A Book of Positive Role Models For 21st Century Boys. . . And the Adults Who Love Them.* Richmond, VA: Brandylane Publishers, Inc.

Kidder, R. M. (2006). *Moral Courage.* New York, NY: Harper Paperbacks.

Lee, G. (2007). *Courage: The Backbone of Leadership*. San Francisco, CA: Jossey-Bass.

Lee, J. L. C., Nader, K. & Schiller, D. (2017). An update on memory consolidation updating. *Trends in Cognitive Science*, 21(7), 531–545.

Lilienfeld, S. O., Watts, A. L. & Smith, S. F. (2015). Successful psychopathy: A scientific status report.*Current Directions in Psychological Science*, 24(4), 298–303.

Luks, A. (1988). Helper's high: Volunteering makes people feel good, physically and emotionally. *Psychology Today*, 22(10), 34–42.

Luks, A. (with Peggy Payne) (1991). *The Healing Power of Doing Good: The Health and Spiritual Benefits of Helping Others*. New York: Fawcett.

Mandela, N. (1995). *The Long Walk to Freedom*. New York, NY: Little, Brown & Company.

Marsh, A. A., Stoyco, S. A., Brethel-Hautwitz, K. M. *et al.* (2014). Neural and cognitive characteristics of extraordinary altruists. *Proceedings of the National Academy of Sciences USA*, 111(42), 15036–15041.

McCain, J. (2004). *Why Courage Matters*. New York, NY: Random House.

Moll, J. G., Krueger, F., Zahn, R. *et al.* (2014). Human front-mesolimbic networks guide decisions about charitable donation. *Proceedings of the National Academy of Sciences USA*, 103(42), 15623–15628.

Ortiz, D. (2001). The survivor's perspective: Voices from the center. In E. Gerrity, T. M. Keane & F. Tuma (eds.), *The Mental Health Consequences of Torture*, pp. 13–34. New York, NY: Kluwer Academic/Plenum Publishers.

Poulin, M. J., Brown, S. L., Dillard, A. J. & Smith, D. M. (2013). Giving to others and the association between stress and mortality. *American Journal of Public Health*, 103(9), 1649–1655.

Quenqua, D. (2013). Seeing narcissists everywhere. *New York Times*, August 5. Retrieved from http://www.nytimes.com/2013/08/06/science/seeing-narcissists-everywhere.html?pagewanted=all

Rachman, S. (1979). The concept of required helpfulness. *Behaviour Research and Therapy*, 17, 1–6.

Raskin, R. & Terry, H. (1988). A principal-components analysis of the Narcissistic Personality Inventory and further evidence of its construct validity. *Journal of Personality and Social Psychology*, 54(5), 890–902.

Reuter, M., Frenzel, C., Walter, N. T., Markett, S. & Montag, C. (2010). Investigating the genetic basis of altruism: The role of the COMT Vall58Met polymorphism. *Social Cognitive and Affective Neuroscience*, 6, 662–668.

Rushton, J. P. (2004). Genetic and environmental contributions to pro-social attitudes: A twin study of social responsibility. *Proceedings of the Royal Society London*, 271, 2583–2585.

Schwartz, C. E., Meisenhelder, J. B., Ma, Y. & Reed, G. (2003). Altruistic social interest behaviors are associated with better mental health. *Psychosomatic Medicine*, 65, 778–785.

Schwartz, C. E. & Sendor, M. (1999). Helping others helps oneself: Response shift effects in peer support. *Social Science & Medicine*, 48(11), 1563–1575.

Shapiro, Y. (1994). A reconsideration of altruism from an evolutionary and psycho dynamic perspective. *Ethics & Behavior*, 4(1), 23–42.

Sherman, N. (2005). *Stoic Warriors: The Ancient Philosophy Behind the Military Mind*. New York, NY: Oxford University Press.

Shermer, M. (2011). The science of right and wrong. *Scientific American*, 304(1): 83.

Stockdale, J. B. (1978). Firing line. *Naval War College Review*, Number 3 (Sequence 266). Georgetown University.

Stockdale, J. B. (1984). *A Vietnam Experience: Ten Years of Reflection*. Stanford, CA: Hoover Institution.

Stockdale, J. B. (1995). *Thoughts of a Philosophical Fighter Pilot*. Stanford, CA: Hoover Institution.

Stockdale, J. B. & Stockdale, S. B. (1990). *In Love and War: The Story of a Family's Ordeal and Sacrifice During the Vietnam Years*, 3rd edn. Annapolis, MD: Naval Institute Press.

Svoboda, E. (2013). *What Makes a Hero? The Surprising Science of Selflessness*. New York, NY: Penguin.

Twenge, J. M. & Campbell, W. K. (2009). *The Narcissism Epidemic: Living in the Age of Entitlement*. New York, NY: Free Press.

Twenge, J. M., Miller, J. D. & Campbell, W. K. (2014). The narcissism epidemic: commentary on modernity and narcissistic personality disorder. *Personality Disorders*, 5(2), 227–229.

Weng, H. Y., Fox, A. S., Shackman, A. J. *et al.* (2013). Compassion training alters altruism and neural responses to suffering. *Psychological Science*, 24(7), 1171–1180.

Werner, E. E. & Smith, R. S. (1992). *Overcoming the Odds: High Risk Children from Birth to Adulthood*. Ithaca, NY and London: Cornell University Press.

Whang, O. (2010). The Giraffe Program. Blog post, The Giraffe Heroes Project. Accessed September 3, 2010 at www.giraffe.org/in-new-jersey-200707266/

Widom, C. S. (1977). A methodology for studying noninstitutionalized psychopaths. *Journal of Consulting and Clinical Psychology*, 45, 674–683.

Zak, P. J., Stanton, A. A. & Ahmadi, S. (2007). Oxytocin increases generosity in humans. *PLoS One*, 2(11), e1128.

Zanon, M., Novembre, G., Zangrando, N., Chittaro, L. & Silani, G. (2014). Brain activity and prosocial behavior in a simulated life-threatening situation. *Neuroimage*, 98, 134–146.

Zimrin, H. (1986). A profile of survival. *Child Abuse and Neglect*, 10, 339–349.

# CHAPTER 5

# Religion and Spirituality: Drawing on Faith

Many people turn to religion or spirituality as a way to cope with hardship or trauma. Some find solace in formal religious services, while others seek inspiration and strength through individual spiritual practices that help them to connect with God or to find their place in the universe.

In her 2009 book *The Journey Home*, psychologist Ann Graber defines religion "as a path to God, the Source of Being" and spirituality "as that essential human endowment in which direct experience of God can take place" (2009, p. 19). She observes: "People may change their religion, but they retain their inherent spirituality." Religion and spirituality are of great importance in American culture and in other cultures around the globe. Among Americans, a 2007 Gallup poll found that 92 percent believe in God or a universal spirit, 81 percent believe in heaven, and 70 percent believe in the devil and in hell (Newport, 2007). The US Army includes the spiritual dimension as one of the core strengths in its Comprehensive Soldier Fitness (CSF) program. A survey of 230 countries and territories by the PRE Research Center found that 84 percent of the world's population identified with a religion in 2010.

After Pakistan's devastating 2005 earthquake, our colleague at New York University, Dr. Samoon Amad, journeyed into the mountains of Pakistan where he interviewed earthquake survivors. There, he found religious belief among survivors to be the single most powerful force in explaining the tragedy and in explaining survival.

Similarly, in our interviews with highly resilient individuals, time and again they told us about the powerful effects of spirituality or religion, particularly during times of high stress. For social worker Elizabeth Ebaugh, it was years of practice in spiritual traditions that saved her emotional life as she faced a life-threatening trauma and its aftermath.

# Will I Live to See the Sun Come Up?

It was 9 p.m., and Elizabeth was returning home from work. The previous day, she had attended a Gestalt therapy training program that focused on synthesizing Eastern spiritual philosophy and Western psychological insights. As part of the experiential training, she was held down by two other participants and then instructed to fight free. The goal of the exercise was to experience a freeing of her personal power which was trapped inside. She had also just completed a 10-day cleansing fast designed to help purify body and soul.

On her drive home, Ebaugh stopped to buy groceries. When she returned to her car with groceries in hand, she noticed a man sitting in a pickup truck in the parking space next to hers. She thought he looked a bit suspicious, so she hurried along, trying to focus simply on getting into her car and driving away. But when she put her grocery bag on the front passenger seat and turned to close the car door, there he was: crouching beside her, holding a hunting knife, ready to take the wheel.

Ebaugh was not new to trauma. As a social worker, she had treated many patients who suffered from symptoms of PTSD. For years, she had volunteered as a counselor for a child abuse and crisis telephone hotline. She knew how to negotiate with angry and hostile clients, so she was not particularly afraid, at first. Besides, the man looked scraggly and homeless; she thought he probably just needed money.

Using her negotiating experience, she began to bargain with her assailant by suggesting that the two of them drive to an ATM where she would withdraw cash for him and then return to the parking lot where he would leave her and go his own way. At first, he seemed agreeable. He drove her car to the bank, she withdrew cash from the ATM, and they headed back to the parking lot. Ebaugh remembers picturing herself sitting at home, telling her friends about her adventure.

However, as they approached the supermarket, Ebaugh's captor had a change of heart. He took a sharp right turn and drove to a remote section of the parking lot. He parked, then cuffed Ebaugh's hands behind her back. Now, she was truly frightened. She screamed and kicked. He told her to shut up. She tried to reason with him, but he ignored her and began to drive. Hours and miles went by, and Ebaugh started to lose hope.

The kidnapper told Elizabeth that he was not going to hurt her and that he would soon let her go.

> And I was holding onto that. Every time he stopped the car, I thought he was going to let me out. So it was hope, disappointment, hope, disappointment throughout the night.

At 1:00 in the morning, after driving aimlessly, he stopped at a convenience store just outside the city limits. At last, Ebaugh thought, she could escape. But the relief quickly turned to fright when he tied her hands to the steering wheel. As he entered the store, Ebaugh pounded the car horn over and over, hoping to attract attention. No one responded. Now she feared that her assailant would punish her for trying to expose him.

Once back in the car, he drove to a motel, forced her inside, and raped her. Then he calmly watched an erotic movie on TV. He lay in bed for awhile, silent. She worried that he was planning how to murder her. She suggested that he handcuff her to the pipes in the bathroom and leave without her.

He did not take her up on that suggestion. Instead, after several hours in the motel room, he dragged Ebaugh back into the car, gagged her, tied her hands, and headed back toward town. Pre-dawn, the roads were deserted. As they crossed a bridge several miles from the supermarket where the man had abducted her, she could only hope he was driving back to his truck and would let her go. But 10 minutes into their drive, her assailant pulled a sudden U-turn and headed back toward the bridge they'd just crossed. Then he stopped the car, looked into Ebaugh's eyes, and told her to get out.

Once she gained solid footing, she felt relieved, believing that her nightmare had ended and that her captor would soon free her. But he had a different plan. He pointed to the bridge. "He wanted me to jump off. That's when I fainted."

Ebaugh woke up when she hit the icy water 40 feet below. Her assailant had thrown her limp body off the bridge and left her to die. Upon landing, she felt no pain – just the shock of the freezing water. Maybe the air pockets in her heavy wool coat had broken her fall. Or, perhaps because she had fainted, her muscles were relaxed enough to absorb the shock.

Rather than panicking, Elizabeth felt an immediate burst of hope. Now she had a chance to get out of this alive. She was an accomplished swimmer, though she'd never tried to swim with her arms tied together. Using only her legs, she rolled onto her back and began to kick toward shore, nearly 100 yards away. Her heavy winter coat began to weigh her down. "I was exhausted and worried that I would get hypothermia." Each time she began to sink beneath the surface, she kicked faster and harder. Miraculously she reached the shore.

The river bank was steep, and the mud was thick. Inch by inch, Ebaugh scaled the slick bank of mud and crawled to a nearby road. After being ignored by several passing cars, she successfully flagged down a UPS truck. The driver took her to the nearest convenience store, called the police, and bought her a cup of hot tea.

Not surprisingly, Ebaugh suffered with symptoms of PTSD. Like many trauma survivors, she felt haunted by memories of her ordeal and lived day in and day out with an overwhelming sense of terror. Even though she knew that her abductor had been arrested, she felt so frightened that she could not stay alone in her house for more than 15 minutes at a time. She moved in with a close friend. When she felt ready to return to work, friends picked her up in the morning and then drove her home at the end of the day. Fortunately, her boss allowed her a flexible schedule; some days she could work, some days she simply couldn't handle it. For months, she recalls, she felt like a helpless infant.

Ebaugh believes that her background in spiritual practices strengthened and helped to protect her during the horrific ordeal and played an enormous role in her recovery. When she regained enough emotional equilibrium to reach out, she looked for spiritual leaders and healers. She meditated, chanted Sanskrit mantras, took various herbal and homeopathic supplements, and studied breathing and movement therapy. Her goal was to reach a higher spiritual plane and, in the process, rise above her trauma. In her pursuit of inner peace, she was relentless.

Several years later, Ebaugh completed additional professional training and left her government job to open a therapy practice focusing on holistic health and well-being. She also forged a loving personal relationship, got married, and became a mother. Despite having lived with debilitating stress, which plagued her for years, Ebaugh believes that her abduction served as a platform for her personal development. It forced her to evaluate her life and gradually change it for the better. She credits her ability to move forward after the abduction to numerous resilience factors, but most importantly her dedication to spirituality. Her path to healing led to a radical change in her world view. Before her ordeal, even though she wasn't a stranger to trauma, Ebaugh had lived with the belief that "it wouldn't happen to me." Now she had to grapple with the truth: life is fragile and can be taken from us in an instant.

> I believe that the only way to find closure is within yourself. It's not about what's happening outside. I could never go back to feeling that it wouldn't happen to me – it did. Studying spiritual philosophy and practicing meditation and chanting helped me experience the spiritual field, or field of awareness, and the interconnectedness of all that is. I am more completely present in my current reality and yet I feel a deep knowing that I am part of something much greater.
>
> When something bad happens, instead of asking how I can fix it or make sure it doesn't happen again, I recognize that suffering and pain can be a part of life. However, I am not stuck in the experience of pain. The experience of pain dissolves, and I can feel completely alive in the face of all that is. This helps me to have faith that every experience, no matter how traumatic, can bring me closer to the essential, to the awakened awareness. This doesn't rule out any reaction of anger that I was raped; however, those moments are only part of the journey to the experience of the essential self.

Ebaugh now feels that she was an "unconscious" person at the time of her abduction. "I think he woke me up. I was so asleep and didn't even know it," she says. When her abductor was in prison, she had her meditation community send him spiritual literature, "hoping his time in jail would be like in a monastery. He would be able to grow that way." Many years later, she recalls, "I went out into the woods with a friend, and I felt his spiritual presence and I turned around and faced his presence and I just thanked him for being a teacher along the path. And then I felt his presence leave."

Ebaugh believes that for survivors of trauma, there is a bridge between victimhood and returning to the world. She believes that she crossed that bridge by turning to spirituality and by deepening her connection with a larger view of reality and with a power greater than herself. Duke University trauma researcher Kathryn O'Connor notes that "a spiritual approach can be helpful in restoring hope, and acquiring a more balanced view about justice and injustice, safety and danger, good and evil... In posttraumatic stress disorder, the acceptance of a spiritual power may lead to a spiritual awakening" (Connor, Davidson & Lee, 2003). This is what Elizabeth discovered. But it was not easy. It took years and it took courage for her to embark on what the great scholar of mythology, Joseph Campbell, called the "hero's journey." Rather than obsess about revenge and hide in the shadows of fear, she gradually chose to confront the "dark night of the soul," what Carl Jung referred to as "the shadow." For Ebaugh, the end result was a spiritual awakening.

## Risking One's Life for Religion

As Americans, we have the luxury of freedom of religion – a freedom only dreamed of by people in other places. When one of us (SS) learned about his own family history, he found that religious convictions caused some of his ancestors to put their lives on the line. This information came to Steve's attention after his father spent most of a decade researching and writing a book titled *Southwick Pioneers in Nebraska* (2005). Through his father, Steve learned about Lawrence and Cassandra Southwick.

Lawrence Southwick sailed across the Atlantic Ocean with several hundred other settlers and arrived in the New World in the late 1620s. He lived in Salem, Massachusetts for a year or so before returning to England. Three years later he sailed back to Salem with his wife, Cassandra, and their four children. A glassmaker by trade, Lawrence was given land by the town of Salem on which to build a glass and earthenware manufacturing company.

Like the other residents of Salem, Lawrence and his family joined a Puritan Church where they attended services every Sunday. Over time, however, the Southwicks gravitated toward a small but emerging faith-based movement known as the Society of Friends, or Quakers.

Quakers are typically known to be peace-loving and modest but determined seekers of the truth. They believe that all individuals possess the light of God within them, and that inspiration and revelation emanate from that inner light. At Sunday meetings, members speak out when God moves them to do so, and their words are believed to be the actual words of God. Consequently, in the

Quaker tradition there is no need for clergy to serve as translators of God's will, since God can speak directly through everyone. Similarly, there is no need for ritual or special sacraments, since life itself is seen as a sacrament.

In 1656, Quakers in the Colony of Massachusetts spelled out their reasons for separating from the Puritan Church. Some of the reasons they gave were:

- "We deem our salvation to be an individual work which we cannot do by proxy or for another."
- "We deem it proper to declare and proclaim to all the world our abhorrence of all wars, and our independence of all despotic rulers, either temporal or spiritual."
- "We deem it proper to declare and protest against the cruel and vindictive persecutions of our (so-called) Christian Church, and we proclaim our independence of the same, and we recognize the true brotherhood of man."

The egalitarian and personal nature of the Quaker tradition threatened the established Puritan Church, with its inextricable ties to politics, social hierarchy, rules of conduct, and rigid doctrine. The Commonwealth of Massachusetts passed laws that punished colonists who identified themselves as Quakers and who failed to attend Puritan Church services. When Lawrence and Cassandra stopped attending services at the First Puritan Church and hosted two Quakers in their home, they were arrested, fined, publicly whipped and eventually jailed, starved, and forced into hard labor.

In poems written two centuries later, the Quaker poet and Massachusetts native John Greenleaf Whittier dramatized the plight of the Southwick family.

> Last night I saw the sunset melt through my prison bars,
> Last night across the damp earth-floor fell the pale gleam of stars;
> In the coldness and the darkness all through the long night-time,
> My grated casement whitened with autumn's early rime.
> All night I sat unsleeping, for I knew that on the morrow
> The ruler and the cruel priest would mock me in my sorrow,
> Dragged to their place of market, and bargained for and sold,
> Like a lamb before the shambles, like a heifer from the fold!
> I cried, "The Lord rebuke thee, thou smitter of the meek
> Thou robber of the righteous, thou trampler of the weak
> Go light the dark cold hearth-stones – go turn the prison lock
> Of the poor hearts thou has hunted, thou wolf amid the flock!"

Upset by how their parents had been treated, the Southwick children also stopped attending Puritan Church services. One son, Joshua, was punished by being tied to an ox cart, stripped to his waist, and paraded through several towns where he was mocked and brutally whipped with the dried intestines of animals. Yet, it is said, a defiant Joshua, with his flesh torn and mutilated, called out to his torturers, "Here is my body. If you want a further testimony to the truth I profess, take it and tear it in pieces; your sentence is no more terrifying to me than if you had taken a feather and blown it in the air."

Two other children, a son named Daniel and a daughter named Provided, were ordered by the General Court of Massachusetts to be sold as slaves in Barbados. However, no merchant captains sailing south from New England would agree to transport them; one captain was reputed to have said he would rather sink his ship than "bear this child away."

While the elder Southwicks were in prison, a new law was enacted calling for banishment or death of Quakers. As a result, upon their release, they were prosecuted retroactively and banished from the Massachusetts colony. Then in their late 50s and having had their land and possessions taken by the colonial authorities, they bought a small boat with the little money they had, said goodbye to their children, and sailed along the New England coast in search of a home. Eventually, they made their way to Shelter Island in Long Island Sound, where they survived the frigid winter but eventually died of exposure and starvation.

In a second poem, Whittier describes their plight.

Safer with winds and waves than human wrath.
With ravening wolves than those whose zeal for God
Was cruelty to man, the exiles trod
Drear leagues of forest without guide or path,
Or launching frail boats on the uncharted sea,
Round storm-vexed capes, whose teeth of granite ground
The waves to foam, the perilous way they wound,
Enduring all things so their souls were free.
When his wife moaned, "Let us turn back," Lawrence said,
"Kneel down and say thy prayers; the Lord himself will steer.
And led by Him, nor man nor Devils I fear."
So the gray Southwicks, from a rainy sea,
Saw, far and faint, the loom of land and gave
With feeble voices thanks for friendly ground
Whereon to rest their weary feet, and found
A peaceful death-bed and quiet grave.

In 1884, a monument was erected on Shelter Island to the memory of Nathaniel Sylvester, the proprietor who gave refuge to the two Quakers. On its eastern end, the inscription reads:

LAWRENCE AND CASSANDRA SOUTHWICK, Despoiled – Imprisoned – Starved – Whipped – Banished, Who fled here to die.

Lawrence and Cassandra knew that they could be released from prison and restored to their previous position in the community if only they would renounce their Quaker faith and return to the Puritan Church. But they chose not to. Their deep faith in God and their profound moral courage provided the strength and resilience that the Southwicks needed to defend their unshakable belief in religious freedom.

# God Comes First

Like Lawrence and Cassandra Southwick, and like Elizabeth Ebaugh, many of the resilient people we interviewed found strength in their spiritual beliefs and practices. This was particularly true among former Vietnam POWs. In fact, in *Honor Bound*, the classic account of American prisoners in Vietnam, Stuart Rochester and Frederick Kiley made the following observation, "There is virtually no personal account in the Vietnam POW literature that does not contain some reference to a transforming spiritual episode" (1998, p. 413).

Major Dick Bolstad is an example of a soldier whose religious faith never wavered. Forty-five years later, Major Bolstad still describes Catholic faith as the foundation of his life.

Dick grew up in a poor family on the south side of Minneapolis. His father worked as a carpenter who spent most of his waking hours laboring to support his wife and their six children. Even though Dick's father did not have time for church, he insisted that the children attend every Sunday.

For Dick, a defining moment in his life came in the sixth grade when he attended a two-week religious summer program at the Saint Albert's School. On the last day, his teacher announced that the student with the best attendance would receive an award, a portrait of Saint Anthony that hung on the wall of her classroom. Dick was the only student who had not missed a class.

> So she gave me that picture. Saint Anthony, he's the saint who helps you find things. If you lose something or if you lose your mind, you know, he's kind of there for the hopeless cases. Ever since then, I have Saint Anthony to help me.

Dick Bolstad enlisted in the Marine Corps Reserves when he was 19 years old. Two years later, during the Korean War, he was called to active duty. As a member of the 1st Marine Division, Bolstad landed at Inchon, Korea, where he fought as an infantryman, was wounded, and received a Purple Heart. Years later he was serving as an Air Force pilot when his plane was shot down and he was imprisoned by the North Vietnamese. Major Bolstad prayed to Saint Anthony to help him find courage, hope and endurance.

> Just give me strength to withstand whatever they were doing to me... During any beating, any time I was being hurt, I'd offer the pain to God... And I always prayed that I could hold my head high when I returned home... I prayed that I would have the

strength to do what was honorable... And, of course, I prayed for other people... I prayed to Saint Anthony and asked him to pray to Jesus for me, to intercede for me, to ask Jesus to grant my request. Saint Anthony, he's got a little more pull than I do.

In prison, Bolstad never felt alone. During his intolerable torture and deprivation, he believed that he was joined by St. Anthony and by Jesus Christ, who had suffered and died on the cross, and who now helped Dick bear his own cross.

When Bolstad was released from prison, he and his fellow POWs were flown to Clark Air Force Base in the Philippines. Shortly after arriving on base, all the healthy prisoners were taken to the mess hall. To a group of POWs who had starved for years, this was a dream come true. But Bolstad had other plans.

My first thought, when we got to Clark, was to get hold of a priest and have him hear my confession before anything else.

When he found a Catholic chaplain, the priest told him that he had to wait for morning Mass.

And I said, "No father, now."
And he said, "Maybe we could do it a little later."
I said, "No, now."
So he set up a room and heard my first confession.
And then I was fine... I figured I was squared away with God.

When asked to list the 10 most important factors that helped him survive in prison, Dick Bolstad ranked religion first.

Oh, yeah. There's no doubt about it. I'm not a religious fanatic; I'm just a normal person but I believe in my faith. I practice my faith... The top ten... I put my family up there and I put my country up there... but (my religious faith) is at the top... There's nothing that's gonna knock that off.

Former POW Colonel Robbie Risner used prayer to connect with absent loved ones. In his book *The Passing of the Night*, Risner describes praying for others:

I was praying a lot, for it was one of the few ways I could occupy the day. I would pray not only for my family but also for each one of the prisoners that I knew of. Then I would go through all of my relatives and friends as well as our government leaders. Mentioning names in prayer gave me a feeling of closeness to them that was very meaningful. (2004, p. 87)

To survive torture sessions, Risner used prayer in two ways. Usually he asked God for "the ability to stand it," but when the pain became unbearable, he prayed for relief.

> I said, "Lord, I have been in long enough. I am half-sick, miserable and cold and hungry. I am asking you to get me out of these stocks, to provide me more clothes, another blanket and some food." (2004, p. 89)

And when his North Vietnamese guards tied both arms behind his back and then gradually lifted them higher and higher until one or both shoulders dislocated, Risner turned to the Bible.

> When the pain started really ripping me I began desperately to pray. I began quoting a scripture verse from the Bible over and over: "My grace is sufficient. My grace is sufficient." I thought that meant God would give me grace to bear whatever I had to bear without giving in. (2004, p. 94)

Another Vietnam POW, Larry Stark, believes that God is always present, that He understands our "situation," and that He will work as a partner to lighten our load, if only we recognize his presence.

> I think that one has to recognize that along the way the Lord is there and He knows your situation. All you have to do is acknowledge His presence. So no matter what, I can handle it. We can handle this thing together. And if you do that, then you don't have that great big burden. You don't have to do it all yourself... without some religion, it [the imprisonment] would have been a lot more difficult and maybe not bearable.

Even during a grueling forced march when he wondered whether he had the stamina to endure, Stark found signs that God was by his side.

> We're going up this mountain, and I could see up above the clouds. In fact, we walked right up through the lower level to where we were actually looking down on the cloud layer. And again I said, "Hey, this is a way for the Lord to say hello. Now this is fantastic beauty."

And in *Honor Bound*, ex-POW John McCain recalls,

> To guard against such despair, in our most dire moments, POWs would make supreme efforts to grasp our faith tightly, to profess it alone in the dark, and hasten its revival. Once I was thrown into another cell after a long and difficult interrogation. I discovered scratched into one of the cell's walls the creed, "I believe in God, the Father Almighty."
> (Rochester & Kiley, 1998)

Ritual and ceremony are central elements in most religious and spiritual practices. Even under circumstances in which formal ceremonies are forbidden, people of faith somehow find a way to worship together. For example, as we mentioned in previous chapters, the North Vietnamese centralized their prison system by housing large numbers of American POWs in one facility, nicknamed the Hanoi Hilton. In 1970, the North Vietnamese brought many more prisoners to Hanoi from outlying locations.

Soon dozens of prisoners, against prison rules, held a formal religious service. Men from all over the prison heard the singing and joined in.

"We agreed that we were going to have a church service and told the Vietnamese, and they said no," recalled former prisoner Bud Day. But on February 12, 1970, the prisoners went ahead anyway, holding a service and singing songs. "The Vietnamese broke in and seized the people who were standing against the wall doing the service," Day said. "They marched them out of the room at gunpoint. So I stood up and started singing 'The Star-Spangled Banner,' 'God Bless America,' 'My Country 'Tis of Thee' and every song we could think of."[1]

Even though the organizers of what was later called the "church riot" knew that the North Vietnamese would punish them severely, they proceeded because they believed that this collective expression of faith would improve morale. After the service, North Vietnamese guards shackled the organizers for 38 days.

Bob Shumaker, one of the most respected senior officers at the Hanoi Hilton, believes in God but does not see himself as devout. However, as a seasoned prisoner, he offered the following advice when a new POW arrived in the cell next to him:

> The first thing you need around here, old buddy, is faith. I'm not a preacher. I'm not gonna try to convert you. I'm just gonna tell you the truth. If you can't tap into a source of strength and power greater than yourself, you're probably not gonna last.

Some of the POWs we interviewed told us that although they embraced religion and prayed frequently during their imprisonment, they had not considered themselves to be religious before their capture. Being subjected to conditions, in which suffering was all around them and death never far away, motivated them to focus on God and to pray far more than they had at any other time in their lives. The authenticity of this so-called "foxhole religion" has been questioned by some religious figures, but for many POWs and other trauma survivors, religion and spirituality, whether long-standing or newfound, played an essential role in their survival.

# What If You Are Not Religious?

Among the former POWs we interviewed, there were a few who did not call upon religion or a belief in God to stay strong and to survive. Al Carpenter is a former Navy fighter pilot who withstood nearly six and a half years of

---

[1] See, for example, http://advanceindiana.blogspot.com/2008/08/mccains-church-riot-in-hanoi-hilton.html accessed August 21, 2009; Zuckman (2008).

isolation, torture, and extreme deprivation in a North Vietnamese prison. Other POWs describe him as one of the tough guys. When we asked if religion or spirituality played a role in his experience as a POW, he replied,

> Not at all. Well, it was a factor, but it didn't influence me in the long term. I was not a religious person. I had had a normal Protestant upbringing, went to church a couple of times a year. When I ended up in prison, I thought I would never have a better opportunity to seriously explore what truly might be important about it [religion] and how it might work in my life. I made a vow that I would pursue it for at least one year no matter how irritated, bored, whatever I might get with it. And I sought out those with different religious backgrounds whom I could get to.

For example, Carpenter tried to learn as much as possible about Catholicism from another prisoner who was devoutly religious.

> I worked on prayer, not to get me out of this situation, but I asked for what I thought was reasonable, to help me cope with my situation and understand better. I really seriously tried. I tried hard and I worked at it all the time. And you know what I concluded? The benefit people get from prayer... is the ability to open up... open up and get a look inside of themselves through verbalization. And I can do the same thing talking to a tree or the wall or whatever. I do not think that a supreme being answered my prayers, giving me comfort. The comfort came from within... and I stopped swearing during this period. I said if you are gonna do this, go whole hog. And that was the toughest thing. That was almost unbearable to not express myself in my old sailor's language. But I did it. I did it for a year. That was tough. But the conclusion I came to was that I can handle things myself. I am very independent.

Even though Carpenter concluded that religion did not enhance his resilience, he did recognize that religion and spirituality helped others to face adversity.

## Special Forces Instructors Also Turn to God for Strength

Given the dangers inherent in their job, it is not surprising that many Special Forces instructors we introduce in this book also spoke about spirituality or religion as a source of strength and an aid for controlling fear. Like the former POWs we interviewed, most believed in God, felt that they had a personal relationship with God, and tended to be idealistic and ethical. In fact, over 50 percent of Special Forces missions are humanitarian in nature.

Mark Hickey has been a member of the Special Forces for most of his adult life. He is a medic who is viewed by his peers as a man of great integrity, strength, and endurance. However, at 5 feet 4 inches tall, he does not derive his stature from his height.

I'm not the typical picture. I'm not the poster boy for Special Forces, a six-foot-four-inch barrel-chested freedom fighter. I don't see myself physically as anything special. I think the only thing I do have going for me is my relationship with God... It's the Bible that drives me. The Bible says, 'Do all things unto the glory of God.' I'm going to do my best, not just for me, but for God as well. He is the one I really want to impress.

When we asked Master Sergeant Hickey about the role that his faith in God played in his success as a Special Forces soldier and instructor, he said,

For me it is the reason. It is *the* reason... I believe in an afterlife so if I die I've got someplace to go. It's just the next step. That lets me do some of the things I do because I don't fear death. I may fear a particular way of dying – I don't want to be eaten by a shark – but the thought of death doesn't really scare me because I have faith that there's something else, my faith in God, that there's something else out there.

Cliff Welch, another Special Forces instructor, has similar beliefs:

The way I look at it, I'm not afraid of dying. And if I do die, I'm gonna be in a better place. So, bring it on. You know, I really don't care. And a lot of people say, "It's not a smart man's way of doing things." But, to me, faith's a big deal. I mean, if you don't have faith, you don't have anything. People say there is no God. Some of them say religion is just for weak-minded people. That's crap. You gotta have faith in something, or you're just a hollow, empty person. And that's pretty much the way I've lived my whole life, even from my earliest recollection of going to church on Sunday. Always, church has been there.

# Faith and Recovery

For some survivors, faith assumes a central role in their lives only after their trauma, when they are trying to recover. Tim Pollock is a young Iraq veteran who was severely injured. According to a *USA Today* interview, an insurgent "blew off half his skull during a reconnaissance operation in 2004" (Swensen, 2009). After returning home to Ohio and retiring from the Army, Pollock suffered from seizures stemming from his injury. He struggled with agitation, anxiety, and other symptoms of PTSD; he "drank hard, bought a gun and considered suicide."

For Pollock, the way back was through studying for the ministry. He found a renewed sense of purpose by getting involved with Point Man International Ministries, a nonprofit whose mission is to connect the suffering veteran with other veterans who are further along in the transition to home. Supported by religious congregations around the country, Point Man coordinates more than 250 veteran-led "Outpost" groups worldwide, as well as "Home Front" groups that are led by mothers, husbands, wives, and friends to provide support for the families of active service members and veterans. Pollock visits wounded soldiers in hospitals and coaches veterans living with PTSD. "I'll always have post-traumatic stress," he observes, "but I'm learning through God how to control that."

There are, of course, many religion-based programs for trauma survivors of all faiths who are not necessarily military veterans. Torah and the Twelve Steps, Inc., for example, focuses on the transformational change needed to overcome addictions, a common problem in survivors of trauma. As the organization's website explains, "Drugs and alcohol *mimic* the essential need for a relationship with the Creator through a 'pseudospiritual' sense of connection and transcendence, and a false sense of 'good' that in actuality leads to greater dissatisfaction, emptiness, despair and eventually death." Although the program is open to people of all faiths, it offers spiritual support through specific Jewish teachings and their applications to 12 steps of recovery; interactive classes, with the study of basic Kabalistic thought, and classical texts on ethics to increase personal character development; and training in leadership skills and methods to increase learning capacity. Another organization, The American Association of Christian Counselors, coordinates a nationwide network of resources for those seeking help in recovering from trauma.

Many survivors who are not affiliated with any formal religion engage in a variety of spiritual practices to deal with trauma and other life challenges. Some practices grow out of the Judeo-Christian tradition while many do not. Examples include yoga, tai chi, qigong, aikido, tantric rituals, sufi mysticism, sadhana, and Native American healing traditions. Research to test the effectiveness of these approaches for trauma survivors is expanding rapidly. In a 2006 scientific study conducted by Boston University researcher Bessel van der Kolk, patients with PTSD participated in either hatha yoga classes or group therapy sessions. The patients who practiced yoga showed significantly greater reduction in PTSD symptoms than those who took part in group therapy. Yoga was also associated with improved heart rate variability, which has been related to emotion self-regulation. Additional recent evidence suggests that yoga may increase levels of gamma-aminobutyric acid (GABA), which is the brain's primary inhibitory neurotransmitter. Drugs that increase GABA availability decrease anxiety and tend to have a relaxing effect (Streeter *et al.*, 2010). Similarly, tai chi, an ancient Chinese mind–body exercise and martial art, has been found to be effective in reducing anxiety and perceived stress. Tai chi incorporates multiple elements known to modulate the stress response and enhance performance, including physical fitness, meditation, and natural breathing techniques (Zheng *et al.*, 2017).

# Faith, Guilt, and Forgiveness

Guilt and forgiveness are complicated topics, particularly in the context of stress, trauma and resilience. Guilt can haunt or even cripple survivors for years, and to forgive a specific person, organization, or society that has intentionally caused great harm may be next to impossible for many of us. However, when left unattended, guilt and the inability to forgive can be painful and emotionally draining (Toussaint, Shields & Slavich, 2016). In a five-week study in which participants reported their levels of forgiveness, perceived stress, and mental and physical health symptoms, Loren Toussaint and colleagues found that forgiveness was associated with decreased stress and better mental health (Toussaint, Shields & Slavich, 2016).

For returning war veterans, spiritually based programs often address the guilt that many veterans carry, consciously or unconsciously. In a study of present and former soldiers, Everett Worthington and Diane Langberg (2012) noted that "being in the military... can create opportunities for self-condemnation" and therefore "soldiers need the skills of self-forgiveness" (p. 274). These researchers view forgiveness of oneself as both a decision and an emotional process. They identify six strategies for people who seek to forgive (pp. 284–285):

- Receive God's forgiveness
- Repair relationships
- Rethink ruminations
- Reach emotional self-forgiveness
- Rebuild self-acceptance
- Resolve to live virtuously

Point Man Ministries president Dana Morgan sums it up when he tells veterans that "everybody else can forgive you, and now it's your turn to forgive yourself because God already has."

For someone who is a victim of crime or abuse, forgiving the offender may be even more difficult than forgiving oneself. In a *New York Times* article, Elizabeth Kadetsky (2009) describes having been mugged in the hallway of her apartment building by a man wearing a ski mask. "In a dream several months later, the man with the mask was sitting in my hallway waiting for me to come home, holding the mask in his hand. At first when I saw him, I was scared, but when I saw his face I also saw that he was human. He told me he was struggling with guilt over having hurt someone. I tried to imagine if I could forgive him."

The question, "Can I forgive?" is a central one. In a 2009 study of more than 100 adults, Nathaniel M. Lambert and colleagues at Florida State University assigned participants to pray for a specific person, or pray about any topic, or think positive thoughts about a specific person every day for four weeks. Those who prayed for the specific person were found to be more forgiving, and showed an increase in selfless concern, compared to the participants in the other conditions. In the process of forgiving, it may be that we develop greater empathy for the other person and his or her perspective, as Kadetsky did when she dreamed about her attacker. Forgiveness involves relinquishing the desire for revenge – a desire that can keep us stuck in a victim frame of mind.

# Faith as It Relates to Physical and Mental Health

Scientific research supports the relationship between faith and resilience that has been so eloquently described by Dick Bolstad, Bob Shumaker, Mark Hickey, and Elizabeth Ebaugh. One of the first resources that many people turn to when faced with adversity or serious illness is their religion or spirituality. For example, in one study of seriously mentally ill subjects, more than 80 percent reported using religion to help deal with their illness, and the majority believed that their religious beliefs and practice helped to reduce their symptoms (Pargament & Lomax, 2013). This turning to religion to deal with adversity is very common among practitioners of all major world religions. Meta-analyses (summaries of all available well-designed and well-conducted studies on a particular topic that have been published in the scientific literature) have concluded that practicing religion is associated with physical and emotional well-being among healthy individuals and with better coping among people who are suffering from medical illnesses. For example, a group of researchers led by Michael E. McCullough at the National Institute for Healthcare Research analyzed 42 published studies that involved 126,000 subjects. They found that those who actively practiced a religious faith lived slightly longer than those who did not (McCullough *et al.*, 2000). Similarly, in meta-analyses involving over 44,000 cancer patients, religion or spirituality was modestly to moderately associated with physical, mental, and social health. The strongest association was for the affective dimension of religion or spirituality, which includes feelings of comfort, peacefulness, and equanimity as well as a sense of reverence and empowerment (Park, 2015). In addition, studies involving patients with rheumatoid arthritis, severe burns, and organ transplants have found that those who consider themselves to be religious tend to see themselves as healthier, require fewer days in the hospital, and report fewer medical complications than those who do not describe themselves as religious (Powell, Shahabi & Thoresen, 2003).

Numerous studies have also shown that higher levels of religiousness are related to lower levels of depression and suicidal ideation. This has been found in elderly people living in the United States and Europe, medically ill older patients, elderly patients recovering from hip surgery, bereaved adults, and college students. In a study of 838 patients over the age of 50 who were admitted to the hospital for medical illnesses, a group of researchers from Duke Medical School found fewer symptoms of depression in those who described themselves as religious (Koenig, George & Titus, 2004). In a study of people with a family history of depression, Lisa Miller and colleagues at Columbia University College of Physicians and Surgeons found significantly lower levels of depression in participants who reported religion/spirituality as an important part of their lives (Miller *et al.*, 2014).

Religion/spirituality has also been linked to resilience, quality of life, and fewer suicide attempts among hospitalized depressed patients (Mosqueiro, da Rocha & Fleck, 2015). Similarly, in a large prospective study of over 89,000 nurses, those who attended religious services at least once per week had a five-fold lower suicide rate compared to other nurses (VanderWeele *et al.*, 2016). Religiousness may even help to protect against depression, anxiety, and PTSD.

As we described earlier in this chapter, religion/spirituality may serve as a source of strength and inspiration for many soldiers. In a study of over 3,000 US military Veterans, those with high Duke University Religion scores had significantly decreased lifetime PTSD and alcohol disorder. High scores on this scale were also associated with greater dispositional gratitude, purpose in life, and posttraumatic growth (Sharma *et al.*, 2017). Further, in a study of Israeli soldiers, those who were religious were less susceptible to the effects of traumatic stress, and in another study among individuals who were at high risk for developing depression, those with higher self-identified religiosity were less likely to develop depression over a period of ten years (Mosqueiro, da Rocha & Fleck, 2015).

A similar relationship has been reported in adolescents: those who are religious are less likely to express suicidal thoughts and behaviors than those who are not. In a study of young adult college students who had been exposed to significant violence during childhood, "aspects of spirituality, such as a connection to a higher power, finding strength and comfort in the divine, and feeling blessed are linked to enhanced resilience" (Howell & Miller-Graff, 2014, pp. 1991–1992).

There is an important caveat: religious coping is not always associated with well-being or resilience. Some researchers have distinguished between positive and negative patterns of religious coping (Pargament *et al.*, 1998; Pargament & Lomax, 2013). Individuals who see God as punitive and judgmental may feel that they "deserve" their troubles, and that their fate is controlled by an unsympathetic all-powerful being, leaving them with little sense of control.

Although it seems clear that religion is associated with positive physical and mental health as well as resilience, it not known exactly why. It appears likely, however, that regular attendance at religious services may foster a number of resilience factors including social support, optimism, altruism, and a search for meaning and purpose. In addition, as a member of a religious congregation, parishioners routinely interact with positive and resilient role models who encourage them to adopt meaningful social roles in which they can give to others through acts of generosity. Religious faith may also protect against destructive habits such as drug and alcohol abuse, because it values and promotes self-regulation and self-restraint. In a variety of studies, religion and spirituality have been linked with lower rates of substance use, delinquency and crime, and sexual promiscuity (Pargament & Lomax, 2013).

By focusing on discrete components of religion and spirituality such as prayer, meditation, and attendance at religious services, science is beginning to uncover which elements of faith and spirituality are most closely linked to psychological well-being and resilience. For example, the relationship between resilience and religion may partly be explained by the social quality of religious attendance. The word "religion" comes from the Latin "religare," meaning "to bind." People who regularly attend religious services may have access to a deeper and broader form of social support than is often available in a secular setting. It is not uncommon for a religious congregation to provide food, money, and emotional and moral support to fellow members who are under duress.

However, the support that practitioners receive may come not only from fellow human beings but also from their belief in God. Many religions focus on the practitioner's relationship with God, often described as a supreme being who provides guidance, strength, and protection. For some people, their relationship with God bolsters their own feelings of inner strength and self-efficacy, and helps them to follow the advice of the Italian Renaissance poet and philosopher Dante Alighieri, "Be bold and the mighty shall protect you." Believing that God is at their side, they have the confidence to tackle challenges that otherwise would seem too daunting. In 2006, mental health researchers Roger D. Fallot and Jennifer P. Heckman (2006) found that survivors who used religious coping strategies at the time of traumatic experiences reported lower subsequent levels of distress than those who did not.

## Faith Strengthens a Challenged Family

Among the resilient people we interviewed are Ron and Barb Garrett, parents of a son with Down syndrome. During the pregnancy, Barb and Ron were excited and hoped the new baby would be a girl. Barb had chosen the name Heidi.

Bryan's birth, then, came as a shock. The Garretts never had any particular reason to learn about Down syndrome, or even to give it much thought. There had been no prior indication that their baby would be born with congenital problems. Without warning, they had to revise their ideas about parenting and "redefine normal." Like most Down syndrome babies, Brian was born with poor muscle tone and had difficulty swallowing. Barb recalls, "Everything that I would normally do, I had to relearn – how to hold him, how to feed him." When Bryan was only six weeks old, he began speech/feeding therapy, occupational therapy, and physical therapy. Barb recalls that during her first three months of maternity leave she cried every day, mourning the normal child she did not have. Some friends seemed to distance themselves, apparently feeling awkward about the idea of a child with such a disability. Barb read a book with the message, "Someday you will be happy again," but she did not believe it. When Bryan was an infant, Barb was invited to have lunch with a group of other women who were mothers of Down syndrome children. While this helped her to feel less alone, she relied more on her faith for strength than on other people. Particularly helpful was the phrase "God gives good gifts," spoken by a missionary whose child had died.

Barb and her husband are evangelical Christians; as Ron explains it, "Our faith gives us strength for everything, including being parents to Bryan." The Garretts never asked, "Why us?" However, Barb struggled with the question of whether Bryan's having Down syndrome was God's doing. As the years passed, she came to believe that God allowed Bryan to have Down syndrome, but that the condition is only temporary. "Once he's in heaven, he will be whole," she explained.

When Bryan was small, the Garretts sometimes watched the television series *Life Goes On*, which stars a teenager with Down syndrome. They found it informative, but also frightening, as it foreshadowed problems that might arise in the future. Life with Bryan continued to present challenges. As he grew older, physically stronger and more active, his mental and emotional development lagged far behind. In adolescence, his behaviors still resembled those of a much younger child with high energy, near-continuous talking, attention seeking, and the tendency to cause messes around the house.

Over the course of many hours of practice using the "Hooked on Phonics" technique, Bryan learned to read. This made an enormous difference in his education. Bryan excelled in the Special Olympics, the international athletic competitions for people with intellectual disabilities. He won numerous medals. Just before his 18th birthday, Bryan graduated from his local public high school, which combines mainstreaming with special education. He subsequently enrolled in a special needs program called STRIVE, which focuses on practical life skills.

Still, parenting Bryan involves major challenges. For example, Bryan has a knack for disappearing: he has been reported missing from school on numerous occasions, sometimes requiring police, school administrators, and teachers to comb the neighborhood. Once Brian wandered away from his parents in a crowded airport. Barb and Ron continually pray, "Lord, help us keep track of him!"

Bryan has a special talent for making friends with strangers. Barb says he is the friendliest person she has ever known. While she considers herself to be somewhat shy, she has learned to socialize more effectively by watching how Bryan relates to others. In fact, Bryan has become a role model for Barb. She does not imitate all of Bryan's social behaviors, however. For example, several years ago at a large "meet and greet" party, Barb spotted Bryan across the room standing behind a bald-headed man. Without warning, Bryan began to rub the man's head. Fortunately, the gentleman did not seem to mind, although Barb was mortified.

Bryan has inspired many people, even influencing the careers of a few who have decided to go into special education after getting to know him. Ron and Barb believe that God has a special role for Bryan to play in promoting friendship and cheering people up when they most need it. They see him as a blessing, a person who has brought joy to their lives. Still, they look toward eternity in the belief that "Someday Bryan will be in heaven and we will enjoy him without anything holding him back."

## Prayer, Meditation, and Mindfulness

Most religion and spirituality practices incorporate some form of prayer, meditation, or mindfulness. These practices have been used for thousands of years to quiet and discipline the mind.

Prayer is, in the simplest terms, talking to God, to a higher power, to the universe. Author Robert Longman Jr. (2002–2009) describes it this way:

> Prayer is, at its heart, the communication that is the fabric of the human being's (and human species) relationship with its Father. When a Jew, Muslim, or Christian prays to God, the very act itself assumes these to be true at the very least:
> - that there's One beyond each and all of us, beyond all that is around us;
> - that this One cares enough to bother with you;
> - that this One cares enough to want your response;
> - that this One cares enough to respond to you;
> - that this One is effective enough for that response to make a difference.

In his book *Letters to Malcolm: Chiefly on Prayer*, the Christian novelist and theologian C. S. Lewis (1963, 1964) refers to sincerity as the essence of prayer: "The prayer preceding all prayers is, 'May it be the real I who speaks. May it be the real Thou that I speak to.'"

The well-known proponent of alternative medicine Dr. Deepak Chopra (2009) broadens this definition further: "Why not consider prayer to be an action in consciousness? It may be too hard for someone in the Judeo-Christian tradition to let go of a personal (and usually masculine) God in favor of something as impersonal as one's own awareness, but I think this is where the focus should lie."

The possible connection of prayer with life satisfaction was explored by Brandon Whittington and Steven Scher (2010) at Eastern Illinois University, who studied 430 individuals with a wide range of beliefs, including atheism. A comprehensive review of clinical studies suggested that "frequent private prayer is associated with a significant benefit for depression, optimism, coping, and other mental health conditions such as anxiety" (Anderson & Nunnelley, 2016). The results were intriguing even though the findings were correlational, like those for most studies cited in this chapter, and therefore do not prove that prayer causes any particular outcome. Using a scale that categorizes prayer into six different types (Laird *et al.*, 2004), participants reported which types of prayer they engaged in. They were also given a battery of assessments related to dimensions of subjective well-being, including spiritual support (Ai *et al.*, 2005), optimism (Scheier, Carver & Bridges, 1994), meaning in life (Steger *et al.*, 2006), life satisfaction (Diener *et al.*, 1985), and self-esteem (Rosenberg, 1965). The researchers found that three kinds of prayer were associated with positive outcomes. These include prayers of adoration focused on the worship of God; prayers of Thanksgiving focused on gratitude to God; and prayers of reception involving an attitude of surrender or receptivity to God's wisdom and guidance. The other three prayer types were associated with negative well-being. These include supplication which asks God to intervene for self or others; confession, which involves asking forgiveness for sins; and obligation, where practitioners recite mostly fixed prayers at regular fixed intervals. The authors also noted that the egoless aspect of some prayer types resembles the egoless mode in some spiritual and meditative practices.

> ...prayers of *thanksgiving* were significant predictors of subjective well being, of self-esteem, and of optimism. Prayers of *reception* [involving an attitude of openness and surrender]... [had] significant effects on self-esteem, optimism, and meaning of life. Finally, prayers of *adoration* had positive effects on both optimism and meaning of life. (Whittingham & Scher, 2010, p. 64)

The researchers theorize that "the prayer types which had positive effects on well-being are distinguished by their egoless nature... This may connect prayer in the Abrahamic faiths [Judaism, Christianity, and Islam] to other religious practices such as Buddhist meditation" (pp. 66–67).

This raises the question: are prayer and meditation different? Most would say yes, though some would also say that one can pray while meditating and vice versa.

Meditation takes a variety of forms. Some are based on mindfulness, which teaches the practitioner to live consciously "in the moment" and to be "fully present" for what is happening right now. With practice, a person who meditates learns to become a "participant-observer" who watches his or her mind as it automatically and repetitively follows the familiar paths of old conditioned responses. One monk explained that, while meditating, we can observe our mind going off on a tangent, and gently bring it back as we would correct a child who has wandered from a path. In his book *The Power of Now*, German philosopher Eckhardt Tolle (1999) underscores this point.

Cultivating present awareness requires long practice. As the *Bhagavad Gita* warns, "The mind is restless, turbulent, powerful, violent" and trying to control it "is like trying to control the wind." Learning to use the mind, as opposed to having the mind use you, is one of life's most challenging tasks. However, many meditative traditions teach that such efforts can increase personal freedom, which grows out of an enlarged capacity to modify thoughts and feelings, and change behaviors. Learning to observe the mind and body, and direct attention to the present moment allows us to "face whatever comes to us calmly and courageously, knowing we have the flexibility to weather any storm gracefully," writes Eknath Easwaran, one of the world's great meditation teachers (Easwaran, 2010, p. 49).

Scientists have begun to investigate neurobiological factors associated with prayer, meditation and mindfulness. We will review some of this research when we discuss brain fitness in Chapter 9.

# Practical Suggestions: Bringing Spirituality into Your Life

There is no single best way to explore the spiritual dimensions of your life or to build a spiritual practice. You may have been raised in a particular religious tradition in which you feel comfortable and find strength and renewal. Or your religious experiences may have been limited or less positive, even negative. You may be, like Elizabeth Ebaugh before she was abducted, a seeker of spiritual enlightenment. Or you may have no particular interest in formal religious or spiritual practices.

Whatever your individual circumstances and inclinations, there are many ways to explore the spiritual dimension of your life and how it might serve as a source of strength. Here are some approaches that may be useful for interested readers.

- Set aside a time for prayer or meditation as part of your daily routine. This is often first thing in the morning, last thing at night, or both.
- Make a regular habit of reading scriptures, sacred texts, or other writings pertaining to your chosen faith or practice.
- Designate a physical place for your daily spiritual practice. This may be a room or smaller space in your home or a location in nature. It might even be in your car.

- Practice a physically active form of spirituality such as walking prayer, yoga, martial arts, or liturgical dance.
- Practice a creative form of spirituality such as chanting; singing or playing sacred music; painting or drawing with the goal of expressing sacred ideals; or writing spiritually inspired poetry.
- Become part of a group that worships or practices together, such as a congregation, a scripture study group, or a prayer or a meditation circle. This community may come together in person or online.

Finally, we would like to share a moving prayer for survivors with PTSD. It was written by Patience Mason, the wife of a veteran who returned from Vietnam with PTSD:

> Higher Power, I know it's not within the harmony of the universe that I be healed from the trauma of remembering without pain.
> Help me through the pain.
> Surround me with the golden light of healing, fill me with the white light of peace and love.
> Help me to bear the pain as I go through the memories.
> Help me to cry.
> Help me to remember.
> Help me to love myself no matter what happened to me or what I did to survive.
> Help me to release and let go of my survival skills, the things such as anger and numbness that helped keep me alive, as I become aware of how ineffective they can be in getting me what I want today.
> Fill me with light and love until I am green and growing again in the harmony of the universe, if it be Thy will,
> AMEN.
>
> (Mason, 1993)

Perhaps more than any of the other resilience factors described in this book, religion and spirituality are deeply personal matters about which people tend to have strong feelings. As a potential source of strength and resilience, religion, spirituality, mindfulness, and meditation are available to billions of people on our planet.

# References

Ai, A. L., Tice, T. N., Peterson, C. & Huang, B. (2005). Prayers, spiritual support, and positive attitudes in coping with the September 11 national crisis. *Journal of Personality*, 73, 763–791.

Anderson, J. W. & Nunnelley, P. A. (2016). Private prayer associations with depression, anxiety and other health conditions: an analytical review of clinical studies. *Postgraduate Medicine*, 128(7), 635–641.

Chopra, D. (2009). Day of prayer: What is it meant to be? *Huffington Post*, May 7. Accessed August 21, 2009 at www.huffingtonpost.com/deepak-chopra/what-is-prayer-meant-to-b_b_199109.html

Connor, K. M., Davidson, J. R. T. & Lee, Li-Ching (2003). Spirituality, resilience, and anger in survivors of violent trauma: A community survey. *Journal of Traumatic Stress*, 16(5), 487–494.

Diener, E., Emmons, R. A., Larsen, R. J. & Griffin, S. (1985). The satisfaction with life scale. *Journal of Personality Assessment*, 49, 71–75.

Easwaran, E. (2010). *Conquest of Mind: Take Charge of Your Thoughts and Reshape Your Life Through Meditation*. Tomales, CA: Blue Mountain Center of Meditation.

Fallot, R. D. & Heckman, J. P. (2006). Religious/spiritual coping among women trauma survivors with mental health and substance use disorders. *The Journal of Behavioral Health Services and Research*, 32(2), 215–226.

Graber, A. (2009). *The Journey Home: Preparing for Life's Ultimate Adventure*, p. 19 Birmingham, AL: LogoLife Press.

Howell, K. H. & Miller-Graff, L. E. (2014). Protective factors associated with resilient functioning in young adulthood after childhood exposure to violence. *Child Abuse & Neglect*, 38(12), 1985–1994.

Kadetsky, E. (2009). The art of defying death. *New York Times*, October 14. Accessed October 21, 2010 at http://opinionator.blogs.nytimes.com/2009/10/14/the-art-of-defying-death/?scp=1&sq=Kadetsky%20The%20art%20of%20defying%20death&st=cse

Koenig, H. G., George, L. K. & Titus, P. (2004). Religion, spirituality and health in medically ill hospitalized older patients. *Journal of the American Geriatrics Association*, 52, 554–562.

Laird, S. P., Snyder, C. R., Rapoff, M. A. & Green, S. (2004). Measuring private prayer: Development, validation, and clinical application of the multidimensional prayer inventory. *The International Journal for the Psychology of Religion*, 14, 251–272.

Lambert, N. M., Fincham, F. D., Stillman, T. F., Graham, S. M. & Beach, S. R. H. (2009). Motivating change in relationships: Can prayer increase forgiveness? *Psychological Science*, 21(1), 126–132.

Lewis, C. S. (1963, 1964). *Letters to Malcolm: Chiefly on Prayer*. New York, NY: Harcourt Brace Jovanovich, Inc.

Lewis, E. & Rhoads, S. (1847). *Friends' Review: A Religious, Literary and Miscellaneous Journal*. Philadelphia, PA: J. Tatum.

Longman, R. Jr. (2009). Prayer. Accessed August 21, 2009 at www.spirithome.eom/prayer.html#whatis

Mason, P. H. C. (1993). *An Explanation of PTSD for 12 Steppers: When I Get Sober I Feel Crazy*. High Springs, FL: Patience Press. www.patiencepress.com

McCullough, M. E., Hoyt, W. E., Larson, D. B., Koenig, H. G. & Thoresen, C. (2000). Religious involvement and mortality: A meta-analytic review. *Health Psychology*, 19(3), 211–222.

Miller, L., Bansal, R., Wickramaratne, P., Hao, X. *et al.* (2014). Neuroanatomical correlates of religiosity and spirituality: a study in adults at high and low familial risk for depression. *JAMA Psychiatry*, 71(2), 128–135.

Mosqueiro, B. P., da Rocha, N. S. & Fleck, M. P. (2015). Intrinsic religiosity, resilience, quality of life, and suicide risk in depressed inpatients. *Journal of Affective Disorders*, 179, 128–133.

Newport, F. (2007). Americans more likely to believe in God than the devil, heaven more than hell: Belief in the devil has increased since 2000. *Gallup News Service*, June 13. Accessed at www.gallup.com/poll/27877/americans-more-likely-believe-god-than-devil-heaven-more-than-hell.aspx

Pargament, K. I., Smith, B. W., Koenig, H. G. & Perez, L. (1998). Patterns of positive and negative religious coping with major life stressors. *Journal for the Scientific Study of Religion*, 37(4), 710–724.

Pargament, K. I. & Lomax, J. W. (2013). Understanding and addressing religion among people with mental illness. *World Psychiatry*, 12, 1, 26–32.

Park, C. L., Sherman, A. C., Jim, H. S. & Salsman, J. M. (2015). Religion/spirituality and health in the context of cancer: Cross-domain integration, unresolved issues, and future directions. *Cancer*, 121(21), 3789–3794.

Point Man International Ministries mission statement. Accessed January 26, 2010 at www.pmim.org/

Powell, L. H., Shahabi, L. & Thoresen, C. E. (2003). Religion and spirituality: Linkages to physical health. *American Psychologist*, 58(1), 36–52.

Risner, R. (2004). *The Passing of the Night: My Seven Years as a Prisoner of the North Vietnamese*. Old Saybrook, CT: Konecky & Konecky.

Rochester, S. & Kiley, F. (1998). *Honor Bound: The History of American Prisoners of War in Southeast Asia, 1961–1973*. Washington, DC: Historical Office, Office of the Secretary of Defense.

Rosenberg, M. (1965). *Society and the Adolescent Self-Image*. Princeton, NJ: Princeton University Press.

Scheier, M. F., Carver, C. S. & Bridges, M. W. (1994). Distinguishing optimism from neuroticism (and trait anxiety, self-mastery, and self-esteem): A reevaluation of the Life Orientation Test. *Journal of Personality and Social Psychology*, 67, 1063–1078.

Sharma, V., Marin, D. B., Feder, A. *et al.* (2017). Religion, spirituality, and mental health of U.S. military veterans: Results from the National Health and Resilience in Veterans Study. *Journal of Affective Disorders*, 217, 197–204.

Steger, M. F., Frazier, P., Oishi, S. & Kaler, M. (2006). The meaning in life questionnaire: Assessing the presence of and search for meaning in life. *Journal of Counseling Psychology*, 53, 80–93.

Streeter, C. C., Whitfield, T. H., Owen, L. *et al.* (2010). Effects of yoga versus walking on mood, anxiety, and brain GABA levels: A randomized controlled MRS study. *Journal of Alternative & Complementary Medicine*, 16(11), 1145–1152.

Swensen, J. (2009). Ministries pave a spiritual path to help veterans with PTSD. *USA Today*, August 5. Retrieved from http://usatoday30.usatoday.com

Tolle, E. (1999). *The Power of Now: A Guide to Spiritual Enlightenment*. Novato, CA: New World Library.

Torah and the Twelve Steps, Inc. Accessed January 26, 2020 at www.torahtwelve steps.org/our_philosophy.html

Toussaint, L., Shields, G. S., Dorn, G. & Slavich, G. M. (2016). Effects of lifetime stress exposure on mental and physical health in young adulthood: How stress degrades and forgiveness protects health. *Journal of Health Psychology*, 21(6), 1004–1014.

Toussaint, L. L., Shields, G. S. & Slavich, G. M. (2016). Forgiveness, stress, and health: a 5-week dynamic parallel process study. *Annals of Behavioral Medicine*, 50(5), 727–735.

van der Kolk, B. (2006). Clinical implications of neuroscience research in PTSD. *Annals of the New York Academy of Sciences*, 1071, 1–17.

VanderWeele, T. J., Li, S., VanderWeele, T. J. *et al.* (2016). Association between religious service attendance and lower suicide rates among US women. *JAMA Psychiatry*, 73(8), 845–851.

Whittington, B. L. & Scher, S. J. (2010). Prayer and subjective well-being: An examination of six different types of prayer. *The International Journal for the Psychology of Religion*, 20, 59–68.

Whittier, J. G. (n.d.). *The Ballad of Cassandra Southwick*.

Worthington, E. L. & Langberg, D. (2012). Religious considerations and self-forgiveness in treating complex trauma and moral injury in present and former soldiers. *Journal of Psychology and Theology*, 40(4), 274–288.

Zheng, S., Kim, C., Lal, S. *et al.* (2017). The effects of twelve weeks of Tai Chi practice on anxiety in stressed but healthy people compared to exercise and wait-list groups – a randomized controlled trial. *Journal of Clinical Psychology*, 74(1), 83–92.

Zuckman, J. (2008). McCain and the POW church riot: GOP presidential candidate talks about the faith that sustained him during captivity. *Chicago Tribune*, August 15, p. 1.

# CHAPTER 6

# Social Support: Learning the Tap Code

In order to thrive in this world, we need other people. We all benefit by knowing that someone cares about our welfare and will catch us if we fall. Even better is having an entire network of family and close friends who will come to our aid at a moment's notice. It is also important for us to give of ourselves to help others. Forming relationships may not seem important when things are going well; we tend to take our friends and family for granted. However, close relationships built during good times protect us when we must endure stress or face danger. Far from signifying weakness, interdependence with others can provide a foundation for resilience.

Former POW Admiral Robert Shumaker appreciates the importance of social networks. Like nearly all of the resilient people we interviewed, both military and civilian, he knew how to capitalize on a basic biological reality: humans are designed to bond with one another. During his eight years in North Vietnamese prisons, Shumaker used creativity to help develop an ingenious method of communication known as the Tap Code. That code provided a critical lifeline that allowed scores of prisoners to connect with one another.

Alone in his dark, sweltering, rat-infested cell at Hoa Lo, Shumaker wondered whether he would ever again see another American. Each day, he spent hours lying on the soggy floor so he could peer through a crack at the bottom of his cell door, hoping and praying to see a fellow prisoner. Three months into solitary, a tall, white, emaciated American, escorted by a North Vietnamese guard, walked past Shumaker's cell on his way to the latrine. Shumaker was elated. But how would he make contact with this prisoner? Bob spent the next several days devising a scheme. The latrine seemed the only possible place to communicate. The guards rarely entered it themselves; the putrid smell of human and rat urine and feces was overwhelming.

Once a day the guards would let me out of my cell and take me to this "shower area" where I emptied my [human] waste bucket. I noticed the other American was getting the same treatment. I'd see him come out of this "shower area," which was maybe 100 feet away – I had good eyesight then – and I took a chance. There was a spot of ink on this wooden table in my area and I put water on it and it turned back into ink. On toilet paper I wrote, "Welcome to the Hanoi Hilton." And I told him to "scratch his balls when he walked out [of the shower area]." And he walks out scratching away. So it was a happy day for me when I made contact. And the name "Hanoi Hilton" stuck.

Soon, other Americans began to arrive. When three new prisoners were added to Shumaker's cell, the four talked nonstop for several days, acutely aware that the North Vietnamese would probably soon separate them to prevent an organized resistance.

We started talking about how we could organize to fight to keep our sanity and maximize survival; and I said, "What we need is some method by which we can communicate."

As the group was brainstorming, one of the cellmates, Air Force Captain Smitty Harris, recalled a conversation that he had overheard years earlier during Jungle Survival School. A former POW in Korea had described how American prisoners communicated by tapping on water pipes and then placing their ears on the pipe to listen for tapping responses coming from another building. It consisted of five rows and five columns of letters from the alphabet; the prisoners in Korea called it the AFLQV Code (from reading down the first column).

Shumaker immediately recognized the importance of Harris's story. Shumaker, who would earn the name "Martini Mixer" for his crucial role in enabling communication among prisoners, had been valedictorian of his high-school class, stood eighth in his class of 686 midshipmen at the Naval Academy, held a master's degree in aeronautical engineering, and had been chosen for the NASA astronaut program. Right away, he understood that what he later called the "Tap Code" could prove to be a life-saver for hundreds of American POWs. This is what it looked like:

|   | 1 | 2 | 3 | 4 | 5 |
|---|---|---|---|---|---|
| 1 | A | B | C | D | E |
| 2 | F | G | H | I | J |
| 3 | L | M | N | O | P |
| 4 | Q | R | S | T | U |
| 5 | V | W | X | Y | Z |

(To understand how the code works, readers will find it helpful to know that the sender taps to indicate the row first, then the column. For example, to send the letter "H," which is in the second row and third column, one would tap twice, pause slightly, and then tap three times. In order to form a symmetrical grid, the letter "K" is omitted from the matrix; "K" is represented by "CC.")

When the four cellmates were separated, each one spread the code to their new cellmates. Then, whenever one of them was transferred from the Hanoi Hilton to a different prison, he would teach the code to a whole new group of prisoners. By tapping with their knuckles and listening with their water cups against the wall, POWs relayed messages to each other. Within months of its adoption, the Tap Code formed the backbone of the prisoners' communication network and resistance efforts at Hoa Lo and beyond.

Here's how Captain Steve Long learned about the Tap Code.

> On one side of me, I had two Navy pilots, and on the other side was an Air Force back seater, a navigator. The first night I was there, the Air Force navigator spoke toward the ceiling so that I could hear over in the next cell.
>
> He said, "Do you know the Tap Code?" I said no. He says, "It's a 25-square matrix, the left side is A F L Q V. We'll tap in the morning." So I had the rest of the night to figure that out. Of course, brevity was a necessity because we needed to speed up communication, so we went by initials. I was S.L. And the S is the fourth row down, third column over and the L is in the third row down, first column. So I tapped that on the wall, and everybody would know that S.L. was in camp. That worked real good until Svede Larsen showed up.

Sometimes, instead of tapping on the wall, prisoners used other noises to send messages. If someone was in solitary and did not share a common wall with another prisoner, he would use coughs or sweeps of a broom to signal numbers. All the prisoners knew that a sniff was 1, a cough 2, clearing the throat 3, a hack 4, and a spit 5.

> Coughing, sweeping with a broom, one, two, three... The one we used that was probably the most ingenious – and we held it as closely as possible so the Vietnamese didn't learn about it – was the voice tap where a sniff and a cough would be a one and a two. Like B is in the first row of the second column and we'd go (sniff, cough) and that's a 1–2 which is a B. A throat clear would be a three and a hack would be a four and a spit would be a five. We shortened everything, like "interrogation" was shortened to "quiz" which was shortened to "Q." When they came to my room and told me that I was going to an interrogation, I wanted to tell the others, so I'd go hack, throat clear (S), throat clear, sniff (L), hack, sniff (Q), and that's SLQ, or "Steve Long Quiz."

Captain Charlie Plumb describes his first exposure to the Tap Code shortly after being tortured and imprisoned by the North Vietnamese. Pacing back and forth, Plumb heard a chirping noise coming from the corner of his cell and at first thought it was a cricket. But when he listened carefully, he noticed a distinct rhythm. And then he spotted a piece of wire moving back and forth through a hole at the base of his prison cell wall. A scrap of toilet paper clung to the end of the wire. On the other end of the wire was Shumaker. Schumaker recalls:

> We were in adjoining cells that were separated by about six feet. Charlie was by himself, and he had a lot of boils. I had stolen some wire – and it was kind of stiff wire, but it wasn't as stiff as a coat hanger – I would hide this wire in the cement wall of my cell. But there was the problem of getting the wire into Charlie's cell, which was about six feet away. Each cell had concrete walls but they also had little drain holes.
>
> He was afraid to pick it up for awhile. And then he finally got the courage up, and he took the note and the wire disappeared, and he read the note and it said, "Memorize this code and eat this note." And he gulps it down. And then every day, I'd slip the wire in. Now, the tap code calls for tapping on the wall. Well, we couldn't do that with a wire, so he would put tension on his end and I would put tension on mine. And then I would go: tug – tug, tug, tug, so this became an extension of the tap code.

Plumb (1992) would later describe his feelings when he realized that the chirping cricket was actually a communiqué:

> Can you imagine what might be going through your mind in an experience like this? Wow! What an opportunity. Somebody wants to network. Somebody wants to team up with me. Somebody wants to communicate!

Other ingenious forms of "tapping" emerged, depending on the demands of the particular situation. For example, Jerry Denton, who later served as a US senator from Alabama, blinked the word t-o-r-t-u-r-e while being video-taped by a Japanese film crew.

Shumaker understood that the Tap Code was an essential tool not only for passing on information and organizing resistance but also for preserving sanity. In times of stress and trauma, few things are more painful or more destructive to a person's mental and physical well-being than isolation. Prisoners used the Tap Code to create a vital social network. Supportive communication was especially important whenever a prisoner returned from being interrogated and tortured. Using the Tap Code allowed the prisoner to unburden himself when beset by worry, guilt, or despair about having "given in" and divulged information, and it provided a way for prisoners to sympathize and reassure one another. Telling his comrades what he had revealed during the interrogation also helped other prisoners keep their stories straight.

Steve Long believes that the Tap Code saved his life. During the Vietnam War, both American and North Vietnamese combat and supply missions spilled over into Laos, even though Laos was not officially involved in the war. Because neither the United States nor Vietnam publicly acknowledged these missions into Laos, when soldiers were killed or captured there, both sides kept the information secret. Prisoners captured in Laos were kept separated from other prisoners, held incognito and always listed as missing in action (MIA). For Steve Long and the others caught in Laos, this was a living nightmare. How could he reassure anyone back home, especially his family, that he was still alive?

> We were treated differently. We weren't given privileges. There was no media, there were no letters home, there was nothing for us. We realized that we needed to communicate with them [the "regular" prisoners] so that if one of them got released, they could get our names out. We took it upon ourselves, as our self-appointed mission, to get our names as widely spread out as possible. So we communicated extensively, probably more than a lot of the other prisoners, because we felt the need for our own safety, for our own lives.

Long's hunch proved to be correct. When the Vietnam War ended in 1975, the Paris Peace Talks called for an exchange of prisoners between the United States and North Vietnam. Waves of relief and joy spread throughout the prisons of North Vietnam, but for Steve Long the exhilaration was short-lived.

> When a North Vietnamese soldier came to our cell, he asked, "What do you think?" We thought, "This is great. We're going home." He said, "No. The Vietnam War is over. The Vietnam prisoners go home. When the Laotian War is over, the Laotian prisoners go home." And that was depressing. It took the wind right out of your sails. We would not be released.

One week after the peace accords were signed, the first cohort of American prisoners was released. They immediately met with intelligence de-briefers, who asked for the names of all known American POWs.

> And, of course, our names, at least the four of us who had been up there for a long time and who had communicated extensively, were some of the first names that they mentioned. Well, the intelligence community gave that to the State Department, and the State Department went back to Paris and said, "Hey, look, Vietnamese, we know that Long, Stischer, Bedinger and Brace are in North Vietnam and if you do not release them, then we will resume bombing North Vietnam with B-52s." The Vietnamese had had enough of that. That's why they decided to end the war anyway, because the B-52s were bombing them. So the Vietnamese came up with not only our four names but six more as well. So it did pay off that we communicated as much as we did.

# Strong Ties Save Lives

It is not surprising that Vietnam POWs found ways to bond with each other despite solitary confinement, because the military strongly emphasizes fostering and sustaining strong personal relationships. Soldiers belong to units: squads, platoons, companies, battalions, and divisions. No one operates in isolation. Groups, not individuals, solve most problems. This esprit de corps is conveyed symbolically from the first day of training, when men's heads are shaved, and men and women are issued military fatigues. The preferences of the individual give way to the needs of the group.

As we saw in Chapter 4 on moral compass, the POWs in the Hanoi Hilton looked up to Admiral James Stockdale as the senior officer among them, and he developed the "BACK US" principle of resistance to their North Vietnamese captors. Stockdale insisted that after a torture session, prisoners never be left alone to ruminate about their perceived fragility and failure. As soon as a prisoner returned from being interrogated, he was to be greeted with supportive messages that fellow prisoners whispered or tapped on the walls of his cell.

Stockdale recognized that humans, like other animals, are biologically "wired" for survival. When confronted with stressful and dangerous situations, a person naturally focuses on his or her own welfare. It is normal to protect oneself and to fight for resources. However, like so many of the literary and philosophical writers Stockdale admired, he believed that resilience, courage, and hardiness involved far more than personal strength, acquisition, and the instinct for survival. True resilience and courage were measured by acts of generosity, compassion, and altruism. As he wrote in *A Vietnam Experience*:

> When you are alone and afraid and feel that your culture is slipping away, even though you are hanging onto your memories... hanging on with your fingernails as best you can, and in spite of your efforts, still see the bottom of the barrel coming up to meet you, and realize how thin and fragmented our veneer of culture is, you suddenly know the truth that we all can become animals when cast adrift and tormented for a mere matter of months. It is then that you start having some very warm thoughts about the only life-preserver within reach – that human mind, that human heart next door... [When people ask] "What kept you going? What was your highest value?" my answer is: "The man next door." (1984, p. 110)

"You are in short, your brother's keeper." This was the "US" in "BACK US": unity before self. This was Stockdale's "life preserver."

Strong connections among soldiers motivate military men and women more powerfully than do abstractions such as patriotism, says General Hugh Shelton. Shelton commanded US Special Operations before becoming chairman of the Joint Chiefs of Staff:

> When you find a high-speed unit in today's Armed Forces, you find that its members are more concerned about the individual on the left and right than they are about themselves. Everybody is there to accomplish the mission of the team. The organizational and social structure recognizes team performance, not what one individual carries out. We know that's why people fight – we like to say people fight for the flag or they fight for the nation, but they really fight for the one on the left and right – their buddies.

The Special Forces provides a strong example of how units foster close ties. For the 12-man team of soldiers, the label "band of brothers" has real meaning.

Optimal unit cohesion and functioning depend on several factors: trust, healthy competition, reciprocal support, and altruism.

After his retirement from the military, when General Shelton gave a talk to corporate managers at Anheuser Busch, he suggested fostering team spirit similar to the kind he had learned and practiced as Commander-In-Chief of the Armed Forces. "This is one team, one fight," he told them. "If we are going to get better, it's all about working together. A rising tide lifts all boats."

Most of the Special Forces instructors we interviewed told us they know they can count on former team members for the rest of their lives. Even members who have never met one another, total strangers, will wholeheartedly welcome fellow SF members into their homes. Gordon Smith feels that he has a "family" of team members scattered all over the world who will be there to help him, his wife, and children at any time, no matter what.

# Social Networks Are a Key Element of Being Human

One need not be a Special Forces soldier or a POW to experience mutual support and helpfulness. Much of our behavior, whether we know it or not, is driven by the need to connect with others and to be understood. Social connectedness and cooperation activate the reward centers in our brains and bolster our mental and physical health (Eisenberger, 2013b; Morelli, Torre & Eisenberger, 2014). Conversely, the threat of rejection activates some of the same brain areas that process physical pain; it is easy to see how this relates to the evolutionary drive to survive (Apicella *et al.*, 2012; Eisenberger, 2013b; Meyer, Eisenberger & Williams, 2015).

Social psychologists Nicholas Christakis and James Fowler (2011) have documented the pervasiveness of social connections, including those that are often unconscious. We may think of ourselves as individualists, but chances are that, consciously or not, we are strongly influenced by other people. For example:

- Each happy friend a person has increases the person's probability of being happy by 9 percent and each unhappy friend decreases the person's probability of happiness by 7 percent.
- Restaurant diners who sit next to heavy eaters eat more.
- Restaurant servers who smile receive better tips.
- College students who have studious roommates study more.
- College students who have depressed roommates become more depressed.
- If a friend becomes obese, you are three times more likely to become obese.
- If a friend of your friend gains weight, you will also be likely to gain weight.
- If a friend's friend stops smoking, you will be more likely to stop smoking.

The point is that these forces are influencing us, whether we know it or not. People not only copy friends, they copy friends' friends and their friends; we imitate others much more than we think. Emotions are contagious; how you feel depends on the feelings of those around you.

We give and receive social support in countless ways throughout our lives. Most of us have "built-in" social connections in the form of family members, classmates, co-workers, and the like. Some of these associates are people we see every day, while others may be more distant, dwelling mostly in the back of our minds as we go about our activities; still, the knowledge that they are "there for us" is valuable. Technology has also given us new opportunities to connect through electronic social networks. Many of us have Facebook friends, Twitter followers, fellow gamers or other online associates, some living nearby and others thousands of miles away. Of course, for generations it has been possible for people to speak by telephone from anywhere on earth, but technologies such as Skype and Facetime have enriched phone conversations by adding the visual dimension. With today's technologies, even people with disabilities who have difficulty leaving their homes can have richly rewarding social lives by participating in online communities.

There are also voluntary organizations of all kinds that provide, among other benefits, the opportunity for social support. For example, the Boy and Girl Scout organizations, although primarily designed for youth, value and encourage service and helping others. And many, if not most, religious denominations view providing help and social support as part of their mission. These are just a few examples of groups that foster a sense of common cause and community.

# Reach Out for Support

Elizabeth Ebaugh, the social worker who was kidnapped, raped, and thrown off a bridge, believes that genuine support from friends and professionals was essential during her arduous recovery. For the first few months after her ordeal, helpers were everywhere.

> One reason I did so well, from that moment throughout my entire healing process, was that I had the best of the best. The police officers were incredibly sensitive, incredibly careful about every word, everything they did. They were so beautifully heartfelt. Plus the UPS driver who drove me to the hospital was like an angel. He couldn't do enough for me. When I got to the hospital, the doctors and nurses were totally on my side.
>
> I really think that [the days and weeks after a trauma] is a crucial time in terms of being able to come through it. To know that you're back into your world and your world is going to rally around you is a huge healing force. At that time, this was the worst crime to happen in this area. I had people calling me 24 hours a day, all my friends, this

> whole community – coming to see me; getting letters from people I didn't know; people were praying for me. I had to turn the phone off. There was no way I could feel like I was alone and isolated and not cared for. My story was on the front page of the newspaper for at least two weeks.

A colleague of ours, Alice, described similar feelings shortly after her husband died:

> I feel terribly sad and hurt over the loss of my husband, but I don't feel depressed. I feel so much support from people all around me, family and friends, neighbors, and even strangers who have no particular reason to be kind to me. Like the woman at the credit card company when I had to call and tell them to close my husband's account, she was very caring. People at church are praying for me. People where I work who hardly know me have sent cards. My mother and sister are calling me all the time. I just feel very lifted up.

After a trauma, it is not uncommon for the survivor to be showered with an outpouring of help and kindness. But once the initial flurry of attention dies down, the real tests of love and friendship begin. Well-wishers typically return to their normal daily routine shortly after a trauma, and sometimes survivors, themselves, may react to even the best intended approaches with coldness or even hostility. For example, Ebaugh remembers feeling distrustful, angry, and filled with rage; feelings that are commonly seen in posttraumatic stress reactions. She no longer felt that she could fully trust anyone. When she met the man who eventually became her husband, forging a relationship was not easy.

> He got the brunt of a lot of my rage. I needed to be in control, and he comes from a background where he wasn't very trusted, so here I was not trusting him. But it wasn't him I didn't trust, it was the world. He hung in there and really was the solidity in my life... My husband and I complement each other. We are both healers. At times when other couples would have broken apart, we meditated together and asked for help in those really dark moments.

Without caring professionals, steadfast friends, and a loving husband and family, Ebaugh believes that she would still be drowning in the psychological aftermath of her horrific ordeal, trapped in the haunting memory of her attack. "We can't do anything without support... The act of leaning in for support opens you," she says. However, she also observes that "supporters need to know not to coddle – there's a difference between supporting and enabling. At some point, we all need somebody to say, 'It's time to get on with it.'"

Our friend Victor Daniels found the same was true after he lost his wife of 42 years to cancer. Victor was a cardiac patient with two stents in his heart when his wife was diagnosed with incurable sinus cancer which was rooted too deeply in her brain to be operable. After three years of treatment, she was admitted to a hospice, where she died a few weeks later. Victor and his wife had no children, and his family members were too busy with their own lives to spend much time with him. Several of his friends and neighbors had also lost their spouses, and most seemed to be trapped in grief for years after being widowed. He did not want to follow their example.

On a visit to his primary care doctor, Victor described feeling listless and having trouble getting out of bed in the morning. She recommended that he attend a weekly bereavement support group sponsored by the cancer center at the local hospital. Victor took her advice and began attending the group, where he met a number of other people who were working toward finding a "new normal" and establishing positive directions for their lives after losing a loved one. With their encouragement, Victor began to look ahead, to reconsider how he wanted to spend the rest of his life, rather than dwelling on what he had lost. He made a list of goals he wanted to accomplish in his "new life." Step one was to resume working part-time at a local golf course, which he did. This gave structure to his days and provided social contact with people who were actively enjoying life. Victor's energy and outlook gradually improved, and with the support of friends and co-workers he continued to achieve his goals. Before long, social networking really paid off: Victor fell in love and remarried. His new wife was a widow whom he had met in the support group.

Finding support requires taking the initiative to seek assistance. It does not mean passively waiting and hoping for someone to rescue us.

## Social Support Protects Against Physical and Mental Illness

Researchers who study health psychology and social epidemiology have consistently found that strong social ties are associated with reduced incidence of mental and physical health problems and death (Eisenberger, 2013b). Strong social support has been linked to a decreased chance of developing depression, an increased likelihood of recovering from depression, improved psychological outcomes after severe traumas such as childhood sexual abuse, and reduced rates of combat-related PTSD (King, 1998, Tsai et al., 2012). Similarly, when patients with cancer (Manne et al., 1999), cardiac illness (Holahan et al., 1995), rheumatoid arthritis (Revenson et al., 1991) or multiple sclerosis (Mohr, Classen & Barrera, 2004) have high levels of social support, they are significantly less likely to be clinically depressed.

Strong social support has also been associated with fewer negative effects of various medical disorders. For example, in recent published studies, adolescents with type 1 diabetes had improved self-care and glycemic control when they received global peer support (as opposed to diabetes-specific support, which tended to be perceived as nagging) (Doe, 2016); adult children of obese mothers were less likely to be obese or overweight if they had strong social support networks (Serlachius *et al.*, 2016); and high level of perceived social support, particularly from friendships, was associated with reduced risk of death among patients experiencing their first heart attack (Netanela Weiss-Faratci and colleagues, 2016).

In contrast, a large body of research supports the finding that social isolation and low levels of social support are associated with high levels of stress, depression and PTSD. For example, in a study of 2,490 Vietnam veterans, researchers found that those with low social support were more than two and a half times more likely to suffer from PTSD than were veterans with high social support (King *et al.*, 1998). Isolation can also affect our physical health and how long we live. For example, well-designed studies have shown that a small social network or inadequate emotional support is associated with a threefold increase in subsequent cardiac events among patients who have already had a heart attack, and a two- to threefold increase in future coronary artery disease among healthy patients (Rozanski, Blumenthal & Kaplan, 1999).

Epidemiologist Teresa Seeman and colleagues (1987) studied mortality over a 17-year period in northern California and found, after controlling for other factors such as age, sex, race, and baseline health status, that social ties were significant predictors of a lower risk of death. While being married lowered the risk of death in younger adults, ties with close friends or relatives were especially significant in reducing mortality among those aged 60 or older. A meta-analysis of 70 independent prospective studies involving over 3 million participants followed for an average of seven years (Holt-Lunstad *et al.*, 2015) found that the likelihood of death increased by 26 percent in those who were lonely, 29 percent in those who felt socially isolated, and 32 percent in those living alone.

There are a number of psychological and behavioral mechanisms that may help to explain why having a strong and supportive social network is associated with resilience, as well as better mental and physical health. When people feel supported by their family and friends, they tend to feel more confident and in better control; more motivated to adopt healthier and less risky behaviors, such as smoking and drinking alcohol; more inclined to use active coping strategies; and less likely to see negative or stressful events as being insurmountable (Holahan, 1995; Rozanski, Blumenthal & Kaplan, 1999).

Overall, high-quality positive social support is associated with resilience to stress, and positive physical and mental health. It may even help you to live longer.

# Is It Better to Give Than to Receive?

Up to this point in the chapter, we have focused on the value of receiving social support from others. However, giving social support is also valuable; perhaps equally so. Dale Carnegie gave good advice in his classic 1936 self-help book *How to Win Friends and Influence People*: "You can make more friends in two months by becoming interested in other people than you can in two years by trying to get other people interested in you" (2009 [1937], p. 56). To make a friend, be a friend.

Befriending people and providing social support both depend on our ability to be "fully present" for the friend. In a world rife with distractions, truly paying attention to someone, even for a few minutes, is easier said than done. A Gallup Panel survey (Newport, 2015) found that most Americans check their smartphones at least a few times per hour – and that doesn't include actually using the phone for answering calls, texting, tweeting, and other functions. To engage in the practice of giving social support, it is crucial to turn off distractions and turn on focus. By doing so you may help not only your friend, but also yourself.

Stephanie Brown and colleagues (2009) conducted a study of more than 3,000 elderly married individuals whose spouse was in poor health, and they found that those who engaged in caregiving at least 14 hours per week had a lower mortality risk than those who did not provide care for their spouses. In another study of older adults (Brown *et al.*, 2003), after filling out a questionnaire that asked about how much social support they received and how much they gave, subjects were followed for five years. At the end of five years, there was no relationship between mortality and receiving social support from others. However, death rates were significantly reduced for individuals who reported *giving* emotional support to a spouse, and for individuals who provided instrumental support (such as material goods, services, or financial support) to friends, neighbors and relatives. In another study called Project MATCH, researchers at Brown University's Alpert Medical School (Pagano *et al.*, 2004) looked at treatment options for recovering alcoholics. They found that helping other alcoholics avoid drinking made a significant difference in reducing the chance that the helper would relapse. In Chapter 4 on moral compass and altruism, we discuss other studies about the benefits of being a helper.

In E.B. White's novel *Charlotte's Web*, the beloved spider at the heart of the story tells the pig whose life she saved: "By helping you, perhaps I was trying to lift up my life a trifle. Heaven knows anyone's life can stand a little of that" (1952, p. 164).

# Social Neuroscience Provides Clues to the Biology of Relationships

The field of social neuroscience investigates how during times of need, various brain regions, neurotransmitters, and hormones help to bind people together – parents with their children, husbands with their wives, friends with friends.

In a review of the literature related to the neural circuitry of rewards, Jamil Bhanji and Mauricio Delgado (2014) noted that social support can come from interactions as small as a smile from a colleague or a word of praise from a teacher; it is also experienced through cooperation, as in sharing a prize won in a game. The researchers found that such socially supportive interactions activate the same brain responses as do nonsocial rewards like food or money.

Naomi Eisenberger (2013a, 2013b; Meyer, Eisenberger & Williams, 2015) finds that when we experience social rejection or loneliness, our brains respond in ways similar to those associated with fear and physical threats: the amygdala, dorsal anterior cingulate, dorsal medial prefrontal cortex, sympathetic nervous system, and HPA axis become activated. Conversely, when we experience positive social support, our fear responses decrease; this is evident in reduced activity of our ventromedial prefrontal cortex, ventral anterior cingulate cortex, right dorsolateral prefrontal cortex, and caudate. Positive social support reinforces our feelings of being safe and secure, and enhances our ability to cope with stress.

Another important component of social support is the feeling of being understood. In a brain imaging experiment in which subjects were artificially induced to feel either understood or not understood, feeling understood activated neural regions related to reward (ventral striatum), while feeling not understood activated neural regions related to negative affect (insula, dorsomedial prefrontal cortex) (Morelli, Torre & Eisenberger, 2014). Similarly, in a study of returning Iraq and Afghanistan veterans, our colleague Robb Pietrzak found that the feeling of being understood was more important than other types of social support (e.g. emotional support; advice) in predicting lower PTSD symptoms (Pietrzak, Harpaz-Rotem & Southwick, 2011).

Social neuroscientists have also found that the hormone oxytocin plays an important role in our relationships with others. Oxytocin improves a person's ability to recognize a familiar face, to correctly classify a facial expression as either positive or negative, and to accurately infer the mental state of another person (Shahrestani, Kemp & Guastella, 2013; Heinrichs, von Dawans & Domes, 2009; Lee *et al.*, 2009; Sippel, Allington & Pietrzak, 2017). Scientists believe that these actions of oxytocin may enhance prosocial behavior by promoting social recognition, trust, and social approach (Heinrichs, von

Dawans & Domes, 2009; Striepens *et al.*, 2011; Sippel, Allington & Pietrzak, 2017). It is also known that during states of fear or stress, oxytocin reduces anxiety by dampening the cortisol system (HPA axis) and inhibiting the amygdala and related sympathetic nervous system activation (Shahrestani, Kemp & Guastella, 2013; Koch *et al.*, 2016).

Some of the most interesting research on oxytocin and vasopressin has investigated how these hormones affect the social behavior of two species of rodents, the prairie vole and the montane vole. Prairie voles tend to be monogamous and form attachments with their mates for life. This is unusual; it has been estimated that only 3 percent of mammals are monogamous. (Humans, obviously, are not on this list.) Montane voles, on the other hand, typically mate with many partners.

Oxytocin and vasopressin bind to specific chemical receptors, and in so doing, set off a cascade of chemical reactions. Thomas Insel and colleagues at the National Institute of Mental Health have found that the pattern and distribution of oxytocin and vasopressin receptors differ in the brains of the two species of voles (Insel & Shapiro, 1992). Prairie vole brains have more oxytocin and vasopressin receptors in several areas of the brain, including the nucleus accumbens and the amygdala. As we noted in Chapter 1, these brain regions are involved in social, emotional, survival, and sexual behaviors. Remarkably, when researchers elevated the number of vasopressin receptors in these brain regions, the previously nonmonogamous montane voles created pair bonds. (Imagine the possibilities for keeping a mate from straying with a simple additive to his or her morning coffee!)

To further understand the effects of oxytocin on behavior, scientists have employed "knockout" techniques in which they bred mice to be identical except for oxytocin genes (Hammock & Young, 2006; Winslow & Insel, 2002). Mice with and without the oxytocin gene were then run through a host of learning and memory tests. They found no differences in learning and memory between normal mice and the knockout mice except for social memory. Oxytocin knockout mice showed deficits in social memory, including failure to recognize mice with whom they had shared a cage. On the other hand, injection of oxytocin appears to facilitate affiliative behaviors such as increased touching and grooming. Similar deficits in social memory occur in knockout rats and mice lacking vasopressin receptors (Bielsky & Young, 2004).

This research may have implications for human behavior because human relationships rely heavily on social interactions, including the ability to recognize other individuals, remember their personal qualities, develop trust, and form friendships. In studies with human subjects, oxytocin has been shown to increase trust (Kosfeld *et al.*, 2005) and to decrease stress.

Oxytocin not only fosters trust but may also protect against potentially harmful chemicals (e.g., cortisol) that are released during stress. For example, researchers led by Markus Heinrichs of the University of Zürich (Heinrichs *et al.*, 2003) studied healthy young men in an experiment that focused on how they handled stress. Some of the men were told to come to the experiment alone, while others were asked to bring a close friend. The subjects were randomized into two groups: one group received a dose of oxytocin (via nasal spray) and the other a dose of placebo. The subjects then participated in two stress tests. Those who had brought a friend were allowed to ask the friend for support before and during the stress tests. The first test involved a mock job interview before a panel of strangers, which most people find highly stressful. In the second stress test, participants were asked to solve an arithmetic problem in their heads. During this test, subjects were constantly pushed by the panel to think faster. Salivary cortisol, a hormone marker of stress, was measured at several points during the experiment.

The lowest levels of cortisol were found in men who brought a friend to the test and received oxytocin. The next lowest levels were observed in those who brought a friend but received a placebo instead of oxytocin. Men who came to the experiment alone and who received placebo had the highest levels of cortisol. The researchers concluded, "The combination of oxytocin and social support exhibited the lowest cortisol concentrations as well as increased calmness and decreased anxiety during stress" (Heinrichs *et al.*, 2003, p. 1389).

More recently, some studies have found that the effects of oxytocin administration may depend on social context. It may be that oxytocin enhances sensitivity to environmental cues and has stress-reducing and prosocial effects in positive social environments, but negative social effects in negative contexts (Shamay-Tsoory & Abu-Akel, 2016). For example, oxytocin administration to individuals who are characteristically aggressive has been shown to increase their inclination toward aggression, not only in general but specifically toward intimate partner violence (DeWall *et al.*, 2014; Ne'eman *et al.*, 2016).

In summary, research has found that oxytocin is released during social situations where it appears to facilitate interpretation of social signals, enhance recognition, increase feelings of affiliation, and promote social approach. Oxytocin's actions in reducing amygdala activation and arousal may help to explain why positive support from others can reduce stress (Heinrichs, von Dawans & Domes, 2009; Lee *et al.*, 2009, Sippel, Allington & Pietrzak, 2017).

Researchers have just begun to examine what happens to oxytocin and vasopressin when people do not have the benefit of a strong social network or a "Tap Code" – when they are isolated, separated from others, or friendless. A study by University of Wisconsin researcher Alison Wismer Fries and colleagues (2005) found lower baseline levels of vasopressin and oxytocin in four-year-old children raised in deprived social settings with deficient caregiving (orphanages in Russia and Romania) compared to levels of children who had received more nurturing. This was true even though the orphans had been adopted by US families, in some cases up to three years before the experiment took place.

# Building Ties That Bind

Clinicians and researchers, including the authors of this book, have not always fully appreciated the importance of social support. In the past, we focused most of our attention on trying to improve one-on-one psychotherapy techniques and searching for medications to reduce painful symptoms. We did not spend much time thinking about the social networks of our patients. But that has changed. Our recent work with patients, our interviews with highly resilient individuals, our reading of the scientific literature, and our discussions with expert social scientists have convinced us that supportive social networks have the power to protect us and strengthen us.

So, how can you assess your own social network, and how can you strengthen that network? Social scientists have developed a number of ways to measure social networks. These methods assess the extent of and/ or the quality of a person's network; they typically include questions like "Whom could you count on to help you if you had just been fired from your job or expelled from school?" and "Who do you feel would help you if a family member very close to you died?" (Sarason *et al.*, 1983). They may also ask the extent to which you agree with various statements such as: "I am carefully listened to and understood by family members or friends," "Among my friends or relatives, there is someone who makes me feel better when I am feeling down," "I have problems that I can't discuss with family or friends," and "Among my friends or relatives, there is someone I go to when I need good advice" (D. W. King, L. A. King & Vogt, 2003; L. A. King *et al.*, 2006). We recommend that you ask similar questions and test similar statements to evaluate your own social networks.

The resilient people we interviewed invest effort in giving and receiving social support. Ron and Barb Garrett, the parents of a son with Down syndrome whom we described in Chapter 5, go out of their way to help neighbors with everyday needs; former Vietnam POWs stay in touch with one another through an active website as well as local and annual meetings. In this way, they remain connected and take care of one another. For instance, Tim Cooper calls upon his extensive national network of fellow Special Forces members for help with problems no matter how large or small. Many groups have formed in recent years to provide social support for veterans of the Iraq and Afghanistan wars.

For example, women veterans established the Service Women's Action Network (SWAN), whose mission is not only to connect female veterans with each other but also to press the Pentagon to improve its treatment of women in the military.

As General Hugh Shelton noted, the resilience-enhancing effects of a strong, supportive and trustworthy social network are by no means restricted to the military. We all can find strength by reaching out and connecting with friends, colleagues, mentors, and family. This is particularly true during times of high stress, fear, and loss.

There are myriad ways to broaden and strengthen the extent and strength of your relationships. Gaining and giving social support is a process, not an event; it does not happen overnight. Nevertheless, even if you feel friendless or isolated, it is important to start somewhere. No matter how small or weak your current network may be, you can take steps to increase its size and strength. For example, you might make a habit of smiling and saying hello to the neighbor at the elevator or the co-worker who sits near you. You might pick up the phone and call a family member who is lonely, send a Facebook message to a distant friend who has suffered a loss, or take the time to have coffee with a classmate who has just done poorly on a test.

For some of us who are shy or lacking in self-confidence, striking up a one-on-one conversation may seem difficult. In that case, try to attend social gatherings of any kind – join a hiking group or a book club, or enroll in a continuing education class; take part in religious services or help out at a community event. Another step might involve joining a committee within an organization. As a committee member, you may be assigned specific tasks and goals, which will allow you to interact in a productive way with other group members.

A third way to build one's social network is to join a support group. Support groups of many kinds – including online support groups where the participants never meet in person, and perhaps do not even know each other's identities – can provide the crucial social support that helps us recover after a trauma, or to endure an ongoing ordeal such as living with cancer or HIV/AIDS, or raising a child with special needs. Members of support groups are likely to understand the challenges that others in the group are facing, and they can learn how other members are coping with problems similar to their own. The range of support groups available is almost limitless, and we encourage readers to seek a group that meets their specific needs. If you can't find one that works for you, start one!

Effective social support typically involves genuine communication that reaches beyond the superficial. In a study of the conversations between college undergraduates, Matthias Mehl and colleagues (2010) at the University of Arizona found that conversations of a substantive nature, as opposed to trivial or "small talk" conversations, were correlated with greater happiness. As the authors note, the findings are purely correlational – they do not show whether in-depth conversations cause happiness, or whether being a happy person might cause one to have more in-depth conversations. Further research on this topic may explore such cause–effect relationships.

In summary, those who know how to build strong positive social networks reap many benefits. Strong positive relationships are associated with better physical health, protection against depression and stress disorders such as PTSD, enhanced emotional well-being, and longer life. In our experience, most resilient individuals take advantage of the profound strengthening effects of positive social networks. In fact, Special Forces soldiers often deny having exceptional personal strength, sturdiness, or resilience. Instead, they believe that they acquire their strength and courage from their squad, from their buddies, from their "family" of fellow soldiers. The same is true for civilians. Elizabeth Ebaugh believes that family, friends, and caring professionals provided a "container" for her healing, and in that container she found strength and courage to endure, and eventually to flourish. But, for most of us, our support network, even if it is extensive and strong, will not automatically reach out to embrace us when we are most in need. Rather, we would be wise to follow the example of the resilient individuals in this book by taking action, reaching out and "leaning into" those who care about us most. Very few resilient individuals go it alone – and neither should you.

# References

Apicella, C. L., Marlowe, F. W., Fowler, J.H. & Christakis, N. A. (2012). Social networks and cooperation in hunter-gatherers. *Nature*, 481(7382), 497–501.

Bhanji, J. P. & Delgado, M. R. (2014). The social brain and reward: Social information processing in the human striatum. *WIREs Cognitive Science*, 5, 61–73.

Bielsky, I. R. & Young, L. J. (2004). Oxytocin, vasopressin, and social recognition in mammals. *Peptides*, 25(9), 1565–1574.

Brown, S. L., Nesse, R. M., Vinokur, A. D. & Smith, D. M. (2003). Providing social support may be more beneficial than receiving it: Results from a prospective study of mortality. *Psychological Science*, 14, 320–327.

Brown, S. L., Smith, D. M., Schulz, R. *et al.* (2009). Caregiving behavior is associated with decreased mortality risk. *Psychological Science,* 20(4), 488–494.

Carnegie, D. (2009, original 1937). *How to Win Friends and Influence People.* Reissue edn. New York, NY: Simon & Schuster.

Christakis, N. A. & Fowler, J. H. (2011). *Connected: The Surprising Power of Our Social Networks and How They Shape Our Lives – How Your Friends' Friends' Friends Affect Everything You Feel, Think, and Do.* New York, NY: Little, Brown & Co.

DeWall, C. N., Gillath, O., Pressman, S. D. *et al.* (2014). When the love hormone leads to violence. *Social Psychological and Personality Science*, 5(6), 691–697.

Doe, E. (2016). An analysis of the relationships between peer support and diabetes outcomes in adolescents with type 1 diabetes. *Journal of Health Psychology*, July 7. [Epub ahead of print]

Eisenberger, N. I. (2013a). An empirical review of the neural underpinnings of receiving and giving social support: implications for health. *Psychosomatic Medicine*, 75(6): 545–556.

Eisenberger, N. I. (2013b). Social ties and health: A social neuroscience perspective. *Current Opinion in Neurobiology*, 23, 407–413.

Fricchione, G. (2011). *Compassion and Healing in Medicine and Society: On the Nature and Use of Attachment Solutions to Separation Challenges*. Baltimore, MD: The Johns Hopkins University Press.

Hammock, E. A. D. & Young, L. J. (2006). Oxytocin, vasopressin and pair bonding: implications for autism. *Philosophical Transactions of the Royal Society of London, Series B, Biological Sciences*, 361(1476), 2187–2198.

Heinrichs, M., Baumgartner, T., Kirschbaum, C. & Ehlert, U. (2003). Social support and oxytocin interact to suppress cortisol and subjective responses to psychosocial stress. *Biological Psychiatry*, 54, 1389–1398.

Heinrichs, M., von Dawans, B. & Domes, G. (2009). Oxytocin, vasopressin, and human social behavior. *Frontiers in Neuroendocrinology*, 30(4), 548–557.

Holahan, C. J., Moos, R. H., Holahan, C. K. & Brennan, P. L. (1995). Social support, coping, and depressive symptoms in a late-middle-aged sample of patients reporting cardiac illness. *Health Psychology*, 14(2), 152–163.

Holt-Lunstad, J., Smith, T. B., Baker, M., Harris, T. & Stephenson, D. (2015). Loneliness and social isolation as risk factors for mortality: A meta-analytic review. *Perspectives on Psychological Science*, 10(2), 227–237.

Insel, T. R. & Shapiro, L. E. (1992). Oxytocin receptor distribution reflects social organization in monogamous and polygamous voles. *Proceedings of the National Academy of Science USA*, 89(13), 5981–5985.

King, D. W., King, L. A. & Vogt, D. S. (2003). *Manual for the Deployment Risk and Resilience Inventory (DRRI): A Collection of Scales for Studying Deployment-Related Experiences in Military Veterans*. Boston, MA: National Center for PTSD.

King, L. A., King, D. W., Vogt, D. S., Knight, J. A. & Samper, R. (2006). Deployment Risk and Resilience Inventory: A collection of measures for studying deployment-related experiences of military personnel and veterans. *Military Psychology*, 18(2), 89–120.

King, L. A., King, D. W., Fairbank, J. A., Keane, T. M. & Adams, G. A. (1998). Resilience-recovery factors in post-traumatic stress disorder among female and male Vietnam veterans: Hardiness, postwar social support, and additional stressful life events. *Journal of Personality and Social Psychology*, 74, 420–434.

Kim, D. A., Hwong, A. R., Stafford, D. *et al.* (2015). Social network targeting to maximize population behavior change: A cluster randomized controlled trial. *Lancet*, 386(9989), 145–153.

Koch, S. B., van Zuiden, M., Nawijn, L. *et al.* (2016). Intranasal oxytocin normalizes amygdala functional connectivity in posttraumatic stress disorder. *Neuropsychopharmacology*, 41(8), 2041–2051.

Kosfeld, M., Heinrichs, M., Fischbacher, U. & Fehr, E. (2005). Oxytocin increases trust in humans. *Nature*, 435, 673–676.

Lee, H. J., Macbeth, A. H., Pagani, J. H. & Young, W. S. (2009). Oxytocin: The great facilitator of life. *Progress in Neurobiology*, 88(2), 127–151.

Manne, S. L., Pape, S. J., Taylor, K. L. & Dougherty, J. (1999). Spouse support, coping, and mood among individuals with cancer. *Annals of Behavioral Medicine*, 21, 111–121.

Mehl, M. R., Vazire, S., Holleran, S. E. & Clark, C. S. (2010). Eavesdropping on happiness: Well-being is related to having less small talk and more substantive conversations. *Psychological Science*, 21(4), 539–541.

Meyer, M. L., Eisenberger, N. I. & Williams, K. D. (2015). Why social pain can live on: Different neural mechanisms are associated with reliving social and physical pain. *PLoS One*, 10(6), e0128294.

Mohr, D. C., Classen, C. & Barrera, M. Jr. (2004). The relationship between social support, depression and treatment for people with multiple sclerosis. *Psychological Medicine*, 34, 533–541.

Morelli, S. A., Torre, J. B. & Eisenberger, N. E. (2014). The neural bases of feeling understood and not understood. *Social Cognitive and Affective Neuroscience*, 9(12), 1890–1896.

Ne'eman, R., Perach-Barzilay, N., Fischer-Shofty, M., Atias, A. & Shamay-Tsoory, S. G. (April 01, 2016). Intranasal administration of oxytocin increases human aggressive behavior. *Hormones and Behavior*, 80(9), 125–131.

Newport, F. (2015). Most U.S. smartphone owners check phone at least hourly. Blog post: Gallup Panel, July 9. Retrieved from www.gallup.com/poll/184046/smart phone-owners-check-phone-least-hourly.aspx

Ozbay, F., Fitterling, H., Charney, D. & Southwick, S. (2008). Social support and resilience to stress across the life span: A neurobiologic framework. *Current Psychiatry Reports*, 10(4), 304–310.

Pagano, M.E., Friend, K. B., Tonigan, J. S. & Stout, R. L. (2004). Helping other alcoholics in Alcoholics Anonymous and drinking outcomes: Findings from Project MATCH. *Journal of Studies on Alcohol*, 65(6), 766–773.

Pietrzak, R. H., Harpaz-Rotem, I. & Southwick, S. M. (2011). Cognitive-behavioral coping strategies associated with combat-related PTSD in treatment-seeking OEF-OIF Veterans. *Psychiatry Research*, 189, 2, 251–258.

Plumb, J. C. (1992). *Overcoming Adversity*. Audio cassette. Calabasas, CA.

Revenson, T. A., Schiaffino, K. M., Majerovitz, S. D. & Gibofsky, A. (1991). Social support as a double-edged sword: the relation of positive and problematic support to depression among rheumatoid arthritis patients. *Social Science and Medicine*, 33, 807–813.

Rozanski, A., Blumenthal, J. A. & Kaplan, J. (1999). Impact of psychological factors on the pathogenesis of cardiovascular disease and implications for therapy. *Circulation*, 99, 2192–2217.

Sapolsky, R. M. (2004). *Why Zebras Don't Get Ulcers: An Updated Guide to Stress, Stress Related Diseases, and Coping*, 3rd edn. New York, NY: Henry Holt & Co.

Sarason, I. G., Levine, H. M., Basham, R. B. & Sarason, B. R. (1983). Assessing social support: The Social Support Questionnaire. *Journal of Personality and Social Psychology*, 44(1), 127–139.

Schwartz, C., Meisenhelder, J. B., Ma, Y. & Reed, G. (2003). Altruistic social interest behaviors are associated with better mental health. *Psychosomatic Medicine*, 65, 778–785.

Seeman, T. E., Kaplan, G. A., Knudsen, L., Cohen, R. & Guralnik, J. (1987). Social network ties and mortality among the elderly in the Alameda County study. *American Journal of Epidemiology*, 126(4), 714–723.

Serlachius, A., Elovainio, M., Juonala, M. *et al.* (2016). High perceived social support protects against the intergenerational transmission of obesity: The Cardiovascular Risk in Young Finns Study. *Preventive Medicine*, 90, 79–85.

Shahrestani, S., Kemp, A. H. & Guastella, A. J. (2013). The impact of a single administration of intranasal oxytocin on the recognition of basic emotions in humans: a meta-analysis. *Neuropsychopharmacology*, 38(10), 1929–1936.

Shamay-Tsoory, S. G. & Abu-Akel, A. (2016). The social salience hypothesis of oxytocin. *Biological Psychiatry*, 79(3), 194–202.

Sippel, L. M., Allington, C. E., Pietrzak, R. H. *et al.* (2017). Oxytocin and stress-related disorders. *Chronic Stress*, February 17. [Epub ahead of print]

Southwick, S. M., Bonanno, G. A., Masten, A. S., Panter-Brick, C. & Yehuda, R. (2014). Resilience definitions, theory, and challenges: Interdisciplinary perspectives. *European Journal of Psychotraumatology*, 5(1), 10.3402/ejpt.v5.25338.

Stockdale, J. B. (1984). *A Vietnam Experience: Ten Years of Reflections*. Stanford, CA: Hoover Institution, Stanford University.

Striepens, N., Kendrick, K. M., Maier, W. & Hurlemann, R. (2011). Prosocial effects of oxytocin and clinical evidence for its therapeutic potential. *Frontiers in Neuroendocrinology*, 32(4), 426–450.

Tsai, J., Harpaz-Rotem, I., Pietrzak, R. H. & Southwick, S. M. (2012). The role of coping, resilience, and social support in mediating the relation between PTSD and social functioning in veterans returning from Iraq and Afghanistan. *Psychiatry*, 75(2), 135–149.

Weiss-Faratci, N., Lurie, I., Neumark, Y. *et al.* (2016). Perceived social support at different times after myocardial infarction and long-term mortality risk: A prospective cohort study. *Annals of Epidemiology*, 26, 424–428.

White, E. B. (1952). *Charlotte's Web*, p. 164 New York, NY: Harper & Row.

Winslow, J. & Insel, T. (2002). The social deficits of the oxytocin knockout mouse. *Neuropeptides*, 36(2), 221–229.

Wismer Fries, A. B., Ziegler, T. E., Kurian, J. R., Jacoris, S. & Pollak, S. D. (2005). Early experience in humans is associated with changes in neuropeptides critical for regulating social behavior. *Proceedings of the National Academy of Sciences*, 102, 17237–17240.

# CHAPTER 7

# Role Models: Providing the Road Map

One of the first psychologists to study resilience, Emmy Werner, followed the lives of children raised in impoverished homes by an alcoholic, abusive, or mentally ill parent. Werner observed that resilient children – the ones who grew up to be productive, emotionally healthy adults – found at least one person who truly supported them and served as an admired role model (Werner, 1993; Werner & Smith, 1992). Our research has found a similar pattern: all of the resilient individuals we interviewed have role models whose beliefs, attitudes, and behaviors inspire them.

Psychiatrist Francine Cournos, a clinical professor at Columbia University's College of Physician and Surgeons, looked to her parents as role models. As a young girl, Francine lived through the deaths of her mother and father, rejection by her extended family, and placement in foster care. Yet the memory of her parents continued to inspire her, particularly her mother's ability to endure hardship:

> I had a really good connection with my mother that I internalized, of someone who had my best interest at heart – a very good role model for how to handle adverse situations. She was very stoic and never revealed vulnerabilities. She never talked about being ill. Any adverse event I had, I always tried to be like her. Even during my episode of major depression, I was smiling, and people were shocked.
>
> My mother was like that. She worked until the day she died. She was a role model for how you function no matter what. I learned from my mother that survival is the most important thing. You must survive first. I admired her ability to get up and go to work no matter how she felt. Toward the end she was very sick: she had metastatic cancer, she couldn't breathe and had pleural effusions removed from her lungs. But she just didn't succumb. I viewed my mother as having tremendous physical toughness, and, by

comparison, psychological pain was nothing. That was my view of it. So I felt that if she didn't give herself any excuses, I certainly didn't have any excuses. I was healthy.

Cournos barely knew her father, as he died when she was only three. Most of what she knows of him has come from newspaper clippings, records of court testimony, and conversations with relatives. As a young man, Alexander Cournos was a member of the Industrial Workers of the World, known as the "Wobblies," a labor group whose goal was to organize all the world's workers into "one big union." In 1917, he was arrested because of his political activism and spent the next six years in prison. He was described as a man with "great strength of character and unbelievable moral stamina, courageous beyond description and uncompromising and unshakeable when it came to matters of his conviction and integrity." In her memoir, *City of One*, Cournos (1999) describes how she has used her picture of her father to orient her own life:

> I held onto the positive image: I now knew that my father believed deeply in a cause, that he had a fighting spirit. Over the years I would feel him watching over me whenever I needed to defend my own beliefs, and I tried to live up to what I imagined he would have expected of me.

Another colleague of ours who was inspired by a strong role model is pediatrician Lisa Satlin. She was raised in a conservative family in which girls were trained to be musicians and expected to defer to their husbands, ideally "nice Jewish doctors." But Lisa was free-spirited and independent. In high school, after discovering that she enjoyed science, Lisa told her violin teacher that she no longer planned to apply to the prestigious Juilliard School of Music. "He took my brand-new violin and threw it across the room – where it shattered into a million pieces – and walked out."

Satlin applied to Columbia Medical School and was accepted. During her first week there, she received overnight mail and telegrams from relatives telling her that although they would love her "anyway," practicing medicine "was no life for a woman." They told Satlin that she didn't know what she was doing and reassured her that "it was not too late" to change her mind and drop out. The only two family members who supported her decision to become a physician were her mother and her grandfather, a neuropsychiatrist who had taken her on rounds to meet his patients when she was a girl. In spite of the intense pressure to leave medical school, Satlin stayed on. She describes how her mother influenced her and her two sisters:

> We are strong women and it is because of her. . . We are all very, very independent. . . My mother would constantly tell us, the three girls, how important is was to have our own careers. She told us to try whatever we could and to try to do it all. . . I was able to watch her own evolution. She raised us with unconditional love and we always felt secure that she was behind us, even when we were in college. She adored us.

With this foundation, Satlin forged her own path. She received her medical degree from Columbia, completed a pediatric nephrology fellowship at the Albert Einstein College of Medicine, and went on to become one of the world's leading pediatric kidney specialists. In 2010, Lisa Satlin was named chair of the Department of Pediatrics at the Icahn School of Medicine at Mount Sinai.

# Who Can Be a Role Model?

In addition to parents (living or deceased), role models can include other relatives, teachers, coaches, or clergy. They may be older or one's own age; they may be friends, siblings, colleagues at work, or military buddies. Role models can even be children – and not necessarily our own children.

Dorinne Naughton, who worked with us for years, was not only a dedicated administrative officer, but also a good friend. She was shocked when she learned that she had cancer: Within the previous 12 months, her fiancé, mother, and father had all died of cancer, and now she, too, faced a potentially lethal form of the disease. Five days a week for more than a month, Dorinne went to the oncology division of the National Institutes of Health for radiation treatment. There, she found an unexpected role model.

> Every day I saw a little boy there in the waiting room. His name was David and he was five years old, with a great attitude. He and I would play checkers or tic-tac-toe while we were waiting. Seeing that little boy made me realize that I was pretty lucky to go through 50 years without ever being sick. He had a brain tumor and had been through surgery, but he was the happiest little kid, not scared a bit. He used to bounce in and say hello to me. He once said, "I'm going to teach you tic-tac-toe so you can beat all of your friends."

Role models may also be people we have never met. Barb Garrett, the mother of a son with Down syndrome whom we describe in Chapter 5, cites Joni Eareckson Tada as one of her heroes. Paralyzed from the neck down in a diving accident when she was a teenager, Tada has dedicated her life to a ministry for the disabled and suffering. From the time Barb was in high school, she has admired Tada's spirit and found inspiration in Tada's radio program, writings, and other creative expressions. Tada is an artist who paints by holding the paintbrush between her teeth. She is also a talented singer; Garrett says she listens to Tada's songs to dispel feelings of self-pity. In one song, Tada describes how she would like to peel potatoes, change a baby's diaper, and do other mundane tasks that most people take for granted. Garrett says, "Listening to that, and knowing she can't move – no matter what I'm facing, I know it can't be that bad!"

In Chapter 2, on optimism, we told the story of Deborah Gruen, the Yale University graduate and Paralympic swimmer born with spina bifida. She sees Franklin Delano Roosevelt as one of her role models:

> Franklin Roosevelt really exemplifies what it's like to be a person with a disability in an able-bodied world. I mean, you don't understand how hard this guy had to work just to walk. When he gave speeches and he was standing up, he grabbed the podium so hard to keep himself steady. He hid the fact that he had a disability, but at the same time it was always with him. And I think having polio really changed him. I feel like that's me, too.

Gruen may not realize it, but she herself has served as a role model, for example, for some of her teammates and classmates at Yale. Her father tells the story of their daughter's first interview with a college swim coach:

> The first time you go to a college visit with this kid, you wonder, how is this ever going to work? How is this kid going to swim on a varsity Division 1 team? So four-and-a-half-foot Deb walks into the coach's office and says, "This is what I want to do here at your college on your swim team."
>
> [The coach] probably thinks, "I'll just glad-hand these people for 20 minutes and get them out the door."
>
> But then Deborah gets into it with him. "I swim 25 to 35 miles per week, that's 1,500 miles per year, and I have been doing that for the past four years, which makes 6,000 miles."
>
> Eventually he says, "So you don't need your own lane? And you don't need special coaching?"
>
> And she says, "No, I don't need my own lane and I don't need special coaching." And then she gets right to the point and asks him, "So can I swim here on this team?"
>
> And you can see him begin to shake.
>
> But then. . . he starts to get it, and all of a sudden you can see the little gears going around and around and the light bulb goes off and he realizes that this kid really can be important to his team.
>
> And he says, "You know I can't help you get into the school."
>
> And she says, "I'm not asking you to help me get into this school." So she shows him her GPA and her SAT scores.
>
> And he says, "Oh, yeah. No problem."
>
> But why would they want her on their team? She is not going to score points for them in their championship. They want her there because some of the other kids are whiners and complainers. And that's just not going to happen with Deb. When this kid walks on the pool deck, she'll be the first one there and the last one to leave. An hour later the coach is recruiting her! What was I worrying about?

During her years at Yale, Gruen fulfilled the expectation that she would model positive attitudes and "can-do" behavior for her teammates. In 2010, she won the Amanda Walton Award, which is given to an outstanding athlete at Yale who has "excelled on the field of play and who has shown spirit and courage in transcending unforeseen challenges." She also received the David Everett Chantler Award, for the graduating senior who "best exemplifies qualities of courage, strength of character and high moral purpose."

In some families, resilient role models span multiple generations. Thich Nhat Hanh, one of the world's great Buddhist teachers, points out that we are each a continuation of our ancestors from both a genetic and a behavioral perspective. You already have those ancestors within you. Resilient grandparents and parents beget hardy sons and daughters, who, in turn, raise their own resilient children.

Perhaps it was coming to understand this that motivated me (SS) to look into my own family heritage from the standpoint of resilience. As described in Chapter 5, I was struck by the account of my seventeenth-century ancestors Lawrence and Cassandra Southwick and the persecution they and their children endured after embracing the Quaker religion against the dictates of the Massachusetts Bay Colony. When faced with adversity in my own life, I can keep them in mind and thereby gain strength.

But what about the vast majority of people, who do not have access to a family history with such detail? Are they bereft of ancestral role models? No; we can consider all of humanity that has gone before us as "ancestors" from whom we can draw inspiration and strength. If we think about the hardships of life in past generations, we might say that just about anyone who lived 200 or even 100 years ago was resilient by today's standards, and we are part of that human continuum.

Lew Meyer, the long-term POW whom we mention in Chapter 2 as being influenced by Norman Vincent Peale's *The Power of Positive Thinking*, remembers two adults who guided him through his difficult childhood years. The first was his truant officer, Ed Rowe, whose job was to catch Lew and bring him back to school whenever he climbed out of the classroom window; he and his best friend Dave made a habit of escaping whenever the teacher stepped out of the room. Although Officer Rowe pursued and reprimanded Lew and Dave, he also looked out for them; he was the one who got them summer jobs with the forestry service that led to Meyer's firefighting career.

Once, when Lew and Dave had no sponsor for their neighborhood baseball team, they stole baseball gear from a well-equipped rival team.

> Our baseball team all of a sudden showed up with catching paraphernalia and bats and balls. . . Officer Rowe, instead of catching us, talked to us and told us if we could find the guys who did it and tell them to return it, then he would get us a sponsor. . . So we went through the fence and under the bleachers and into the lockers and returned the stuff. Then the police sponsored our team, and we went to our games in police cars and everything. The local patrols would stop to watch us while we were playing. I think that's how he started turning us around.

Lew Meyer's second role model was Captain Herman Shawver, the strict but patient local fire captain. Shawver took a liking to Lew, caring enough about him to intentionally break firehouse rules by allowing the boy to hang around the station. Lew stuck close to the captain, watching how he ran the firehouse, how he inspired his men, how he sized up a fire and then, without hesitation, marched into the flames. Lew Meyer followed in Captain Shawver's footsteps and eventually became a fire chief himself.

As he grew older, Meyer continued to look for sturdy adult role models. During his late teens, while playing on a military football team, Meyer turned to his coach. This coach expected a great deal of Meyer and never let him take the easy path, despite the fact that he was the smallest player on the squad. During one game against a particularly rugged team, Meyer remembers being called to the sideline for a quick breather. Beaten up and bruised, he turned to his coach and said, "Coach, they're killing me in there."

Meyer never forgot his coach's reply: "I know it. Now get back in there."

Role models do not necessarily have to be older and wiser. Sometimes our peers can guide and inspire us. Air Force pilot Steve Long was 25 years old when, on a flight out of Thailand, he was shot down over Laos. Throughout his ordeal, he drew inspiration from his fellow POWs.

> The routine is they beat you and torture you until they get the information that they want. . . and then if you live through that, they'll give you medical treatment.
>
> But the role models we had were just fantastic. People referred to us as heroes, and I don't think any of us consider ourselves as a hero. But those guys are my heroes, the ones who got us through these ordeals. You'd hear stories, sometimes you'd hear some guy being beaten down the cell block from you and just resisting. And you felt really bad for him, but it pumped you up to know that you were just proud to be serving in the same military with a guy like that. There was always somebody there to set a standard.

At the top of Steve Long's list was Ernie Brace, a civilian pilot whose plane was shot down over Laos in 1965. Long describes how Brace spent the next three years in the jungle on the side of a mountain, strapped inside a bamboo cage.

> Talk about solitary confinement! Three-and-a-half years in a bamboo cage! He escaped three times and was beaten horribly. The last time he escaped, they buried him in a hole for a week. He lost all control of his body from his chest down. When they pulled him out, he couldn't walk. He was paralyzed. So he got around dragging his body by his elbows. And I guess out in the jungle, he got to the point where he could sit up. They brought him into Hanoi and put him in one of the cells next to John McCain. But Ernie was able to crawl over to the corner and by holding on to two walls, he could stand up. And eventually, he regained the ability to walk. . . And you know what, Ernie was one of those guys who never complained.

Jerry White never served in the military. Still, one of his role models was a wounded Israeli soldier. As an 18-year-old foreign exchange student to Israel from the United States, Jerry was hiking in the Golan Heights when he stepped on a landmine. He lost his foot. White was taken to a hospital in Tel Aviv, where he became depressed and discouraged.

> The guy in the next bed wanted to die after losing both legs. I needed to distance myself from that. Then an Israeli soldier came for a peer visit. He walked up to my bed and said, "I stepped on a landmine, too. Can you tell which leg I lost?" He had a perfect gait. I said I couldn't tell and he said, "That's the point. The battle isn't down there." He pointed to his legs. "It's up here." He pointed to his heart. When he found out that I still had my knee, which meant that I wasn't that bad off, he said, "What you have is a nose cold. You'll get over it."
>
> He tapped into my spirit. Could I engage or not? I got the message very clearly. This was peer support with a kick in the pants. The soldier was saying, "I've been through it, and if I can do it, you can too. Get on with it."
>
> He wasn't the typical peer supporter, but better, a role model. No pity. Don't enable and fuel people's victimhood with pity and condescending sympathy. He modeled for me, and today I am a good peer role model. It's not about the thing, it's about you. You can make of this what you want. It's your choice.

White went on to co-found and serve as CEO of the Landmine Survivors Network. The organization shared the 1997 Nobel Peace Prize, which honored the work of the International Campaign to Ban Landmines.

Role models need not be perfect. Everyone has strengths and weaknesses, and we believe that searching for the perfect role model is futile. Years after his amputation, through his work with the Landmine Survivors Network, Jerry White became a friend of Diana, Princess of Wales, and he learned to emulate the strengths he saw in her. Princess Diana used her high-profile position to bring attention to landmine survivors and to advocate for an international treaty banning landmines. On a trip to Bosnia with Diana, White began to appreciate the complexity of her personality.

> In working with Diana, I learned you could be all of these things: You can be catty and competitive and crazy at times, and insecure, but also have a true gift of compassion... Isn't that great, you can be all of these things? What's more interesting than a range of personality traits with virtues and vices and real gifts, where you try to play to your best self? In that last year of her life, she was coming into her own, blossoming and calling her own shots. She understood that every survivor we meet has a date, the date of their trauma. She said to me, "I'm July 29, 1981," and then burst out laughing. That was the day she got married. Her gift was compassion and dignity in the face of raw suffering. Her gift was the way she could touch people. One of the classiest peer supporters I've ever seen. She cared enough to show up, and she listened. "Relax," she said. "Play to your best self. Don't give in to the demons but feed the angels."

Long before he met Diana, when White was struggling to adapt to the loss of his leg, he recognized that his parents served as role models. His parents, a business owner and a homemaker, believed in education and in striving to reach one's potential. They also believed in social justice and reaching out to others.

> My father was a role model because he never changed, but was always kind and good. He made sure things were taken care of, phone calls covered. No fanfare, but solid and good and generous. He was the old-fashioned kind of father. My mother gave me the kick in the pants, the fire of social justice. She said I had an obligation to serve, to fight for justice and to get it right.

White considers himself lucky because both his parents helped to shape his response to trauma. Like his father, Jerry remained solid, good, and generous even during the most trying times. And like his mother, he refused to let the fire of social justice die out. In fact, his tragedy became fuel for a life devoted to helping others.

# The Negative Role Model: What Not to Imitate

Although we generally think of role models as providing positive examples to admire and emulate, sometimes a person stands out by embodying traits we emphatically do not want to adopt. We can think of such a person as a negative role model.

Laurie Harkness, a clinical professor of psychiatry at the Yale University School of Medicine and a national leader in psychiatric rehabilitation for the VA Connecticut Healthcare System, was in her early 50s when she was diagnosed with leukemia. While undergoing treatment, she encountered a number of other cancer patients, one of whom seemed to be "giving up," resigning himself to the idea that he would never get better. Laurie clearly remembers the moment she thought, "I will *not* be like that." Throughout her treatment and recovery, whenever she felt discouraged, she would remember this "negative role model" and use that memory as a motivation to fight the disease and strive for a positive outlook. And that is exactly what she did. Despite feeling weak and nauseated for weeks at a time, Laurie never gave up. If anything, she picked up the pace. In the eight years after receiving her diagnosis, she worked tirelessly to develop vocational and housing opportunities for individuals and families who are homeless or who are at risk of homelessness. She partnered with community agencies to collect over $50 million in federal and state funds and from private and foundation grants to develop more than 500 new units of permanent housing for homeless veterans.

During our work with various clients, we have often encountered people who were mistreated in childhood by one or both parents. Such individuals are often fiercely determined to live a life different from that of their abusers. Rather than imitate the negative behavior, they make a great effort to learn new, more positive behaviors. Like Laurie Harkness, they use the example of the abuser as a guidepost for what not to do and what not to become. This becomes a mission that they carry out as they develop relationships and raise their own families.

## Being a Role Model

In addition to recognizing and benefiting from the role models in our lives, we can also make an effort to serve as a role model for others. Medical school professor Lisa Satlin feels that thinking of herself as a model for others adds meaning to her daily life.

> What I love most is mentorship. It is why I agreed to take the chairmanship [of pediatrics] in the first place. I love the idea of encouraging young people and trying to help them figure out their strengths. How can I help them build on their strengths so that they can enjoy a more fulfilling life? So this is my purpose: helping, in whatever way I can, to guide the next generation of pediatric clinical researchers.
>
> The young people I have been privileged to mentor, they are my extended family in a way. I just like looking out for them, whether it's writing a letter of support for someone's promotion or grant application, or helping someone think through a career decision. For me it's so much fun to stay connected with people who I really care about all over the world. It's fabulous. I am so lucky.

And what do students learn from Satlin? They learn about the science and art of pediatric medicine, how to care for children and their families, how to design and carry out innovative medical research. They also learn about many of the resilience factors described in this book by watching how Satlin negotiates her way through life: by embracing the attitude that "I am just going to do it."

## Everybody Needs Resilient Role Models, Especially Children

Abundant research shows that parents and other adult mentors can help a young person develop the ability to handle trauma and to overcome adversity. Parents often ask, "How can I be a strong role model for my child or teenager?" One answer is to practice the resilient behaviors that we outline in this book, and to give your child ample opportunities to do the same.

Children who are resilient and well-adjusted typically receive support and encouragement from committed mentors and resilient role models. As we mentioned at the beginning of this chapter, psychologist Emmy Werner found that even children who have suffered neglect or abuse can do well if someone truly cares about them and gives unconditional support and encouragement.

Ideally, mentors help to foster resilience through both words and actions: words that teach and actions that demonstrate how to live well. Good mentors inspire, motivate, provide reliable support, and foster self-esteem. By imitating their mentors, children and adolescents learn right from wrong, how to handle challenging situations, and when and how to control their impulses, delay gratification and soothe themselves. They learn about moral and ethical integrity and about courage. They begin to take responsibility for their actions and their lives.

Research has shown that teens with dedicated mentors have more positive attitudes toward school, better grades and attendance, greater maturity, and less depression and anxiety. They also are less likely than teens without mentors to begin drinking alcohol and using illegal drugs. This is particularly true of young people whose mentors come from their natural social environment – that is, relatives, neighbors, teachers, and coaches. These kinds of mentors tend to be more effective than volunteers who come from outside the child's natural social network. Especially effective are non-parental relatives, such as grandparents or uncles and aunts, who know and understand the child's story and his or her personal, family and cultural history (reviewed in Southwick *et al.*, 2006).

Volunteer mentors from outside the child's natural social network tend to be less effective because often they limit their investment of time and energy and because they tend to have only a superficial understanding of family and cultural issues. This does not mean, however, that volunteer mentors cannot be helpful. The mentoring program Big Brothers Big Sisters, for example, has experienced impressive success over the years, but the chances for success increase when the mentor–mentee relationship lasts for at least one year. In fact, the longer the mentor–mentee relationship, the greater the likelihood of success.

Of course, modeling continues to be an important form of learning well into adulthood and even old age. We are never too old to learn from the example of others.

## How Role Modeling Works

Imitation is a powerful form of learning, and it shapes human behavior. Throughout our lives, each of us learns by imitating the attitudes, values, skills, and patterns of thought and behavior of those around us, even though we are often unaware that we are doing so. How do we actually learn from a role model?

It depends, in part, on *observational learning*: learning that takes place not because someone teaches us, but simply because we watch what someone is doing. According to a Buddhist proverb, "A child learns more from his mother's back than from her face." Thus, without intending to teach her child, the mother is providing opportunities for observational learning all day long simply by being where the child can watch her.

Even as adults, we benefit from observational learning. For instance, if we were traveling in a foreign country for the first time, we might be unfamiliar with subtleties of the local culture, such as the particular way in which people wait for a table in a restaurant, summon a taxi, or greet one another. Rather than asking a native how to go about these behaviors, we could simply observe and then "do as the Romans do." In this case, we would learn by observing.

Albert Bandura, one of the most influential psychologists of the twentieth century, believes that learning from a model often involves more than simple imitation (Bandura, 1977, 1986, 2006). Instead, it involves learning rules of behavior that can guide future action. For example, the traveler might absorb and then apply the rules for how to greet people in a given culture: by shaking hands, by kissing, or by nodding or bowing. By developing such rules, the learner is able to incorporate thoughts, values, behaviors, and emotional reactions that resemble those of the role model but that also fit the learner's particular personality and circumstances.

Here's another example: Suppose that you enjoy golf and you want to improve your putting stroke. With modeling in mind, you might first watch your instructor putt the ball from different angles and from short and long distances; you would then carefully analyze his or her putting technique and subdivide it into natural segments; finally, you would transform what you noticed in each segment into a rule designed to guide that aspect of the putting stroke. Such rules would be essential, because no two putting situations are identical.

As you watch your instructor putt the ball on numerous greens, you notice that the instructor zeros in on the ball and stares at it during short putts, long putts, uphill putts, and downhill putts. You the learner can now transform your observations into a rule that will apply whenever you putt, no matter the circumstances. Your rule: whenever I putt, I will continuously keep my eye on the ball.

Observation can help you develop more abstract rules as well. For instance, suppose you have a longtime friend who always seems to handle stressful situations with relative ease. You admire this friend and wonder how she does it, so you begin to study her behavior. When her mother dies, you notice that she reaches out to friends and family, and actively solicits their support. A year later, she is laid off from work; she immediately calls former and current fellow employees and asks if they can help her find a new job. On another occasion, she falls ill with pneumonia. Rather than staying at home alone, she moves in with her sister until she has recovered. Watching how your friend handles these stressful situations, you notice a pattern: during periods of high stress, she reaches out to others and asks for help. You can now turn this pattern into a rule that you can adopt for yourself during a wide variety of your own stressful situations. The rule: to enhance resilience, actively reach out to family, friends and colleagues for advice, assistance, and emotional support. By formulating this rule, you have constructed a guiding principle that you can apply to a myriad of challenging situations.

# Is There a Neuroscience to Learning from Role Models?

The ability to imitate appears to be inborn. Even in the first days of life, infants can imitate rudimentary facial expressions (Meltzoff & Moore, 1989). This ability to imitate persists throughout life and plays an essential role in acquiring behaviors, skills, mannerisms, social bonds, empathy, morality, cultural traditions, and even language.

Researchers have used experiments to explore how imitation works. As early as 1975 – before brain imaging methods such as MRI or positron emission tomography (PET) scans became standard research tools – Seymour M. Berger and Suzanne W. Hadley at the University of Massachusetts, Amherst, examined movements of the arm, hand, and mouth by attaching electrodes to the arms, palms, and lips of research participants. These electrodes allowed the researchers to measure muscle activity while the participants watched a video of someone stuttering and a separate video of two men arm-wrestling. The highest level of muscle activity in the lips was recorded as participants watched the video of the person stuttering, while the highest muscle activity in their arms was recorded while they watched the video of the men arm-wrestling. That is, while observing muscle activity in another person, muscle activity was recorded in the analogous muscles of the observers.

Further advances in neuroscience illuminated possible brain mechanisms that underlie imitation. In the mid-1990s, researchers from the University of Parma in Italy discovered "mirror neurons" in monkeys, in areas of the brain that control movement. Later research with humans has implicated a far broader network of neurons involved in processing movement, perception, emotions, and language. Researchers found that when humans observe the behavior of another person, the observers activate many of the same brain regions that are being activated in the person who they are observing. Thus, it appears that some of the same brain regions that fire when we catch a Frisbee also fire when we watch someone else catch one. Perhaps we are able to understand and, in a sense, vicariously experience the movements and actions of others because we have our own neuronal template for similar movements and actions.

Even reading about a behavior may activate areas of the brain responsible for carrying out the behavior (Aziz-Zadeh *et al.*, 2004). In an experiment at the University of California, Los Angeles, Lisa Aziz-Zadeh and colleagues (2006) used fMRI to observe areas of the brain known to control hand movement while participants read sentences such as "Grasp the banana."

They compared this to brain activity when the same participants watched video clips of someone grasping an apple. The brain areas associated with hand movement became activated under both conditions. Similarly, both reading sentences such as "Bite the peach" and watching a video of someone biting an apple activated areas of the brain known to control movement of the lips and mouth.

In addition to simulating movement and action, some evidence suggests that mirror neurons may help us to understand and empathize with the emotions of another person. In *Mirroring People: The New Science of How We Connect with Others* (2008), Marco Iacoboni at the University of California, Los Angeles, hypothesizes that when we observe the facial expression of another person, our own analogous facial muscle mirror neurons become activated. These cortical mirror neurons then send signals to the emotion center of the brain, causing us to experience the emotion that we are observing in the other person.

A 2003 fMRI study by a team of European researchers led by Bruno Wicker provides another example of this connection between observation and emotion. The research team found that the same areas of the brain became activated when participants either experienced feelings of disgust themselves or observed another person experiencing feelings of disgust. Perhaps, to understand the feelings of others, we must literally activate the analogous brain regions in ourselves.

This research suggests that mirror neurons may play a role in facilitating social interactions by promoting shared understanding and perhaps even empathy. In other words, it may be that mirror neurons internally simulate the movements and emotions of others (Rizzolatti & Fogassi, 2014).

Much remains to be learned about this fascinating and relatively new area of research. For example, when mirror neurons fire in response to watching the actions of another person, how does the brain automatically inhibit the observer from taking the same action – such as biting when watching someone eat an apple? (Bonini, 2016). It is important to note that scholars and researchers have cautioned against overly enthusiastic and exaggerated popular science accounts of the role that mirror neurons play in human behavior (Lamm & Majdandzic, 2014).

# How Can I Use Role Models to Become More Resilient?

Modeling our behavior on that of a resilient person can increase our own resilience. During his POW experience, Rod Knutson preserved his integrity while enduring torture sessions by emulating the moral strength and discipline of his father; while struggling to find his identity as a young man, Lew Meyer looked to the maturity and leadership of Fire Captain Herman Shawver; during his 49 months in a North Vietnamese prison, Steve Long turned to his peers to find inspiration and to observe how they resisted the enemy. And after losing his leg to a landmine, Jerry White emulated the no-nonsense "kick in the pants" approach of an Israeli amputee in order to "get on with it."

You can also do this in your own life; for example, you might choose to learn from those who came before you. Thich Nhat Hanh describes how Buddhists often set up an ancestor shrine in their homes that they contemplate every day. The shrine and the act of contemplation are reminders that we are not separate; we are each here for a short period of time as a link between those who came before and those who follow us. Lisa Satlin, similarly, surrounds herself with physical reminders of her mother and grandparents.

> In my bedroom, I have a couple of my mother's favorite paintings. To me they are absolutely beautiful. When I wake up in the morning, I look at them. Then I make coffee and there are a few more of her canvases in the kitchen. And in my living room and my exercise room I have my grandmother's art. I look at those canvases and every time I imagine both of them painting. [My mother and my grandmother] put everything into those paintings, their feelings and emotions.

Walking into Satlin's living room, the first thing a visitor notices is a massive antique samovar – an ornate metal container traditionally used to boil water – that does not fit with the style of the room's other furniture. "It's completely not 'me'," Satlin explains, "but I placed it in the most prominent spot in the apartment because it's part of my life. I hang all sorts of little things on it, and I look at it every morning." When Lisa and her sister were young girls, their grandparents took them on a trip to what was then the Soviet Union. They purchased the bulky antique there.

"I think about my grandmother and grandfather lugging this huge thing as we traveled through the Soviet Union. They had to pay for extra seats on air flights for this piece because they didn't want to check it."

For Satlin, the samovar and the paintings are continual reminders of her family role models.

> I still feel like my mother and grandmother are always here with me, even though they are not alive. There's not a day goes by that I don't think about them. They are part of my fabric. People ask me if I go to the cemetery to see them, but that doesn't make sense to me. Physically, what's remaining? There's so much more. They are part of me. I feel them constantly surrounding me.

Another way to benefit from role models, as mentioned earlier in this chapter, is to imitate the social behaviors of a resilient friend. In thinking of your friends, perhaps you identify one who is particularly resilient. You notice that during times of high stress, he not only solicits help from others, but he also makes every effort to eat well, get enough sleep, and exercise. Now you have two potential rules to enhance resilience during times of high stress: First, actively reach out to others for advice, assistance, and emotional support. Second, make every effort to eat nutritious food, stay hydrated, and get ample sleep and exercise.

Over the years, researchers have conducted experiments to determine the most effective and efficient ways to learn from role models. We have summarized the following principles based on our understanding of these findings. When trying to imitate another person's behavior, the following steps are helpful:

1. Observe the skill in a variety of settings. You will need to observe the skill numerous times.
2. Break the skill into simple segments: if you want to use modeling to learn a complex skill, it helps to subdivide the complex skill into simple natural segments and then focus on one segment at a time. If, on the other hand, you try to learn the entire complex skill (e.g., putting a golf ball, or trying to become more resilient) without breaking it into segments, you will likely be bombarded with too much information, will make many errors, and will have great difficulty mastering that skill. Breaking the skill into simple segments will take time and concentration.
3. Transform the simple natural segments into rules designed to guide behavior in differing situations.
4. Practice: you will find it helpful to practice in between observations. You may do this by imagining that you possess a particular attitude, personality style, or behavior that resembles that of your role model, or by actually enacting the desired attitude, style, or behavior in your own life. Both forms of practice appear to be effective, although real-life enactment is eventually required for successful imitation.
5. Obtain feedback: whenever possible, ask an expert, or someone with a trained eye, to point out similarities and differences in your behavior and the behavior that you are attempting to emulate. This expert can then recommend steps to correct deviations from the model.

Obviously, most people are less than scientific in the way they benefit from seeing how others behave. It is entirely possible to learn from role models without even being aware of it.

As we have seen from a number of the examples in this chapter, most people typically have more than one role model. This makes good sense, because it is rare, if not impossible, for anyone to be exemplary in every area of life. We are all human, with our own strengths and weaknesses. Thich Nhat Hanh suggests that each of us try to internalize the best qualities of family members who came before us, even those whom we have never met. If my mother is depressed but courageous, then I can imitate her courage. If my father is dedicated but punitive, then I can imitate his dedication. As the landmine survivor Jerry White might say, "Search for resilient role models, imitate their best qualities and then play to your best self." By emulating what is best in multiple hardy role models, we can weave for ourselves a resilient tapestry.

# References

Aziz-Zadeh, L., Iacoboni, M., Zaidel, E., Wilson, S. & Mazziotta, J. (2004). Left hemisphere motor facilitation in response to manual action sounds. *The European Journal of Neuroscience*, 19(9), 2609–2612.

Aziz-Zadeh, L., Wilson, S. M., Rizzolatti, G. & Iacoboni, M. (2006). Congruent embodied representations for visually presented actions and linguistic phrases describing action. *Current Biology*, 16, 1818–1823.

Bandura, A. (1977). *Social Learning Theory*. Englewood Cliffs, NJ: Prentice-Hall.

Bandura, A. (1986). *Social Foundations of Thought and Action: A Social-Cognitive Theory*. Englewood Cliffs, NJ: Prentice-Hall.

Bandura, A. (2006). Toward a psychology of human agency. *Perspectives on Psychological Science*, 1, 4(2), 164–180.

Berger, S. M. & Hadley, S. W. (1975). Some effects of a model's performance on an observer's electromyographic activity. *The American Journal of Psychology*, 88(2), 263–276.

Bonini, L. (2017). The extended mirror neuron network: anatomy, origin, and functions. *Neuroscientist*, 23(1), 56–67.

Conrad, J. (2016). *The Fragile Mind: How It Has Produced and Unwittingly Perpetuates America's Tragic Disparities*. Bloomington, IN: AuthorHouse.

Cournos, F. (1999). *City of One: A Memoir*. New York, NY: W. W. Norton.

Iacoboni, M. (2008). *Mirroring People: The New Science of How We Connect with Others*. New York, NY: Farrar, Straus and Giroux.

Kilner, J. M. & Lemon, R. N. (2013). What we know currently about mirror neurons. *Current Biology*, 23(23), 1057–1062.

Lamm, C. & Majdandzic, J. (2014). The role of shared neural activations, mirror neurons, and morality in empathy – a critical comment. *Neuroscience Research*, 90, 15–24.

Meltzoff, A. N. & Moore, M. K. (1989). Imitation in newborn infants: Exploring the range of gestures imitated and the underlying mechanisms. *Developmental Psychology*, 25, 954–962.

Rizzolatti, G. & Craighero, L. (2004). The mirror-neuron system. *Annual Review of Neuroscience*, 27, 169–192.

Rizzolatti, G. & Fogassi, L. (2014). The mirror mechanism: Recent findings and perspectives. *Philosophical Transactions of the Royal Society B*: 369: 20130420.

Southwick, S. M., Morgan, C. A., Vythilingam, M. & Charney, D. S. (2006). Mentors enhance resilience in at-risk children and adolescents. *Psychoanalytic Inquiry*, 26(4), 577–584.

Werner, E. E. (1993). Risk, resilience, and recovery: Perspectives from the Kauai Longitudinal Study. *Development and Psychopathology*, 5, 503–515.

Werner, E. E. & Smith, R. S. (1992). *Overcoming the Odds: High Risk Children from Birth to Adulthood*. Ithaca, NY and London: Cornell University Press.

Wicker, B., Keysers, C., Plailly, J. *et al.* (2003). Both of us disgusted in my insula: The common neural basis of seeing and feeling disgust. *Neuron*, 40(3), 655–664.

# CHAPTER 8

# Training: Physical Fitness and Strengthening

It is no secret that physical training is good for our health. Scientific studies have repeatedly shown that becoming physically fit enhances general health and can help to prevent or reduce the debilitating effects of high blood pressure, cardiovascular disease, stroke, diabetes, arthritis, and a variety of other chronic medical disorders.

Physical training and mastering physical challenges can also improve mood, cognition, and emotional resilience. Many of the resilient individuals we interviewed have a regular habit of exercise and believe that staying fit has helped them, both during their traumatic ordeals and as they recovered. In fact, some of them credit physical exercise with saving their lives.

## Surviving with the Air Force 5BX and the "Daily Dozen"

Korean War veteran Lew Meyer, who is mentioned earlier in the book, was a civilian firefighter working for the military in South Vietnam when his post in Hue was overrun by North Vietnamese soldiers during the 1968 Tet offensive. After three days of fighting, Meyer and 12 others were captured and force-marched through the jungle for an arduous five months, ultimately reaching Skid Row Prison, not far from Hanoi. There Meyer was imprisoned in a dark 8-by-4-foot cell, where he remained alone for the next 22 months. By the time of his release on March 27, 1973, he had spent more than five years as a POW; only then did he find out that he had been listed as missing in action (MIA) the entire time.

Meyer exercised in prison whenever possible, even when he felt tired or weak. Sometimes he jogged in tiny circles around his cell and sometimes he did isometric exercises, but at other times it was as many sets as possible of the Air Force 5BX, Army "daily dozen" or "JFKs" (exercises recommended by President John F. Kennedy's Council on Physical Fitness). These widely known callisthenic routines contain a variety of exercises such as sit-ups, push-ups, squat jumps, and jumping jacks. Meyer's cell was so small that his fingernails would strike the wall leaving scratch marks when he did jumping jacks.

Lew continued to exercise even while shackled in leg locks that were embedded in the concrete floor of his tiny cell.

> In the morning, I asked them to take my legs out of the locks. I wanted to do my JFKs, my exercises. But they didn't listen. So I started doing sit-ups. Then they pushed me back, yanked my leg locks off, removed them from the cell, and never put the leg locks on me again because the locks helped me do more sit-ups.

When transferred to a larger cell with roommates, Meyer increased the intensity of his workout routine and included his cellmates in practicing the Air Force 5BX and the Army daily dozen. They started with one repetition of each exercise and then progressed to two, three, and four repetitions. Devotion was matched with creativity: the routine often included "weight-lifting," using the smallest prisoner as a weight.

When we interviewed Meyer, we asked how many push-ups he could do at the height of his prison training. He responded, "One arm or two arms?" Anyone who has ever tried to do one-arm push-ups knows how difficult they are and how much strength and balance are required. Even people who can do numerous two-arm push-ups often cannot do even one of the one-arm variety. Meyer could do 64.

One year into his captivity, Meyer acquired a cellmate named Jim Thompson, a Green Beret who had been held in primitive camps in the mountains of South Vietnam and Laos for five years, where he was starved, brutally tortured, and subjected to years of solitary confinement. When Thompson was finally transferred to Skid Row, he weighed less than 100 pounds. Mike O'Connor, a fellow POW, couldn't believe what he saw when Thompson first arrived.

> He was standing right next to me. This guy is dead, I thought. As part of some cruel joke, I thought, they had stuck a corpse up against the door. Then I realized he was moving. He looked like something out of Auschwitz. . . I didn't know how he stood up, how he breathed, how he did anything. His features were so distorted. . . I could literally see his entire skeleton and the balls of his joints around his knees and elbows. . . His stomach was completely wrapped under his rib cage. . . It took him half an hour to stand. . . Talk about a gutsy guy. (Philpott, 2002, p. 159)

On their first morning together, Meyer began the day with his customary exercise routine. When he got to push-ups, Thompson tried to join him but was so weak that his arms gave way and his face struck the concrete floor. He couldn't do a single push-up.

Meyer began to coach Thompson back to health. Each morning, the two started their day with exercise. At first, Thompson could tolerate only deep breathing exercises and gradually some bending and stretching. Every day, Meyer would patiently coach his cellmate, and within six months, Thompson could complete the daily dozen. That was just the beginning.

With time, Thompson's health improved enough that the two men devised an escape plan. Success would depend on preparation and on their ability to navigate the dense surrounding jungle. For over a year, they planned and trained for the extreme physical demands that lay ahead. Their exercise routine became more and more challenging. For aerobic conditioning, they stacked their beds on top of one another and ran laps around their tiny cell, first in their rubber-tire Ho Chi Minh sandals, and eventually barefoot to build up calluses. At the height of their training, Meyer ran for 24 hours, only stopping when he noticed blood in his urine. Remarkably, Thompson ran for 15 hours.

Like Lew Meyer, fellow prisoner Rod Knutson believes that rigorous exercise fosters physical and psychological resilience.

> I worked hard to stay in shape. In 1969, when I lived in a cell with seven guys, we had – I forget what we called it – an Iron Man Contest or something. It involved sit-ups and push-ups, and they had to be regulation style push-ups, regulation style sit-ups. A guy by the name of Cole Black won the push-up contest at 501 push-ups. I won the sit-up contest at 1,615. I was in bad shape after I did that, because I wore all the hide off my tailbone, and I got boils.
>
> Most of us did keep an exercise regimen. And it depended on the cell block you lived in, because sometimes you couldn't exercise. I lived in one cell block without floorspace. All there was were the two pallets. And so if you wanted to walk, it was two paces to the end of your pallet, a turn, and then two paces back to the other end of your pallet. But there was always room to do sit-ups or push-ups or deep-knee bends, or something like that.
>
> Another thing. We had a guy who loved to walk on his hands, so he would teach us to walk on our hands. I frequently did handstand push-ups or walked on my hands. When I got to the States, to a hospital in Oakland, the morning coffee show was to watch me come out of my room walking on my hands, walk down to the coffee urn and get a cup of coffee, and then come back.

For these POWs, rigorous exercise in prison was not a hobby or a way to pass the time; it was a necessity. It helped them feel better and sleep better. Exercise gave structure and purpose to their days and provided them with a routine that enhanced confidence. It saved lives: Meyer described knowing four or five prisoners who made no effort to preserve their physical well-being. In his words, they said "they were planning to take a pill" to restore themselves to health when they got back to the States. Instead, he said, "all of them ended up dying within a few years after release."

Because American POWs had been through boot camp and many other advanced military training exercises, they were accustomed to physical challenges. They understood the value of making the effort to stay fit, even under adverse conditions. Retired sergeant Bruce Norwood describes the rigorous physical training in the military Ranger Indoctrination Program.

> You'd get up at four, go on a 12-mile run, come back and eat breakfast, do two hours on a very hard obstacle course... It is a very organized type of training with continuous and constant feedback, both positive and negative. They first teach you to crawl, then walk, and finally run. It's a great way to teach a new skill set. If you do something wrong, you're held accountable and told to correct it, or you might have to drop and give them 50 push-ups.

## Exercise Makes Civilians Tougher Too

For civilians in far less stressful circumstances, physical exercise can improve physical and mental hardiness and self-esteem. A 2016 report by the Mayo Clinic describes seven benefits of regular physical activity:

- helps control weight
- combats health conditions and diseases
- improves mood
- boosts energy
- promotes better sleep
- puts the spark back in your sex life
- can be fun and social!

Deborah Gruen, who was born with spina bifida, began team swimming when she was six years old because her sister Michele swam, and it looked like fun.

> The coaches treated me like I wasn't anyone different. I didn't kick as well as everyone else, and I was slower than kids in my own age group. But, every once in a while in a swim meet, I do beat able-bodied kids, and if you've never swum before I'll totally blow you away; it's not even close.
>
> I've always been really comfortable in the water; I had a disability that impaired my walking but I always found that water leveled the playing field a little bit. I could keep up with everyone else. I really liked that and plus I didn't need to use any sort of helping device, to help me swim. I could just do it on my own... I could master the full turns, I could play on kickboards, I could swim across the pool; I could keep up with other kids during games.

As a member of the US Paralympic team, Gruen practiced eight times a week, swimming an average of 26 miles. By pushing herself far beyond her own initial expectations and the expectations of others, Deborah has discovered an inner reservoir of power that carries over into other areas of her life.

Swimming has also helped Gruen understand the fortifying effects of support from others, including coaches and teammates.

> We're all on the same boat. It's January and it's like zero degrees outside, the pool is cold, it's dark, and your coach is there and he doesn't want to be there either and I'm going, "Oh this is really bad." But then you come together and realize we have two hours, we're clearly not going home, and you just get in and you do it. That's when it really helps, when you have support from other people. When you have to go it alone, that's when it becomes really difficult.

Finally, like many people, Gruen came to see swimming as a good prescription for reducing stress. When we interviewed her while a student in high school she told us:

> I don't worry because I have a disability. I worry about whether my term paper is going to be late, is my paper good enough? I swim it out. Swimming is so good for that. Really gets your mind off it. That's why I love sports. I think everybody should learn to compete. It just takes out all the stress.

## Training Boosts Recovery After Trauma

General Hugh Shelton, the former Ranger, Green Beret and Chairman of the Joint Chiefs of Staff whom we have mentioned earlier in the book, has been a physical fitness advocate ever since he joined the Army as a young man. Shelton looks the part of a general. He is 6′ 5″ with close-cropped silver-gray hair. He is thoughtful and articulate and speaks with a soft Southern accent. General Shelton is passionate about the military, about its mission to promote stability and peace throughout the world, about its focus on high ethical and moral standards, and about the unwavering dedication and superior quality of its members. He is goal-oriented and shares his vision with exquisite clarity.

After retirement from the military, General Shelton became a highly successful business leader. As before, he continued to push himself physically, running an average of four miles each day and doing his own home repairs and heavy yard work. On a Saturday morning in March of 2002, Shelton had an accident of the kind that could happen to anyone. While he stood on a ladder trimming trees in his yard, a branch struck the ladder. As he fell toward the ground, Shelton saw that he was about to be impaled by the chain-link fence that bordered the house, so he instinctively pulled his feet together, as he had so many times while parachuting, and twisted his body to avoid it. However, the fence snagged his feet, forcing his head to strike the ground first.

Although he felt no pain, he initially could not breathe and, for a moment, he thought he would die. He could not move his head, his arms, or his legs. As he lay motionless, knowing that he was seriously injured, he thought about the dangerous jumps he had survived as an Army Ranger paratrooper. Some jumps had been at night from 20,000 feet with an oxygen mask and no light to see what lay below. What an irony, he thought, if after surviving 246 life-threatening assignments in the Army, he were to perish from a 10-foot fall in his back yard.

Forty minutes later, a neighbor finally heard his cries for help and alerted Shelton's wife, who called an ambulance. At the hospital, doctors braced his neck and scanned his spinal cord. The results were not good. According to one doctor, the general would never walk again and might never regain the use of his hands. Shelton later learned that he suffered from "central cord syndrome," in which several cervical vertebrae compress the spinal cord, causing paralysis.

When Major General Hal Timboe, commander of Walter Reed Army Medical Center, learned what had happened, he immediately sent two surgeons from the prestigious Medical Center to examine Shelton. His prognosis improved, but the military surgeons told him they needed to get him to Walter Reed immediately, and that time was critical. His best chance for recovery would be to elevate his blood pressure to a level that would put him at risk for a heart attack or stroke, but it would get a much-needed blood supply to the damaged area of the spinal cord. Several weeks later, surgeons operated to decompress the spinal cord.

Fortunately, Shelton did not appreciate the severity of his injury and refused to give up. Until he was discharged from Walter Reed after nearly three months, he did not know that the medical staff believed he would remain a quadriplegic for life, and that on the day he was admitted to the hospital, his surgeon gave him a very low chance of ever walking again.

> At the time, I didn't realize how bad it was. It helped not knowing the extent of trauma. It wasn't until the 83rd day at Walter Reed, the day before I walked out, that an assistant neurosurgeon came to my bed around five in the morning and said, "General, I'm out of here today and you'll be walking out tomorrow. I gotta tell you, we never thought we'd see the day you'd walk." That's when the hair on the back of my neck stood up. That's when I realized how bad it had been. That's when it came back to me: during the second week of my stay, the OT and PT people came in and started talking about long-term rehab hospitals in New York and Texas. I kept thinking, "What's wrong with Walter Reed?" I never realized I wasn't expected to recover.

Shelton says that he owes much of his recovery to a physical therapist, Lieutenant Zack Solomon, who believed that Shelton would walk again one day. Solomon was a soldier's soldier: disciplined, determined, positive. Solomon worked with Shelton twice a day in the hospital gym and swimming pool. And even though physical therapy was tiring and painful, neither of them backed down. In fact, Shelton often volunteered to do more. The two were a team. Solomon's loyal determination exemplifies the military ethic to "never leave one of your own behind."

These days, General Shelton gives speeches all across the country, continues to support his alma mater, North Carolina State University, and serves as a board member for numerous corporations. He not only walks without assistance, but he also exercises regularly. He remains mentally and physically tough.

Another individual who has recovered from trauma through physical training is Rose Long, winner of the Collegiate Cycling National Criterium Division 2 in 2013. Having grown up in a family she describes as "outdoorsy," Rose was a distance runner, a cross-country skier, and a cyclist during high school and college. However, at the age of 22, she met with a serious accident that could have ended her career – both athletically and academically – not to mention threatening her life. She was hit by an SUV while bicycling, and the impact broke most of the bones in her face. It also injured her brain and caused her lung to collapse. Over the course of months, she underwent several elaborate surgeries to reconstruct her palate, jaw, and teeth. Once her brain had stabilized, she also had eye surgery.

Rose felt devastated when she realized that she would not only have to withdraw from her graduate studies, but that she would be unable to race in the 2008 collegiate mountain bike nationals. She suffered from posttraumatic stress in the form of insomnia, nightmares, and feelings of fear when around cars. She sought psychological help and did eye-movement desensitization and reprocessing therapy, which helped to reduce her nightmares.

In retrospect, Long said,

> You have no choice but to recover, but how much you recover is your choice... I had a vision in my mind [of] what I expected my recovery to be... I didn't think that I would be winning a national championship ever, but I did think that I'd be able to put a lot of effort into gaining enough energy to walk and then gaining enough energy and gaining my balance back so I could ride.

For the first four months after the accident, she was not physically able to ride. Once she had recovered enough strength and balance, she started to take easy bicycle rides, "just cruising around." However, she found that being on a bike brought up "intense recollections" of the accident. She stopped riding.

This might have been the end of the story, had it not been for a fortuitous career move. Long's academic work in mechanical engineering led to a position in the Dynamics Summer School at the Engineering Institute at the Los Alamos National Laboratory, and she was subsequently hired as a post-bac student. She found that after work hours, there was not much to do in Los Alamos, especially for a young single person. In addition, the country roads nearby were virtually deserted. As she recalls, she started riding regularly because of "a combination of there's nothing to do and there were not a lot of cars."

After a few years at Los Alamos, Long was accepted into a Ph.D. program at The Icahn School of Medicine at Mount Sinai in New York City. When she found that the school did not have a cycling team, she started one. "It's not an NCAA sport; it's governed by the cycling national governing body, so any fulltime student can race collegiate." The team consisted of "a few other students, some med students, some grad students. We got funding mostly from the graduate school and from the Department of Orthopedics... and we would go to races." She began to ride competitively again: "Competing as part of a team is a powerful motivator," she says, as you do not want to let your teammates down.

Long had believed that the car accident meant giving up her dream of competing in a major race. But she eventually got the chance to enter the Collegiate Cycling National Criterium. And she won! Preparing for the race, she scoped out the course, planned her meals and sleep schedule, and visualized herself going across the finish line ahead of the other cyclists. "I knew what my strengths were: I'm quite good at going fast around corners... I knew that's what I was going to use to win the race... that is what made me get to the finish line first." However, all the preparation and planning in the world would not necessarily have made her the winner. Contenders in a race have to assume that every other competitor has also prepared, planned, and visualized. Long sums it up: "Winning is not the 99% of preparation; winning is that extra 1% that it takes to be better than everyone else."

# Physical Exercise Improves Physical and Mental Health

It may seem obvious that physical exercise improves physical health, but do we know specifically how? A 2009 article in *Scientific American* (Ballantyne, 2009) summarized findings by a US Department of Health and Human Services committee on physical activity chaired by William Haskell of Stanford University. A committee member, Jonathan Meyers of the Palo Alto Veterans Affairs Health System in California, explains:

...when a person exercises, the heart muscle contracts forcefully and frequently, increasing blood flow through the arteries. This leads to subtle changes in the autonomic nervous system, which controls the contraction and relaxation of these vessels. This fine-tuning leads to a lower resting heart rate (fewer beats to pump blood through the body), lower blood pressure and a more variable heart rate, all factors that lower the risk of developing cardiovascular disease.

In its 2008 report, *Physical Activity Guidelines for Americans* (US Department of Health and Human Services, 2008), the committee found strong evidence that physical activity in adults lowers the risk of:

- early death
- stroke
- type 2 diabetes
- high blood pressure
- adverse lipid profile
- metabolic syndrome
- colon and breast cancer

Further, the committee found that three to six months after starting an exercise program, on average, formerly sedentary people had experienced a 30 percent drop in levels of C-reactive protein (a marker for inflammation often used to assess risk of cardiovascular disease) – as much as would occur if they had taken a statin drug. There was also moderate evidence for lower risk of hip fracture, bone density loss, and lung and endometrial cancer.

The National Cancer Institute Cohort Consortium pooled findings from six longitudinal studies that included data about exercise habits of over 650,000 Americans and Swedes who had been followed for about ten years. Mild to moderate exercise such as brisk walking was correlated with longer life, such that those who exercised for approximately an hour per day lived four and a half years longer than those who were sedentary (Moore *et al.*, 2012). In addition, a recent analysis of 12 scientific studies with a total of 1.44 million participants reported that those who engaged in high levels of leisure-time physical activity had a significantly lower risk of developing 13 types of cancer compared to participants with low leisure-time physical activity (Moore *et al.*, 2016; *Time* Magazine, 2017).

Aerobic exercise can also help in reduce symptoms of depression. In a study of 156 middle-aged men diagnosed with major depression, James A. Blumenthal and colleagues (1999) found that 16 weeks of aerobic exercise was as effective in reducing symptoms of depression as 16 weeks of treatment with the antidepressant drug Zoloft. Although over 60 percent of participants in both groups had good responses, there were differences. Those who took Zoloft tended to respond faster, while those who exercised responded more gradually but were less likely to experience a return of depression symptoms. Many other studies have found that exercise is substantially effective in easing symptoms of mild to moderate depression (Barbour, Edenfield & Blumenthal, 2007; Schuch *et al.*, 2016). In a review of the literature by the highly regarded Cochrane Collaboration, a meta-analysis of 35 clinical trials (with 1,356 participants) found that exercise was moderately effective for treating depression; in seven clinical trials with a total of 189 participants, exercise was as effective as psychotherapy; and in four trials with 300 participants, exercise was as effective as medication. Furthermore, for patients who receive psychotherapy or medication, exercise may be a valuable adjunct. Exercise even appears to lessen mild symptoms of depression and sadness in people who do not suffer from major depression.

In addition, aerobic exercise has been shown to decrease anxiety. This is true in healthy individuals without established anxiety disorders and among those with anxiety and stress-related disorders, such as generalized anxiety disorder, panic disorder, and social phobia (Stubbs *et al.*, 2017). Exercise may be particularly helpful for people with "anxiety sensitivity," which refers to misinterpreting and catastrophizing the physical sensations that generally accompany anxiety, such as perspiration, rapid heart rate, and rapid breathing. People with anxiety sensitivity often imagine that these symptoms are actually being caused by a serious life-threatening illness such as heart failure. Researchers believe that during vigorous aerobic exercise, the "anxiety-sensitive" person is forced to tolerate many of the same symptoms (that is, rapid heart rate, sweating, and rapid breathing) that frighten him or her during periods of anxiety. Over time, the "anxiety-sensitive" individual who continues to exercise vigorously can learn that these symptoms of arousal are typically not dangerous, and the fear that these symptoms trigger gradually decreases in intensity (Salmon, 2001).

Exercise may even enhance your sex life. In 2009, Benson Hoffman and his colleagues at Duke University Medical Center reported on 200 depressed adults, age 40 or older, who were sedentary and generally overweight. They divided the participants into three groups, assigning one group to exercise by walking, running, or biking, for 30 minutes a day, three days a week, to 70 to 85 percent of their heart rate reserve. The other two groups received either an antidepressant (Zoloft in its generic form) or a placebo pill. After four months, the participants took the Arizona Sexual Experiences Questionnaire (ASEX). The survey results indicated that the group that exercised reported better sex than the placebo group, and marginally better sex than the Zoloft group.

# Exercise, Resilience and the Brain

Abundant scientific evidence shows that physical exercise can also improve brain function and cognition, which includes thinking and memory (Cotman & Berchtold, 2002). Researchers from the University of Illinois at Urbana-Champaign recently reviewed findings from 111 animal and human studies and concluded that aerobic exercise can improve attention, planning, decision-making, and memory. These positive effects of exercise may be related to a number of recent findings: exercise training has been shown to increase the size of the hippocampus and serum levels of brain-derived neurotrophic factor (BDNF), and increase brain volume (prefrontal cortex) in older adults (Erickson *et al.*, 2011). In fact, exercise in midlife has been associated with decreased risk of developing dementia and Alzheimer's disease (Jackson *et al.*, 2015; Andel, Hughes & Crowe, 2005). Among patients already diagnosed with dementia, and even among normal elderly individuals, exercise may slow age-related memory decline.

Most of us want to do whatever we can to remain mentally sharp as we age, and to reduce our risk of developing age-related memory loss and dementia. Yet the fact is that the hippocampus, a key brain area associated with memory, shrinks an average of 1 to 2 percent each year in healthy older adults, likely beginning around the mid-50s. Kirk Erickson and colleagues (2011) conducted a randomized trial with 120 older adults. For one year, the experimental group performed moderate aerobic exercise three days a week while the control group did "stretching and toning exercise." The aerobic group increased their hippocampal volume by 2 percent; over the same period, the control group lost 1.4 percent in hippocampal volume. In addition, the aerobic group demonstrated a correspondingly significant improvement in performance on a memory task.

Exercise has even been shown to reduce aging in mice with a genetic disorder that causes premature aging. In a five-month study of mice with a genetic disease that causes premature aging, Mark Tarnopolsky and colleagues at McMaster University kept some mice sedentary and had others run on a treadmill three times a week. While the treadmill mice exhibited almost no symptoms of the premature aging disease, the sedentary mice lost much of their fur and had poor muscle tone and thinned skin, weakened hearts, and impaired hearing (Safdar *et al.*, 2013).

A number of different neurobiological mechanisms may help to explain the antidepressant, antianxiety, and cognitive-enhancing effects of exercise. First, exercise has been shown to increase concentrations of chemicals that are known to improve mood (e.g., endorphins) and that lessen depression (e.g., serotonin and dopamine).

Second, regular exercise helps to protect against the hormonal effects of chronic stress. During stress, the hypothalamic–pituitary–adrenal (HPA) axis releases high levels of the stress hormone cortisol, which over time can damage neurons in the hippocampus. The good news is that this response may be dampened in exercise-trained individuals. Dampening of the HPA axis would most likely mean lower cortisol production, less brain exposure to cortisol, and therefore less damage to neurons in the hippocampus.

A third potential neurobiological mechanism involves neurogenesis, the making of new brain cells by "turning on" relevant genes. Aerobic exercise enhances the growth of neurons in the brain by increasing production of neurotrophic (growth) factors such as BDNF. ("Neuro" means "brain" and "troph" means "nourish.") BDNF is a protein that is known to promote the growth and repair of brain cells. BDNF and other growth factors play an important role in cell survival, formation of connections between neurons based on how these neurons are used, the repair of damaged nerve cells, and learning (Duman, Malberg & Nakagawa, 2001; Krishnan & Nestler, 2008; Huang *et al.*, 2014). Stress, especially when chronic, is known to reduce the production of these neurotrophic factors.

Aerobic exercise may even protect against the effects of future stress and depression. Carl Cotman and Nicole Berchtold at the University of California, Irvine (2002) assessed the level of depression in 19,000 adults at the beginning of their study and again eight years later. They found that regular exercise over the eight-year period predicted freedom from depression. More recently, Amanda Griffiths and colleagues (2014) studied more than 26,000 working women assessed at various intervals over a period of several years. They found that the greater the level of physical activity, the lower the likelihood of future mental ill-health, including anxiety and depression. This relationship remained after controlling for health and body mass index as well as lifestyle and work-related factors that are known to be associated with mental health.

In studies with laboratory rats (Greenwood *et al.*, 2003), one group was given access to voluntary wheel running for six weeks while another group was kept sedentary, deprived of access to wheel running. Both groups were later exposed to uncontrollable stress in the form of random electric shocks. The sedentary (running-deprived) rats reacted with exaggerated fear and "freezing" behavior, reduced social exploration, increased levels of the stress hormone cortisol, and greater susceptibility to the rewarding effects of morphine. The rats that had been running – the ones in better athletic condition – fared better on all of these measures. These protective effects have been replicated in numerous studies (Fleshner *et al.*, 2011).

The beneficial effects of physical fitness on brain function, cognition and learning are also well documented in children. In a study of 12,000 Nebraska school children in grades 4–8, better physical fitness (measured by a well-known test, PACER) was clearly associated with higher academic achievement as measured by standardized English and math scores. It may even be true that the more difficult something is to learn, the more physical fitness may aid children in learning it. A study by Raine and colleagues suggests that "higher levels of fitness have their greatest impact in the most challenging situations" (Raine *et al.*, 2013) that children face intellectually. Physical activity also probably helps children sit still and pay attention in school or at home, with salutary effects on academic performance.

# How Can You Use Exercise to Increase Your Resilience?

For most of human history, people have spent their waking hours engaged in the physical demands of daily life. The human body evolved for living as gatherers, scavengers, toolmakers, hunters, and artisans. Like our hunter-gatherer ancestors, we as modern humans evolved with physical activity and the capacity to respond rapidly to relatively short bursts of physical stress at its core. However, over the past few centuries, with the advent of the industrial revolution and advances in technology, we have adopted a dangerously sedentary lifestyle. In developed countries, relatively few people engage in physically demanding work, and many of us sit for hours in front of computers or television screens. We are more likely to drive, or ride a bus or train, than to walk. Writing in *The Lancet*, German researchers Rainer Hambrecht and Stephan Gielen (2005) reported that modern humans, per kilogram, use only about one-third of the energy expended by our Paleolithic ancestors. In fact, in 2009, Steven Blair of the University of South Carolina reported that its Aerobics Center Longitudinal Study found that 25 percent to 35 percent of American adults were living very sedentary lives (i.e., worked at sedentary jobs, did no regular physical exercise, and were inactive around the house) (American Psychological Association, 2009). This kind of sedentary lifestyle has many drawbacks; in the context of this book, we can say that it does not foster resilience.

While many Americans do exercise with some regularity, building resilience typically goes beyond "routine maintenance" exercise; to become more resilient, we need to push ourselves. One strategy relevant to physical training is known as "stress inoculation" (Lyons & Parker, 2007; Brockhurst *et al.*, 2015), which involves continually extending the healthy limits of strength and endurance. In order to maximize the growth-enhancing effects of stress inoculation, one must first learn to accurately assess the upper and lower limits of optimal stress exposure. As we have said, stress that is too mild leads to no growth. The result is merely maintenance or even decline. However, too much stress that is unmanageable or overwhelming can also lead to weakening or sometimes even to physical and/or emotional breakdown.

In *Toughness Training for Life*, Jim Loehr, co-founder of the Human Performance Institute, explains: "Stress that toughens falls between maintenance stress and excessive stress." He distinguishes between "insufficient stress and maintenance stress and also between adaptive stress and excessive stress" (1993, p. 48). In another book, *The Power of Full Engagement*, Loehr goes on to say:

> Growth and change won't occur unless you push past your comfort zone, but pushing too hard increases the likelihood that you will give up. Far better to experience success at each step of a progressive process. Building confidence fuels the persistence to pursue more challenging changes. (Loehr & Schwartz, 2003, p. 179)

The *US Army Combat Stress Control Handbook* describes a similar program for building physical fitness:

To achieve greater tolerance or acclimatization to a physical stressor, a progressively greater exposure is required. The exposure should be sufficient to produce more than the routine stress reflexes. Well-known examples of acclimatization are heat acclimatization, cardiovascular (aerobic) fitness, and muscle strength... you can become aerobically fit only by exerting yourself to progressively greater degrees of physical effort... In other words, you must stress the system. After doing that for several days, the same effort raises the heart rate and sweating only a little. You become less short of breath and the effort seems much easier. To become more aerobically fit, you have to increase the work stressor even more until the body again shows the stress of increased heart rate, shortness of breath, and sweating... The issue for master fitness trainers is how to keep the physical work stressors and stress in the positive range, which increases strength and fitness. They must control the stressors and stress so they are not extreme – too little or too much. (Department of the Army, 2003, pp. 29–31)

Cliff Welch, a Special Forces instructor, describes it this way: "If you do things in incremental steps, you know, harder and harder, the person will get better. They'll get stronger and they'll get harder. And that starts from day one of basic training, and it never really ends the whole time you're in the service."

Of course, most people reading this book are not aspiring to become world-class athletes or elite soldiers. But how much exercise is enough to enhance resilience? And what type of exercise is best for your physical health? How about for your mental health? Is it best to exercise alone or with others? Should you consider hiring a trainer to teach you proper exercise techniques? What about cross-training?

These are complex questions that we will not cover in this book. However, bookstores and libraries are filled with excellent books that outline sensible and scientifically sound exercise programs geared toward maintaining good health. At the most basic level, panels of experts agree that most adults should exercise for at least 30 minutes at a moderate level of intensity nearly every day of the week.

A note of caution is also in order: this material is not intended to take the place of medical advice. Before beginning any exercise program, it is always wise to check with your doctor, who can assess any conditions you may have that would limit the amount and types of exercise that are appropriate for you.

# Physical Resilience Requires Recovery

Rose Long believes that competitive cycling contributes to her resilience in everyday life.

Endurance training is essential for the stamina and perseverance required for a Ph.D. and pursuing a research career... The methodical building of power and endurance through training gives me a structure to follow in my professional career where grants aren't won and papers aren't written overnight, but instead through years of careful and methodical research.

Long also notes the benefits of the mutual social support of training and racing with other cyclists, with whom she has developed deep friendships. But Dr. Long also recognizes the importance of recovery. As she puts it, "You can experience a pathological state of stress if you train too hard... Physical recovery is really important."

Dr. Long's observation is strongly supported by exercise physiologists who emphasize that we do not build strength, agility, and coordination only by exercising. Instead, we need to alternate periods of exercise with periods of rest. This is true both for an individual workout and in the longer view of a weekly fitness routine, so you should give your body more challenges on some days than others. Without the opportunity to recover, the body becomes exhausted and worn down.

Dr. Rose Long acknowledges this. Recovery includes proper nutrition: the old adage "you are what you eat" applies. Most experts in nutrition and diet recommend a diet composed predominantly of a variety of fruits, vegetables, and whole grains (US News and World Report, 2010) The guidelines call for modest amounts of lean meat, legumes, and low-fat dairy products and sparing use of fats and sugars. USDA daily calorie recommendations range from 1,600 to 2,400 for women and 2,000 to 3,000 calories for men. Younger adults generally need more calories than older adults because metabolism tends to slow with age. Still, the more physically active you are, the more calories you need to maintain your weight. A healthy diet also involves limiting intake of alcohol – for some people, abstaining altogether – and avoiding tobacco, as well as other substances of abuse.

Sleep is another component of recovery, one that is essential to good health and well-being. For most adults, this means about eight hours of sleep every night. It has become increasingly clear that the benefits of sleep go far beyond just feeling alert and rested. Among other benefits, adequate sleep optimizes coordination and reaction time, according to Harvard Medical School physiologist Martin C. Moore-Ede, whose 1993 book *The Twenty-Four-Hour Society* remains a classic. In his 1998 book *Power Sleep,* Cornell University psychologist James B. Maas points out that many of us go through years of our lives at less than peak performance because we are chronically mildly sleep deprived.

In an experiment in which participants memorized foreign vocabulary words, Stéphanie Mazza and colleagues (2016) found that having a night's sleep between practice sessions significantly reduced the amount of practice time needed to attain peak performance. Sleep also increased how much subjects retained of the material learned, even six months after they learned it. Inadequate sleep, on the other hand, has been shown to impair performance. Researchers in Australia and New Zealand found that many road accidents involve sleep deprivation, and that impairments in performance typically begin as early as 17 hours after waking. In fact, after being awake for 17–19 hours, drivers' performance on some tests (e.g., simple response speed test, hand–eye coordination) were equivalent to performance with a blood alcohol concentration of 0.05 percent. In many countries this degree of impairment is considered to be incompatible with safe driving. Longer periods without sleep were associated with even greater impairments in speed and accuracy (Williamson & Feyer, 2000). At the 2009 annual meeting of the Associated Professional Sleep Societies, researchers presented evidence of the association between sleep deficits and weight gain. Also in 2009, the American Heart Association reported a study headed by Lisa Rafalson of the University at Buffalo that linked the onset of type 2 diabetes to inadequate sleep (less than six hours per night) (American Heart Association, 2009).

Medical practitioners are also recognizing the value of sleep in healing and recovery from illness. In a statewide initiative that began in 2013, hospitals in Connecticut made changes to maximize the ability of patients to sleep. Some modifications included painting and furnishing patient rooms to be more homelike, installing blackout window shades, and using sound-muffling materials in hallways. Hospitals moved nurses' stations and put up signs asking visitors to speak softly. Protocols were also changed so that, for patients who were in a stable condition, nurses would do visual checks at night rather than waking patients to take their vital signs (Weintraub, 2016).

For people who are healthy and busy, getting enough sleep is easier said than done, given our hectic schedules and the rapid pace of our society. Getting sufficient sleep is still more problematic for people who suffer from insomnia, sleep apnea, or other sleep disorders. Although diagnosing and treating sleep disorders is beyond the scope of this book, there are many good resources for sleep "hygiene." What we wish to emphasize in this chapter is that the right amount of sleep enhances recovery, physical and emotional health, and resilience.

There are many neurobiological factors associated with recovery, optimal performance, and resilience. The neurobiology of optimal performance and recovery is complex. One important area of investigation involves regulation of the sympathetic nervous system (SNS). For example, in 1989, Richard Dienstbier from the University of Nebraska reviewed a series of studies showing that people tend to perform best when their SNS activity is low at baseline, accompanied by a robust increase of norepinephrine and epinephrine during stress, and followed by a relatively rapid return of these neurotransmitters to baseline levels once the stress is over. We believe that resilient individuals, who perform well under stress, are likely to fit Dienstbier's description: they maintain the SNS within an adaptive window of activation, not so high as to cause incapacitating anxiety and fear, but high enough to respond appropriately to danger.

One of the neurochemicals that contributes to SNS functioning is neuropeptide Y (NPY). NPY helps to modulate the norepinephrine response to stress. When norepinephrine is released during periods of high stress, NPY is released with it. As described briefly in Chapter 1, NPY helps to decrease anxiety and restore calm after stress, in part by inhibiting the further release of norepinephrine. This helps to keep the SNS from "overshooting." Support for the stress-modulating effects of NPY has come from an innovative series of studies conducted by Yale University and National Center for PTSD researcher Charles A. Morgan, MD (Morgan *et al.*, 2000, 2004). Morgan, an expert in the neurobiology of resilience, found that Special Operations soldiers with high levels of NPY performed better during extremely stressful training procedures than did soldiers with lower levels of NPY. Some researchers have referred to NPY as a neurobiological resilience factor.

As noted in Chapter 1, the parasympathetic nervous system (PNS) has almost the opposite effect of the SNS. Rather than activate the body, the PNS tends to calm and slow down our stress response systems. As such it plays an important role in our capacity to recover and bounce back from adversity and challenges. One of the easiest ways to increase PNS activity is through voluntary regulated breathing. For thousands of years, breathing practices have been a fundamental component of meditative and spiritual practices. As noted by Columbia University researcher Richard Brown and colleague Patricia Gerbarg:

> What do Mahatma Gandi, the martial arts, Bruce Lee, Buddhist meditators, Christian monks, Hawaiian kahunas, and Russian Special Forces have in common? They all used breathing to enhance their physical, mental, and spiritual well-being. (Brown & Gerbarg, 2012, p. 2)

Brown, Gerbarg, and others have conducted numerous studies showing that changing patterns of breathing can help to relieve symptoms of anxiety, depression and PTSD, as well as improve endurance and performance in a variety of activities. While there are hundreds of different breathing practices, those that tend to have a calming effect train the individual to deepen their breaths and slow their rate of breathing. For example, coherent breathing, a form of slow paced breathing, generally involves learning to breathe five to six breaths per minute with equal length of inhalation and exhalation. Coherent breathing has been associated with increases in PNS activity and reductions in stress, anxiety, anger, exhaustion, and depression, as well as improved quality of life.

Level of PNS activity is commonly assessed by measuring heart rate variability (HRV), which reflects the natural variation in the interval between our heartbeats. In general, reduced HRV has been associated with anxiety, depression, exaggerated stress responsivity, aggression, and cardiovascular disease, while increased HRV has been associated with healthier cardiovascular function and improved modulation of the stress response. HRV can be increased by breathing deeply and slowly.

Of note, there is evidence that altered functioning of the autonomic nervous system contributes to vulnerability to PTSD. For example, autonomic biomarkers, such as heart rate vulnerability, predict subsequent development of PTSD (Minassian *et al.*, 2014). This suggests that interventions which change autonomic system function may help to prevent or effectively treat PTSD. Research supporting the efficacy of this approach, include a breathing based meditation intervention – Sudarshan Kriya Yoga – that has been shown to significantly reduce PTSD symptoms in veterans of the Iraq and Afghanistan war (Seppälä *et al.*, 2014) and a 12-week yoga program that was found to increase HRV and parasympathetic tone and reduce perceived stress and depressive symptoms in women (Chu *et al.*, 2017).

Another neurochemical that has been linked to stress recovery, performance during stress, and resilience is dehydroepiandrosterone (DHEA). This adrenal steroid is released under stress and helps to protect against the potentially damaging effects of cortisol. In his studies with Special Operations soldiers, Morgan found that a higher ratio of DHEA to cortisol was associated with better performance during intensive survival training and stressful underwater navigation.

The notion that resilience and recovery go hand in hand has been strongly supported by the research of Rockefeller University professor Bruce McEwen and Stanford University researcher Robert Sapolsky. Repeated failure to shut off our own stress response can damage our body and brain. For example, stress that is chronic and inadequately regulated can lead to changes in neurons located in the amygdala, the hippocampus, and the prefrontal cortex. These changes may be accompanied by anxiety, memory impairment, increased sensitivity to alcohol and drugs, diminished mental flexibility, and depressed mood (Sapolsky, 2004; Sarina, Ledoux & Sapolsky, 2009; McEwen, 2006, 2012, 2017).

# Building Physical Fitness Habits

While many types and intensities of exercise have medical and psychological benefits, to enhance physical and emotional resilience, we recommend an exercise regimen that is manageable but challenging. In 2008, the Department of Health and Human Services recommended two sessions each week of muscle strengthening activities plus at least 2 hours and 30 minutes of moderate-intensity aerobic exercise (e.g., walking fast or pushing a lawn mower) or 1 hour and 15 minutes of intense aerobic activity (e.g., jogging or swimming laps). In general, exceeding those basic guidelines provides even greater health benefits. The US Government's 2018 Physical Activity Guidelines Advisory Committee is actively working on updating the guidelines.

We believe that such a regimen should incorporate the following elements.

1. Learn as much as you can about how physical fitness can improve your health and well-being.
2. Consult your physician before beginning a physical fitness program.
3. Try different forms of exercise. Cross-training has many benefits.
4. Develop a set of well-defined goals for your physical exercise regimen and try to stick to those goals. Record the details of your workouts to ensure that you are achieving them.
5. Consider working with an experienced trainer or coach as you build your fitness.
6. Reward yourself as you meet your goals.
7. Gradually increase the intensity of your cardiovascular and strength training. Repeating the same comfortable routine with the same level of intensity each time you exercise may help to ward off some medical illnesses. However, it will not do as much to enhance your physical resilience as exercising out of your comfort zone. To increase your physical, mental and emotional strength, you need to stress yourself and your body beyond that comfort zone, though not to the point of damage.
8. After each workout, allow your body to recover adequately before beginning your next session.
9. Practice healthy eating and sleep habits.
10. Find friends or family members who will support your physical training. Even better, train with a friend or family member who shares your goal of becoming more resilient.
11. Notice and focus on the positive feelings and greater sense of self-esteem and mental toughness that typically accompany increases in physical resilience.
12. Try to reach the point at which being physically fit becomes integral to your sense of self, a part of who you are.

Researchers are continually seeking more answers about how best to exercise, and more to the point, how to get maximum benefits from the least possible expenditure of time and energy. For example, studies of the effectiveness of interval training compare it favorably to other forms of exercise that require a greater time commitment. In a study of sedentary men, three weekly ten-minute sessions of sprint-interval training (all-out cycling efforts alternated with low-intensity cycling) compared favorably with 150 minutes per week of continuous moderate cycling on measures such as increased glucose tolerance, cardiorespiratory fitness, and skeletal muscle mitochondrial content (Gillen *et al.*, 2016). Although it is premature to judge how well these findings can hold up in the general population over periods of years, they are intriguing and may lead to a better understanding of the link between physical training and psychological resilience.

As we all know, there is no easy way to become physically fit and resilient. It takes planning, desire, drive, consistency, perseverance, and the willingness to live with discomfort. But the benefits are many. For Hugh Shelton, being physically resilient prepared him to face and overcome possible paralysis. For Deborah Gruen, it leveled the playing field. For Lew Meyer, it meant living to see another day.

# References

American Heart Association (2009). Short-sleepers" may develop blood sugar abnormality that can lead to diabetes" Press release, March 11. Accessed December 3, 2009, at http://americanheart.mediaroom.com/index.php? s=43&item=693

American Psychological Association (2009). Sedentary lives can be deadly: Physical inactivity poses greatest health risk to Americans, expert says. *Science Daily*, August 10. Retrieved July 20, 2010, from www.sciencedaily.com/releases/2009/ 08/090810024825.htm

Andel, R., Hughes, T. F. & Crowe, M. (2005). Strategies to reduce the risk of cognitive decline and dementia. *Aging Health*, 1(1), 107–116.

Ballantyne, C. (2009). Does exercise really make you healthier? We examine five claims about the benefits of weight lifting and aerobics to see which carry the most. . . weight. *Scientific American*, January 9. Retrieved from https://www .scientificamerican.com/article/does-exercise-really-make/

Barbour, K. A., Edenfield, T. M. & Blumenthal, J. A. (2007). Exercise as a treatment for depression and other psychiatric disorders: A review. *Journal of Cardiopulmonary Rehabilitation and Prevention*, 7(6), 359–357.

Blumenthal, J. A., Bayak, M. A., Moore K. A. *et al.* (1999). Effects of exercise training on older patients with major depression. *Archives of Internal Medicine*, 159, 2349–2356.

Brockhurst, J., Cheleuitte-Nieves, C., Buckmaster, C. L., Schatzberg, A. F. & Lyons, D. M. (2015). Stress inoculation modeled in mice. *Translational Psychiatry*, 5(3), e537.

Brown, R. P. & Gerbarg, P. L. (2012). *The Healing Power of the Breath*. Boulder, CO. Shambhala Publications.

Chu C., Xie B., Qiu M. *et al.* (2017). Cortical folding in post-traumatic stress disorder after motor vehicle accidents: Regional differences in gyrification. *Psychiatry and Clinical Neurosciences*, 71(4), 247–253

Colcombe, S. J., Erickson, K. I., Scalf, P. E. *et al.* (2006). Aerobic exercise increases brain volume in aging humans *Journal of Gerontology A. Biological Science and Medical Science*, 61(11), 1166–1170.

Cooney, G. M., Dwan, K., Greig, C. A. *et al.* (2013). Exercise for depression. *The Cochrane Database of Systematic Reviews*, 9, CD004466.

Cotman, C. W. & Berchtold, N. C. (2002). Exercise: A behavioral intervention to enhance brain health and plasticity. *Trends in Neuroscience*, 25, 295–301.

Department of the Army (2003). *U.S. Army Combat Stress Control Handbook.* Guilford, CT: The Lyons Press.

Dienstbier, R. A. (1989). Arousal and physiological toughness: Implications for mental and physical health. *Psychological Review*, 96, 84–100.

Duman, R. S., Malberg, J. & Nakagawa, S. (2001). Regulation of adult neurogenesis by psychotropic drugs and stress. *Journal of Pharmacology and Experimental Therapeutics*, 299(2), 401–407.

Erickson, K. I., Voss, M. W., Prakash, R. S. *et al.* (2011). Exercise training increases size of the hippocampus and improves memory, *Proceedings of the National Academy of Sciences USA*, 108(7), 3017–3022.

Ericsson, A. & Pool, R. (2017). *Peak: Secrets from the New Science of Expertise.* New York, NY: Houghton Mifflin Harcourt.

Fleshner, M., Maier, S. F., Lyons, D. M. & Raskind, M. A. (2011). The neurobiology of the stress-resistant brain. *Stress (Amsterdam, Netherlands)*, 14(5), 498–502.

Gillen, J. B., Martin, B. J., MacInnis, M. J. *et al.* (2016). Twelve weeks of sprint interval training improves indices of cardiometabolic health similar to traditional endurance training despite a five-fold lower exercise volume and time commitment. *PLoS One*, 11(4), e0154075.

Gould, D. C. II (2000). *Do Sports Build Character? A Study of the Intramural Sports Program of the United States Air Force Academy.* Master's Thesis. Ft. Leavenworth, KS: Army Command & General Staff College.

Greenwood, B. N., Foley, T. E., Day, H. E. *et al.* (2003). Freewheel running prevents learned helplessness/behavioral depression: role of dorsal raphe serotonergic neurons. *The Journal of Neuroscience*, 23(7), 2889–2898.

Griffiths, A., Kouvonen, A., Pentti, J. *et al.* (2014). Association of physical activity with future mental health in older, mid-life and younger women. *The European Journal of Public Health*, 24(5), 813–818.

Hambrecht, R. & Gielen, S. (2005). Essay: Hunter-gatherer to sedentary lifestyle. *The Lancet*, 366(Suppl. 1: S60–1), 560–561.

Hirshkowitz, M., Whiton, K., Albert, S. M. *et al.* (2015). National Sleep Foundation's updated sleep duration recommendations: final report. *Sleep Health*, 1(4), 233–243.

Hoffman, B. M., Babyak, M. A., Sherwood, A. *et al.* (2009). Effects of aerobic exercise on sexual functioning in depressed adults. *Mental Health and Physical Activity*, 2(1), 23–28.

Huang, T., Larsen, K. T., Ried-Larsen, M., Møller, N. C. & Andersen, L. B. (2014). The effects of physical activity and exercise on brain-derived neurotrophic factor in healthy humans: A review. *Scandinavian Journal of Medicine and Science in Sports*, 24(1), 1–10.

Jabr, F. (2016). Head strong. *Scientific American Mind*, 28(1), 26–31.

Jackson, P. A., Pialoux, V., Corbett, D. *et al.* (2015). Promoting brain health through exercise and diet in older adults: A physiological perspective. *The Journal of Physiology*, 594(16), 4485–4498.

Jarrett, O., Waite-Stupiansky, S. & Welteroth, S. (2009). Recess – it's indispensable! *Young Children*, 64(5), 66–69.

Krishnan, V. & Nestler, E. J. (2008). The molecular neurobiology of depression. *Nature*, 455, 894–902.

Loehr, J. (1993). *Toughness Training for Life: A Revolutionary Program for Maximizing Health, Happiness and Productivity*. New York, NY: Dutton.

Loehr, J. & Schwartz, T. (2003). *The Power of Full Engagement: Managing Energy, Not Time, Is the Key to High Performance and Personal Renewal*. New York, NY: Free Press.

Lyons, D. M. & Parker, K. J. (2007). Stress inoculation-induced indications of resilience in monkeys. *Journal of Traumatic Stress*, 20, 423–433.

Maas, J. B. (1998). *Power Sleep: The Revolutionary Program That Prepares Your Mind for Peak Performance*. New York, NY: Harper Paperbacks.

Mayo Clinic Staff (2009). Exercise: 7 benefits of regular physical activity. Online article from www.mayoclinic.com/health/exercise/HQ01676

Mazza, S., Gerbier, E., Gustin, M-P. *et al.* (2016). Relearn faster and retain longer: Along with practice, sleep makes perfect. *Psychological Science*, 27(10), 1321–1330.

McEwen, B. S. (2006). Protective and damaging effects of stress mediators: central role of the brain. *Dialogues in Clinical Neuroscience*, 8, 367–381.

McEwen, B. S. (2012). Brain on stress: How the social environment gets under the skin. *Proceedings of the National Academy of Sciences USA*, 109(Suppl. 2), 17180–17185.

McEwen, B. S. (2017). Neurobiological and system effects of chronic stress. *Chronic Stress (Thousand Oaks)*, April 10. [Epub ahead of print]

Metzl, J. D. & Zimmerman, M. (2016). *Dr. Jordan Metzl's Workout Prescription: 10, 20 & 30-Minute High Intensity Interval Training Workouts for Every Fitness Level* New York, NY: Rodale Books.

Minassian, A., Geyer, M. A., Baker, D. G. *et al.* (2014). Heart rate variability characteristics in a large group of active-duty marines and relationship to posttraumatic stress. *Psychosomatic Medicine*, 76, 292–301.

Moore, S. C., Lee, I. M., Weiderpass, E. *et al.* (2016). Association of leisure-time physical activity with risk of 26 types of cancer in 1.44 million adults. *JAMA Internal Medicine*, 176(6), 816–825.

Moore-Ede, M. D. (1993). *The Twenty-Four-Hour Society: Understanding Human Limits in a World That Never Stops*. Reading, MA: Addison-Wesley.

Morgan, C. A. III, Wang, S., Southwick, S. M. *et al.* (2000). Plasma neuropeptide Y concentrations in humans exposed in military survival training. *Biological Psychiatry*, 47(10), 902–909.

Morgan, C. A. III, Southwick, S. M., Hazlett, G. *et al.* (2004). Relationships among plasma dehydroepiandrosterone sulfate and cortisol levels, symptom of dissociation and objective performance in humans exposed to acute stress. *Archives of General Psychiatry*, 61, 819–821.

Paruthi, S., Brooks, L. J., D'Ambrosio, C. *et al.* (2016). Recommended amount of sleep for pediatric populations: A consensus statement of the American Academy of Sleep Medicine. *Journal of Clinical Sleep Medicine*, 12(6), 785–786.

Philpott, T. (2002). *Glory Denied: The Saga of Vietnam Veteran Jim Thompson, America's Longest-Held Prisoner of War*. New York, NY: Plume Books.

Raine, L. B., Lee, H. K., Saliba, B. J. *et al.* (2013). The influence of childhood aerobic fitness on learning and memory. *PLoS One*, 8(9), e72666.

Rauner, R. R., Walters, R. W., Avery, M. & Wanser, T. J. (2013). Evidence that aerobic fitness is more salient than weight status in predicting standardized math and reading outcomes in fourth- through eighth-grade students. *The Journal of Pediatrics*, 163(2), 344–348.

Safdar, A., Bourgeois, J. M., Ogborn, D. I. *et al.* (2013). Endurance exercise rescues progeroid aging and induces systemic mitochondrial rejuvenation in mtDNA mutator mice. *Proceedings of the National Academy of Sciences USA*, 108(10), 4135–4140.

Salmon, P. (2001). Effects of physical exercise on anxiety, depression, and sensitivity to stress: A unifying theory. *Clinical Psychology Review*, 21, 33–62.

Sapolsky, R. M. (2004). *Why Zebras Don't Get Ulcers*. New York, NY: Henry Holt and Company.

Sarina, R. M., Ledoux, J. E. & Sapolsky, R. M. (2009). The influence of stress hormones on fear circuitry. *Annual Review of Neuroscience*, 32, 289–313.

Schuch, F. B., Vancampfort, D., Richards, J. *et al.* (2016). Exercise as a treatment for depression: A meta-analysis adjusting for publication bias. *Journal of Psychiatric Research*, 77, 42–51.

Seppälä E. M., Nitschke J. B., Tudorascu D. L. *et al.* (2014). Breathing-based meditation decreases posttraumatic stress disorder symptoms in U.S. military veterans: a randomized controlled longitudinal study. *Journal of Traumatic Stress*, 27(4), 397–405.

Stubbs, B., Vancampfort, D., Rosenbaum, S. *et al.* (2017). An examination of the anxiolytic effects of exercise for people with anxiety and stress-related disorders: A meta-analysis. *Psychiatry Research*, 249, 102–108.

*TIME* Magazine (2017). *The Science of Exercise* (Special edn). New York, NY: TIME Magazine.

US Department of Agriculture (2005). *Dietary Guidelines for Americans 2005:* Chapter 2, Adequate nutrients within calorie needs. Available online at www.health.gov/dietaryguidelines/dga2005/document/html/chapter2.htm

US Department of Health and Human Services Committee on Physical Activity (2008) *Physical Activity Guidelines for Americans*. Washington, DC: US Department of Health and Human Services. Available at http://www.health .gov/paguidelines

US News & World Report (2010). Best diets. Retrieved from http://health.usnews .com/best-diethttp://health.usnews.com/best-diet

Weintraub, K. (2016). Connecticut hospitals wake up to the need for sleep. *Hartford Courant*. Retrieved from http://www.courant.com/health/hc-connecti cut-hospitals-patients-sleep- -20160906-story.html

Williamson, A. & Feyer, A. (2000). Moderate sleep deprivation produces impairments in cognitive and motor performance equivalent to legally prescribed levels of alcohol intoxication. *Occupational Environmental Medicine*, 57, 649–655.

# CHAPTER 9

# Brain Fitness: Challenge Your Mind and Heart

In challenging situations, it helps to be mentally sharp. That edge allows us to focus on the problem, process information quickly, remember what we already know about coping with related challenges, find strategies to solve the problem, make wise decisions, and learn new information. It also helps to regulate our emotions: to control them rather than being controlled by them. These mental and emotional abilities equip us to face challenges, find solutions, and recover from setbacks – in essence, to be more resilient.

Just as we can train our body to become fit and resilient, so can we train our brain. The brain has extraordinary abilities to learn. In our experience, resilient people tend to be lifelong learners, continually seeking opportunities to become more mentally fit. We never know when we will be called upon to meet a challenge that requires mental sharpness and keen regulation of our emotions.

On the afternoon of January 15, 2009, US Airways pilot Chesley Sullenberger was captain of a routine flight departing from New York's LaGuardia Airport when, just seconds after takeoff, the plane collided with a large flock of geese. The collision disabled both engines (*New York Times*, 2009). Suddenly the 150,000-pound aircraft was coasting like a glider over one of the most densely populated areas in the nation. Lacking the speed and altitude he needed to return to the airport, Sullenberger quickly weighed alternatives and realized that his best option was to attempt a water landing on the Hudson River. This would mean the loss of a multi-million-dollar aircraft, but it might save lives. Seconds later, Sullenberger and copilot Jeffrey Skiles succeeded in making the emergency landing – an extremely difficult maneuver that required the plane to make contact with the water at a precise angle and precise rate of speed. Not only did the pilots narrowly miss hitting the George Washington Bridge and successfully land on the river without crashing, but the aircraft continued to float long enough for all aboard to evacuate. Not a single person died, and no one suffered serious injuries.

As Sullenberger describes in his book *Highest Duty*,

> What I focused on, extremely quickly, was that this situation was dire. This wasn't just a few small birds hitting the windshield... I heard the noise of the engines chewing themselves up inside as the rapidly spinning, finely balanced machinery was being ruined, with broken blades coming loose. (Sullenberger, 2009, p. 209)

Sullenberger credits his own training and that of the crew for their successful emergency landing. He reflected, "I did not think I was going to die. Based on my experience, I was confident that I could make an emergency water landing that was survivable. That confidence was stronger than any fear" (p. 237). Sullenberger displayed the power to disengage his attention from the emotions of the moment (anxiety and fear: "Can I do this?" "What if I crash the plane and we all die?") and focus it on the task at hand.

Sullenberger's response to the crisis resembled the reactions of the Vietnam pilots we have described in earlier chapters. They also often reported relying on their training when they were shot down or otherwise disabled. You may recall that in Chapter 3, Facing Fear, we related the story of Al Carpenter being shot down; at one point he stated, "Then your training kicks in and you determine what you're going to do next." That training demands that a combat pilot acquire a battery of technical skills and the emotional stability to respond to emergencies such as enemy fire, aircraft malfunctions, and crashing.

Another Vietnam pilot, Steve Long, describes how training saved his life:

> We got into the target area and took a hit. The airplane started coming apart. I saw about two feet of the left wing separate and the rocket pods were falling off. When I realized that the airplane was no longer flyable, it went into a nosedive and I decided to get out. And when I released my seatbelt to go out the door, I hit my head on something and it knocked me out. I was thrown out of the airplane, unconscious. But I guess the fresh air rushing by revived me enough so that I was able to get to my D-ring in time. And about the time that the chute popped open, I slammed into the ground pretty hard.

How many of us would be well-enough trained to pull the D-ring of a parachute while falling through the air after having been briefly knocked unconscious?

## The Power of the Human Brain

The capabilities of the human brain are indeed remarkable. In a world full of distractions, many of us tend to rush through our lives, not really focusing on details and rarely being "fully present" in the moment. Psychologists refer to this distracted state as the "default mode," because our mental processes tend to revert to it in the absence of a task that requires concentration (Tang, Hölzel & Posner, 2015). In default mode, our mind wanders. We ruminate about things that happened to us in the distant or recent past – sometimes with regret – and we worry or daydream about things that we imagine may occur in the near or distant future – often without any concrete plan for how to avoid a feared event or attain something we desire. Default mode is "disorderly – and occupied by a stream of inner chatter" (Ricard, Lutz & Davidson, 2014). It is the opposite of focusing fully on what is occurring in the moment.

When we do find ourselves in a situation in which we are forced to pay full attention, we notice the rich details of life around us and are often able to solve problems, make constructive associations, and recall complex information. Many of the POWs we interviewed learned to appreciate the scope and power of the brain during months or years in solitary confinement, when few outside distractions intruded. Prisoners were often astonished with the brain's extra-ordinary capacity to access previous memories and to remember large volumes of new information. Many of them reconstructed whole chapters of their lives with the precision of diarists and were able to retrieve distant moments and trivial details with exquisite clarity.

In Chapter 2, on optimism, we described how Lew Meyer remembered passages from *The Power of Positive Thinking* by Norman Vincent Peale. Similarly, Paul Galanti recalled, "When I was in solitary my memories would go way back. . . I started going through algebra and calculus. . . I remembered the periodic table and started chemical equations in my head." Bob Shumaker spent 12 to 14 hours a day building a house:

> I built a house in my mind. I would buy all the lumber and materials and everything for it. I knew how many bricks were in it; how much it weighed; the square footage. . . So, it kept me busy, but I think even more than that it kept me hopeful, you know, that someday I would actually build this house. . . Which I did.

Charlie Plumb (1973) reported that one POW sports enthusiast, Galand Kramer, "memorized the names of over 750 baseball players, and after that the list became tiresome and he memorized it in reverse." Jack Fellowes replayed whole ball games and reproduced team rosters, including "the entire lineup for both teams in the 1946 World Series" (Plumb, 1973, p. 179).

These accomplishments are minor when compared to those of a young Navy apprentice seaman, Douglas Hegdahl. The self-effacing 19-year-old South Dakotan was in the Navy less than six months when he was captured in the pre-dawn hours of April 6, 1967. During a night of bombardment, he had gone topside on the guided missile cruiser *USS Canberra* without authorization and had been knocked overboard by the concussion of the ship's giant guns. After staying afloat for six hours, he was picked up by a fisherman, turned over to the North Vietnamese army, and force-marched to Hoa Lo – the Hanoi Hilton.

Most of the POWs were offered early release, but they refused because of their Code of Conduct and the strength of their unity. However, the senior ranking officers selected Hegdahl to accept the offer of early release. Why? Because Hegdahl had been able to memorize the first, middle, and last names of 256 POWs along with each person's capture date, method of capture, and personal information (dog's name, child's name, and Social Security number). He was also able to recite the names of their next of kin, their hometowns, and telephone numbers. How did he do it? He memorized all the information to the tune of "Old MacDonald Had a Farm"!

When Hegdahl was released from the Hanoi Hilton after 28 months in captivity, the first thing he did was to travel around the United States, from west coast to east coast, north to south. He visited each hometown whose name he had memorized, spoke to each prisoner's relatives, and told them that their loved one was alive. In 1970, Hegdahl testified at the Paris Peace Talks, where he confronted the North Vietnamese about the torture and other maltreatment of prisoners he had witnessed.

We have found many examples of the power of memory, even if few are as remarkable as Hegdahl's. In 1987, Anglican church envoy Terry Waite was kidnapped and held hostage by Shiite fundamentalists in Lebanon for 1,763 days (almost five years). During his captivity, Waite mentally "wrote" his autobiography. *Taken on Trust* was published soon after his release in 1991.

Another example of the power of memory involves the reconstruction of music by women held captive on the Indonesian island of Sumatra during World War II. As the Japanese invaded the islands of the South Pacific, they rounded up thousands of Dutch, British, and Australian women and children into overcrowded internment camps with deplorable conditions: food was scarce, disease rampant, and discipline harsh. Among the women imprisoned in one of these camps were Norah Chambers, a graduate of the Royal College of Music in London and wife of a civil engineer; and Margaret Dryburgh, a Presbyterian missionary with musical training. Using scraps of scrounged paper, the women not only composed songs but also reconstructed from memory the orchestration of classical music compositions. As the Australian music critic Neville Cohn recounts in *OzArts Review* (2008), these included the first movement of Beethoven's *Moonlight* Sonata, Chopin's *Raindrop* Prelude, Dvořák's "Largo" movement from his *New World* Symphony, Grieg's "Morning" from *Peer Gynt*, and Ravel's *Bolero*. Lacking musical instruments, the women in the camp formed a vocal orchestra, singing the various parts. Survivors later related how the activity of singing increased their resilience. When they sang, said one survivor, "we experienced a wonderful surge of optimism and hope – and that was a real comfort." The story of this musical achievement inspired the 1997 movie *Paradise Road*.

To this point, we have been talking about mental feats by people who were imprisoned, but there are also many examples in our everyday world of people who have developed their cognitive capacities to an impressive degree.

Recall that in Chapter 2, on optimism, we described how Helen Keller had to learn an entire new set of Braille symbols before taking her exam in mathematics to graduate from Radcliffe. Leaving the exam aside, attending college was a profound accomplishment in itself. Helen could neither see nor hear her professors; very few of the assigned course books had been translated into Braille; and nearly all of her time was consumed in preparation for her classes. Keller described her experience:

> In the classroom I am of course practically alone. The professor is as remote as if he were speaking through a telephone. The lectures are spelled out on my hand (by Anne Sullivan) as rapidly as possible, and much of the individuality of the lecture is lost to me in the effort to keep in the race. Words rush through my hand like hounds in pursuit of a hare which they often miss... I cannot make notes during the lectures, because my hands are busy listening. (Keller, 1903, Chapter 20)

Although few of us will ever face circumstances as grueling as those of a POW or of one who is both deaf and blind, we can all challenge our brains and increase our mental fitness. Doing so may help us to build resilience and the capacity to cope well under stress.

# Brain Plasticity: A Possible Key to Brain Fitness

One of the most exciting findings of brain research over the past decade has been the observation that we can enhance brain fitness. This means that through a series of brain exercises, we may be able to improve our cognitive abilities. The vast majority of us do not reach our full brain potential.

As we noted in Chapter 1, the brain is far more plastic than scientists previously believed. Neurons that are actively used tend to make more connections with other cells and transmit their messages more efficiently. This "use-dependent" neuroplasticity has been observed in animals and humans. For example, in a much-heralded study, Edward Taub and colleagues from the University of Konstanz (Elbert *et al.*, 1995) reported that violinists, who constantly shift the fingers of their left hand in precise movements across the strings of the violin, have greater cortical brain space devoted to fingers of the left hand than to fingers of the right hand, which hold the violin bow and engage in fewer precise movements. Moreover, cortical space associated with fingers of the left hand was much greater in the violinists than in a group of non-musicians, although there were no differences in cortical space dedicated to fingers of the right hand. While violinists who learned to play before the age of 12 had the largest areas of cortical tissue allocated to fingers of the left hand, even violinists who learned to play as adults had similar but less pronounced expansion of cortical brain space. These findings provide strong support for activity-dependent neuroplasticity and brain reorganization. Greater activity enhances the growth of brain cells and increases the allocation of brain space to the processing of that activity. Similarly, researchers have found enlargement in areas of the brain responsible for lip movement among musicians who play wind instruments (Choi *et al.*, 2015). In a series of experiments on use-dependent cortical reorganization, Alvaro Pascual-Leone and colleagues (2001) found that volunteers who practiced a five-finger exercise on a piano keyboard, two hours per day, for five days showed a modest expansion of the brain region that controls movement of the fingers. To the surprise of many scientists, another group of volunteers who simply imagined practicing these five-finger exercises for an identical period of time also showed an expansion of this brain region. Evidently, it is possible that even thinking about movement, like movement itself, can stimulate neurogenesis and reorganization of the cortex.

Recently published brain-imaging studies have found that training in other skills, including juggling (Scholz *et al.*, 2009) and golf (Bezzola *et al.*, 2011), also leads to enlargement of task-relevant brain regions. Researchers at the University of Michigan have offered the following tentative conclusion: "Structurally, training has consistently been associated with volumetric increases in brain structures thought to be critical for performance of the trained task" (Lustig *et al.*, 2009).

# Brain Plasticity After Traumatic Injury

For individuals who have suffered a bodily or brain injury, brain plasticity is especially good news because it allows the brain to reorganize and regenerate itself to a degree. If a person loses a finger or limb, the brain region dedicated to controlling the lost body part undergoes changes. In the case of a lost finger, for example, researchers have found that the neurons associated with the lost finger "learn" to act upon a neighboring finger (Karl *et al.*, 2001). Similarly, the brain has the ability to compensate for brain injury or damage, such that other areas may take over some of the injured area's functions. These sorts of adaptations likely occur through the generation of new synapses and new connections among neurons (Wittenburg, 2010; Iacoviello, personal communication, 2016).

Examples of brain plasticity are abundant among civilians and veterans who have suffered traumatic brain injuries resulting from events such as car crashes, falls, sports injuries and explosions. In January 2006, ABC News correspondent Bob Woodruff was injured in a roadside bomb explosion in Iraq. As described in a *New York Times* story, Woodruff suffered severe brain trauma and spent more than a month in a medically induced coma (Stelter, 2009; Southern Methodist University, 2008).

In a 2008 interview with Alvaro Fernandez, co-author of *The SharpBrains Guide to Brain Fitness*, Woodruff's wife, Lee, described her husband's recovery process.

> . . .rehab is a long process. Doctors told me that Bob, despite the severity of his injuries, had better chances to recover than other victims, because of the reserve of neurons and connections he had built thanks to an intellectually stimulating and diverse life, including living in China for several years and traveling to dozens of countries, having worked as a lawyer and as a journalist, and his overall curiosity and desire to learn. It seems that more and more research shows how people who are mentally active throughout their lives, either through their jobs, or doing puzzles, Sudokus. . . are, of course up to a point, better prepared to deal with problems such as TBI [traumatic brain injury].
>
> Still, recovery is a long process. Bob had six months of structured cognitive therapy focused on speech and languages areas, because that was the part of his brain that had been most damaged. The therapist identified the main tasks for him to work on in a challenging, yet familiar way, usually asking Bob, for example, to read the *New York Times,* then try to remember what he had read, and write a short essay on his thoughts and impressions. . . I am amazed to watch in real time how, even today, how he gets better and better. To give you an example of his motivation to recover: he recently took on Chinese lessons to see if working on that also helped him. (Fernandez, 2008)

Just 13 months after being wounded, Woodruff was able to return to television, hosting an hour-long prime-time documentary, *To Iraq and Back*, which chronicled his recovery and what it means to suffer a traumatic brain injury. He went on to continue his full-time career as a correspondent at ABC News, and also served as anchor for *Focus Earth*, a weekly series on Discovery Communications' Planet Green cable network.

"I have wanted to 'get back on the horse again' since my recovery," Woodruff wrote in a July 2009 blog post. "This will be a different horse, probably not as big, not as fast and without running outside the 'wire.' This means that I will stay on the US military bases without going out on the streets or battle zones like I have in the past."

# Mental Exercises to Enhance Brain Function: Do They Work?

All of us would like our brains to work more effectively. Just as Woodruff challenged himself by taking Chinese lessons and writing a summary of a news article he had read, most of us can find ways to challenge our brains. In recent years, scientists have begun to develop "mental exercises" to improve brain function and, they hope, to stave off the decline in mental capacity that we often associate with aging. These exercises are of special interest to millions of people approaching old age, who worry about developing memory problems, particularly dementia.

Responding to such concerns, a number of commercial products, or "mind games," have been developed that claim to improve cognitive performance (Rochman, 2010). These approaches, which have become immensely popular, are based on neuroplasticity and the idea that repeated "exercise" of brain systems involved in learning and memory will be beneficial. Nintendo markets a series of Brain Age games with the slogan, "Train your brain in minutes a day!" Even though it is described as an entertainment product, Brain Age was developed in collaboration with neuroscientist Ryuta Kawashima, who prompts and guides the user in many of the exercises. In the United Kingdom, MindWeavers markets MindFit, as "Based on science, proven in practice, fun to play." The US company Posit Science, co-founded by the distinguished University of California neuroscientist Michael Merzenich, advertises its games as "clinically proven to help people think faster, focus better, and remember more." Another brain-training platform, Lumosity, has been aggressively marketed and claimed some 50 million subscribers as of 2014 (Hambrick, 2014).

The mental exercises in these products include mathematical challenges such as calculations, verbal challenges including word lists, and spatial challenges such as mazes. The exercises appear to target specific skills such as:

- mnemonic strategies (organization, visualization, association) to enhance memory
- reasoning training (strategies for finding patterns in letter or word series) to enhance decision-making
- speed of processing training (identifying an object on a computer screen at increasingly brief exposures) to promote rapid processing of information.

Some also aim to build accuracy and strengthen retention. In the case of Posit Science, by 2010 three different programs were available: one focusing on auditory input (processing sounds), a second on visual input, and a third on improving the user's driving skills.

The available evidence on cognitive training is increasingly controversial. Research clearly suggests that when a person practices mental tasks, performance improves on those specific tasks. However, the appeal of consumer products in this area is based on the idea that such skills will transfer to other, more general areas of functioning, such as concentration, speed of processing, memory, decision-making, and ability to learn challenging material. In a comprehensive review of research on brain-training products, Daniel Simons and colleagues (Simons *et al.*, 2016) found support for such claims to be weak at best. In a 2014 study by the Stanford Center on Longevity and the Berlin Max Planck Institute for Human Development, 70 leading cognitive scientists concluded that "the scientific literature does not support claims that the use of software-based 'brain games' alters neural functioning in ways that improve general cognitive performance in everyday life, or prevent cognitive slowing and brain disease" (Hambrick, 2014). In 2016, two brain-training consumer products, Lumosity and LearningRx, were sued for deceptive advertising claims, resulting in settlements of $2 million and $200,000 respectively (Federal Trade Commission, 2016; Morran, 2016).

Emerging research is examining the possibility of using brain-training exercises to address mental or emotional problems. The idea is to affect regions of the brain that are known to be involved in such problems. Brian Iacoviello and colleagues at the Icahn School of Medicine at Mount Sinai worked with patients suffering from major depression, having them perform tasks combining emotion identification and working memory. Through repetitive training on the tasks, the intervention was intended to harness neuroplasticity to make changes in those brain regions associated with major depression. They found that participants in the intervention group had a significantly greater reduction in major depression than control participants (Iacoviello *et al.*, 2014; Iacoviello & Charney, 2014).

So, what can we recommend at this point? Making a habit of challenging your intellect can't hurt, although you may be equally able to boost your cognitive fitness and resilience by learning new things on your own as by buying a brain fitness product. You are never too old to learn new information and develop new skills. Indeed, a 2004 study by Cathie Hammond at the University of London concluded that lifelong learning was associated with

> . . .a range of health outcomes; well-being, protection and recovery from mental health difficulties, and the capacity to cope with potentially stress-inducing circumstances; . . .self-esteem, self-efficacy, a sense of purpose and hope, competences, and social integration. Learning developed these psychosocial qualities through extending boundaries, a process which is quintessential to learning. (Hammond, 2004)

# Training the Emotional Brain

The ability to regulate emotions is an essential life skill that takes years to develop. Children and adolescents typically struggle with their unruly emotions for years. Even in adulthood many of us find it difficult to tame our impulses and contain our feelings. In fact, much of psychotherapy is designed to help clients deal with emotions such as sadness, grief, anxiety, anger, and fear.

Emotions are charged with psychic and physiological energy. If we underreact emotionally, we may allocate too little energy to solve the problem at hand. If we overreact emotionally, we may become flooded with too much energy, which disrupts our ability to process information and make good decisions. By learning to recognize our emotions, and then regulate their intensity, we can channel energy into productive cognitive and behavioral responses, which has great utility when dealing with stress and adversity.

One effective technique that can help regulate emotions is the practice of mindfulness, which we discussed earlier in Chapter 5 on religion and resilience (Kabat-Zinn, 1990). "Mindfulness means paying attention in a particular way: on purpose, in the present moment, and non-judgmentally" (Kabat-Zinn, 1994). The practitioner of mindfulness learns to develop calm and accepting awareness of thoughts, emotions, perceptions, bodily sensations, and functions such as breathing. Through this practice, we can learn to tolerate negative emotions better without impulsively acting upon them. Just as with the brain-training platforms mentioned above, mindfulness training apps and websites are available to consumers. One such app is HeadSpace, which sets forth a mindfulness meditation exercise regimen for the user that keeps them engaged and challenged. The exercises start out relatively easy, and become more challenging over time. The exercises also change once the user has mastered them. Users report that this app, and other similar apps, are helpful in structuring a mindfulness meditation practice to enhance mindfulness for thoughts and emotions.

Another approach to emotion regulation during times of high stress involves focusing on the specific task at hand. In Chapter 3 on facing fear, we mentioned the book *In Extremis Leadership: Leading as if Your Life Depended on It* by Col. Thomas Kolditz, head of the Department of Behavioral Sciences and Leadership at the United States Military Academy at West Point. In this book, he writes,

> Don't try to control your emotions... You can learn to sharpen your focus and skills, to turn outward and make sense of the environment, in periods of high risk rather than getting emotional, dysfunctionally excited, and self-absorbed. (2007, pp. 132–133)

As we described earlier in this chapter, pilot Chesley Sullenberger focused most of his attention outwardly on the technical procedures needed to land his plane safely after both engines were disabled. However, even though he appeared calm to others, he later described the emotional reaction that hit him when the engines went silent.

> I felt abnormal, severe vibrations... I'll never forget those awful, unnatural noises and vibrations... It was shocking and startling... I knew that this was the worst aviation challenge I'd ever faced. It was the most sickening, pit-of-your-stomach, falling-through-the-floor feeling I had ever experienced. (Sullenberger, 2009, p. 210)

This is a powerful example of observing one's emotions but not allowing them to interfere. Sullenberger *felt* the emotion, but did not *become* the emotion. He did this by inwardly observing his emotions as well as by focusing on the precise behavioral tasks needed to land his plane safely.

As we mentioned in Chapter 1, both of your authors have tried to apply the principles of resilience in our own lives. For us, athletic competition, particularly competitive kayak racing, has provided a consistent venue for practicing many of these principles. Several years ago, we decided to compete in a 90-mile, three-day kayak race in the Adirondacks. For a competition of this length, it is vital to train for many months in advance. But one of us (SS) didn't start training until about five or six weeks before the race.

> The day before the race, I realized I wasn't in good enough shape to do it justice. I almost called Dennis to tell him that I needed to back out, but I just couldn't do it. Here we were writing a book about resilience and I was about to quit before we had even started. Not good. Not possible. Fortunately, perhaps as a desperate attempt to reframe the upcoming race, I began to think about mindfulness, a discipline that I had been practicing for several years. I remember thinking, "This will be great. I can turn the race into a self-experiment in mindfulness and resilience."
>
> When we got to the race, there were about 500 competitors. The course covered the last 90 miles of an old Native American trade route through the lakes and rivers of the Adirondacks. I was a little nervous at first, but when the starting pistol fired, I began to paddle furiously. I immediately forgot all about my mindfulness experiment and within minutes was gasping for air wondering how I would ever make it through the first day. No one else looked like they were breathing that hard. In fact, to me they looked relaxed and comfortable.
>
> Soon my neck began to hurt. An almost unbearable pain gripped the right side of my neck from my ear all the way down to my shoulder blade. "You complete idiot," I thought. "You've got 85 miles left and you're already in excruciating pain. What were you thinking? What are you trying to prove? You're not in shape. Now you're gonna have to quit and look like a real jerk."
>
> But then, thankfully, I remembered my intention to turn the race into an experiment in mindfulness. For most of the next 85 miles, to my amazement, I thoroughly enjoyed the race, and I paddled faster than I had anticipated. Somehow, for much of the time, I was able to remain in the "present moment" and observe my thoughts and emotions without constantly judging them. I even spent time marveling at the beauty of the Adirondacks and feeling invigorated by nature. It was pouring with rain on the second day, but I didn't care. On the last day as I was churning along, I passed one guy who looked totally exhausted. He asked, "Do you know how many miles we have left?" I told him I didn't know – which was true – and privately thought, "Who cares? I'm just enjoying every minute of this!"
>
> (I should disclose that by the end of the race my shoulders were so inflamed that I could not touch them; I was unable to kayak for 6 weeks afterwards.)

Interestingly, this kayaking experience relates to a line of research on the effects of spending time in natural surroundings. Attention restoration theory (ART) proposes that when our cognitive "muscles" become fatigued, a highly effective way to rest and recover is to "unplug" by taking a walk in a park or along a body of water, or even just by contemplating a mural of a natural scene (Kaplan, 2001; Goleman, 2013). Although we did not enter the three-day kayak race with the goal of refreshing our mental capabilities, some research has found positive mental effects from spending extended periods of time in nature. In a 2012 study, Ruth Ann Atchley and colleagues assessed participants on a creativity, problem-solving task either before or after four days of wilderness hiking without access to Internet or cell phones. The results were striking: after four days in the wilderness, participants scored a full 50 percent higher than their before-hike group peers (Atchley, Strayer & Atchley, 2012).

Suppose, however, that you lack convenient access to a wilderness, or time off from work for a multi-day excursion. In his book *Deep Work: Rules for Focused Success*, Cal Newport suggests that we can increase our focus and thereby accomplish more in our lives by setting definite times to concentrate (Burkeman, 2016). Many of us live with distraction as our default mode, juggling a million distractions and only turning off our email and smartphone for half an hour when we really, really need to finish a complex task. Newport suggests that the better strategy is to make deeper, complex tasks the default, and only attend to distractions on a limited, periodic schedule.

## Attentiveness, Emotions and Brain Activity

The neurobiology of attentiveness and emotion regulation is highly complex. Here we briefly discuss emerging neuroscience findings related to two promising approaches, meditation/mindfulness and real-time neurofeedback. In most studies, but not all, mindfulness meditation has been shown to help individuals cope with symptoms of stress, anxiety and depression (Newberg, 2011; Goyal *et al.*, 2014; Canadian Agency for Drugs and Technologies in Health, 2015). Mindfulness meditation has also been associated with improved ability to focus attention, increased flexibility of thinking, more rapid speed in processing visual information, and improved verbal memory, as well as greater feelings of psychological well-being (Newberg, 2011).

Researchers are making progress in understanding the neurobiological mechanisms associated with meditation/mindfulness. Richard Davidson, Director of the Waisman Laboratory for Brain Imaging and Behavior and the Center for Investigating Healthy Minds at the University of Wisconsin-Madison, has proposed an elegant model to describe how brain activity moves from one region to another as our focus of attention shifts. In the default state (i.e. mind wandering) the posterior cingulate cortex is active. When we become aware that our mind is wandering or distracted, activity in the salience network increases. That network, which helps us determine whether something is worth paying attention to, involves the anterior insula and the ACC. Finally, activity in the dorsolateral PFC increases when we disengage from what is distracting and refocus on being in the present moment (Ricard, Lutz & Davidson, 2014; Marchand, 2014).

As we've indicated earlier in this chapter, mindfulness meditation is closely related to emotion regulation. A number of studies have reported an association between mindfulness meditation and increased activation of the PFC along with decreased activation of the amygdala (Creswell *et al.*, 2007; Hölzel *et al.*, 2011). Richard Davidson explains in his book *The Emotional Life of Your Brain* (2012) that this effect means the PFC is able to more quickly respond to emotion and quiet the amygdala. Modulation of the amygdala by prefrontal cortical systems is thought to play an important role in emotion regulation (Oschner & Gross, 2005; Martin & Ochsner, 2016). Similarly, researchers have recently observed greater activation and cortical thickness (i.e. increased neuronal cell bodies, etc.) of the ACC among experienced meditators compared to novice meditators. This suggests that mindfulness might lead to "enhanced white-matter integrity" in the ACC, meaning that the neural signals travel faster and more effectively (Tang, Hölzel & Posner, 2015, p. 217; Grant *et al.*, 2010).

Meditation has also been associated with increased concentration of gray matter in the right hippocampus (Hölzel *et al.*, 2011). In addition to being a key brain structure for memory, the hippocampus aids in turning down the stress response; therefore, enhanced function of the hippocampus might help to reduce excess arousal and anxiety under stressful circumstances. Richard Davidson raises a fascinating question:

> Might meditation strengthen the cortical circuitry that modulates the activity of the limbic system, like a thermostat regulating this furnace of emotions? Might mental training rewire the brain's emotion circuits and alter forever the sense of well-being and contentment? . . .Just as people now see the value of exercising the body consistently and for the rest of their life, it's similar with emotional skills. . . training is seen as important for strength, for physical agility, for athletic ability, for musical ability – for everything except emotions. The Buddhists say these are skills, too, and are trainable like any others. (Begley, 2007, pp. 230–231)

Davidson believes that repeated practice in techniques of emotion regulation (e.g. cognitive behavioral techniques and meditation) can lead to enduring changes in brain activation, such as increased activation in the left PFC (Ricard, Lutz, & Davidson, 2014; Schwartz & Begley, 2002).

Is mindfulness meditation too "touchy-feely" for the American military? Traditionally one might think so, but in 2014 the Marine Corps conducted an experiment in which platoons of new personnel undergoing nine weeks of Infantry Immersion Training were randomly assigned either to receive the usual training or to receive Mindfulness-Based Mind Fitness. This approach "emphasizes interoceptive awareness [recognition and monitoring of one's emotional states and bodily sensations], attentional control, and tolerance of present-moment experiences" (Johnson *et al.*, 2014, p. 1). Compared to marines in the control platoons, those who received mindfulness training recovered more rapidly after exposure to stress. The effects included reduced stress-related activation of the anterior insula and ACC. Since these brain areas are involved in controlling heart rate, breathing, and other basic bodily functions that respond to stress, the changes suggest that mindfulness may build up the brain's ability to help us recover from stress (Johnson *et al.*, 2014).

Another promising approach to regulating emotions, real-time neurofeedback, involves training yourself to increase or decrease activity in various brain regions. The advent of real-time fMRI makes it possible to observe the biology of one's own brain while thinking, feeling, and acting. It appears that people can learn to control activation in localized brain regions, with corresponding changes in their mental operations, by observing information from their own brain while inside an MRI scanner.

Researchers from Wales and the Netherlands have used real-time fMRI to record the activation of the amygdala, the subgenual ACC, and other brain areas in response to two different forms of negative stimuli (Johnston *et al.*, 2009). First, the researchers measured fMRI activity while participants looked at a series of standard pictures that have been pre-tested and rated as negative. Next, participants were asked to think of negative imagery or memories from their own personal lives that would activate the same brain areas that the negative pictures had. As they did this, the participants looked at a "thermometer" representing the amount of activity in the target brain area, so that they could see the results of different strategies, such as imagining terrifying scenes, thinking of people they disliked, and so forth. Their goal was to activate these brain areas as much as they could. This research represents another step in understanding how people can learn to regulate the activity of brain areas related to specific emotions.

While Johnson and colleagues demonstrated that healthy subjects could activate brain regions such as the amygdala by imagining negative scenes, our team of researchers led by Michelle Hampson Ph.D. at the Yale School of Medicine and the Veterans Administration National Center for PTSD, asked subjects to do the opposite – to decrease amygdala activation that had just increased by recalling a personally traumatizing combat memory. In this small pilot study, Hampson found that subjects with PTSD could reduce amygdala activity which was accompanied by a reduction in PTSD symptoms. Before meaningful conclusions can be drawn from this research, a larger sample of individuals with PTSD will need to be tested.

Other fMRI studies have focused on a brain structure called the anterior insula, located in the fold of the cerebral cortex marking the boundary between the frontal and temporal lobes. The anterior insula is involved in many functions related to emotions, and it appears to play a key role in representing one's own and others' emotional states. For example, in a 2004 experiment led by Tania Singer at University College of London, activations in the insula were associated with the affective (emotional) but not the sensory components of pain.

A 2007 study by a team of European researchers led by Andrea Caria found that healthy participants could voluntarily gain control over right anterior insular activity. Using real-time fMRI, participants were provided with continuously updated visual feedback showing the level of activation of their insula. While in the scanner and receiving this feedback, they were instructed to recall memories of personal events with positive or negative emotional significance. Within three feedback sessions of just four minutes each, participants were able to successfully regulate blood flow in the right anterior insular cortex.

Another brain structure important in the regulation of emotion is the subgenual anterior cingulate cortex (sACC) (Hamilton *et al.*, 2008). Ian Gotlib and colleagues from Stanford University recently demonstrated that healthy (non-depressed) individuals were able to use neurofeedback from real-time fMRI to modulate activity in the sACC. This suggests that people prone to depression might be able to use real-time fMRI neurofeedback to decrease sACC activation and, potentially, decrease symptoms of depression.

Researchers have also explored the possibility of teaching self-regulation to patients with obsessive compulsive disorder (OCD). OCD is a debilitating mental illness which, is classified as an anxiety disorder. (A person with OCD repeatedly experiences intrusive thoughts and impulses, and feels driven to repeat behaviors like hand-washing, counting, and checking that doors are locked.) Using brain imaging techniques, researchers have found that OCD is characterized by overactivity of the orbital frontal cortex and the striatum, two regions that are involved in worry, anxiety, and detecting errors.

In a study at the University of California at Los Angeles, Lewis Baxter, Jeffrey Schwartz and colleagues used cognitive behavioral therapy with OCD patients in combination with PET brain imaging. The goals were to enable the patients (1) to observe and experience the symptom without reacting to it emotionally – something we might describe as mindfulness – and (2) to realize that the feeling that "something is amiss" is the result of nothing more than a "wiring defect" in the brain. The study found that by viewing their own PET scans, patients were able to achieve both of these goals. Moreover, PET scans after treatment showed significant decreases in orbital frontal cortical activity in 12 of the 18 patients. "Therapy had altered the metabolism of the OCD circuit," Schwartz said (Begley, 2007, p. 147). Thus, subjects who learned to re-label the anxiety-related symptoms as a wiring defect actually appeared to change regional brain activity. The researchers observed that these changes in brain activity resembled those that are typically observed after successful treatment of OCD with medication (Baxter *et al.*, 1992).

Another approach to brain training that is currently being studied involves cognitive-emotional training exercises that specifically target activation of some of the important brain regions mentioned above. With repeated exercise, the functioning of prefrontal cortices can be enhanced, resulting in more control over exaggerated amygdala activity and better emotion regulation. In summary, these brain regions can be modified through activity-based plasticity. It is important to note that this research is still in its infancy, but preliminary results suggest that such cognitive-emotional training exercises could allow people to improve emotion regulation and reduce their symptoms of anxiety and depression (Iacoviello *et al.*, 2014).

With the advent of these laboratory techniques, it may soon be possible to add a whole new dimension to treatment which will allow the patient to correlate his or her thoughts and feelings with actual brain activity. This information should provide a powerful tool for regulating emotions.

# Cognitive and Emotional Training Work Hand in Hand

Even though we have organized this chapter into sections that focus on intellectual training on the one hand and emotional training on the other, in fact the two are closely linked when it comes to brain activity. Increasingly, researchers are finding that mental training increases activity not only in the brain's cognitive circuits, but also in its the emotional circuits. Through mental training, it may be possible to increase our capacity to regulate emotions.

Cognitive behavioral therapy has been referred to as a form of mental and emotional training. For example, in Chapter 2 on optimism, we mentioned that optimists tend to have a positive explanatory style (i.e., they explain events to themselves in ways that promote hopefulness and satisfaction), whereas pessimists tend to have a negative explanatory style. Cognitive behavioral therapy teaches people to recognize their typical explanatory style, test it against reality, and decide whether it is dysfunctional. Patients are then taught to reappraise their understanding and explanation of the situations in which they find themselves.

Sleep provides a good example of the interdependence of mental and emotional functioning. Most of us have observed how children often become cranky – less able to regulate their emotions – when they have not slept enough. As adults, we too can become irritable and emotionally volatile when we are tired. Both behavior and brain function show the effects of sleep deprivation. For example, in a study titled "The human emotional brain without sleep: A prefrontal amygdala disconnect," researchers from Harvard Medical School and the University of California at Berkeley (Yoo *et al.*, 2007) used fMRI to examine participants as they viewed a series of emotionally positive and negative images after they had either slept normally or been kept awake for 35 hours. The sleep-deprived participants had much stronger reactions to the emotionally negative stimuli than did those who were well-rested. The researchers concluded that sleep loss leads to emotionally irrational behavior and overreaction to negative events because it impairs the prefrontal cortex's capacity to regulate emotions (Contie, 2007). U.C. Berkeley researcher Matthew Walker explained, "Sleep appears to restore our emotional brain circuits... sleep is not a luxury that we can optionally choose to take whenever we like. It is a biological necessity, and without it, there is only so far the band will stretch before it snaps, with both cognitive and emotional consequences" (Science 2.0 News Staff, 2007).

It is also well known that sleepy children do not learn or perform well in school. The same is true of adult workers. In his book *Power Sleep*, Cornell University psychologist James B. Maas (1998) outlines the many ways in which inadequate sleep impairs emotional and cognitive performance: it causes mood shifts; increased irritability; loss of sense of humor; anxiety; loss of coping skills; reduced ability to concentrate, to remember things, to handle complex tasks, and to think logically and critically; and less capacity to assimilate and analyze new information.

In our own field, sleep deprivation among medical residents is known to reduce the quality of patient care, because it impairs thinking and emotion regulation. In 2006, a landmark study by Charles Czeisler at Harvard found that when "residents worked 5 marathon shifts in a single month, their risk of making a fatigue-related mistake that harmed a patient increased 700 percent, and the risk of making an error that resulted in a patient's death shot up by 300 percent" (Fackelmann, 2006; see also Barger *et al.*, 2006). This research provides a powerful argument for the importance of sleep, and it has helped to shape graduate medical education policy and the number of consecutive hours that residents are allowed to work without sleep.

# Physical, Mental, and Emotional Conditioning: A Win–Win Effect

In the previous chapter, we emphasized the benefits of physical exercise on our health. What is less appreciated, however, is that physical conditioning can also have a positive impact on our capacity to think clearly and to handle emotional stress. Mastering physical challenges can improve confidence and self-esteem, and overcoming physical adversity can help to foster mental toughness.

General Hugh Shelton makes the connection between the physical, cognitive, and emotional in this way:

> The physical is not separate from the mental. A tremendous amount of mental toughness comes from having endured physical challenges. The best thing I've ever done – the thing that provided me with the confidence to know that no matter what I faced, I could probably overcome it, was Ranger school... It was the mental toughness that I developed out of that course, knowing that no matter how adverse the conditions, I could keep going. I had to keep going for the team around me, going

for prolonged periods of time, being run ragged to the point of exhaustion, pushing you to the limit, where you didn't think you could do one more repetition of whatever it was – one more pull-up – and then being required to do even more, or suffer the consequences, which usually was additional push-ups. The physical piece was important. At the same time, you were developing this mental attitude of "I can do it. I can beat them at their own game."

# Training Requires Discipline

Once the skills have been taught, it takes discipline to maintain and improve upon them. This is true for cognitive training, emotion regulation training, mindfulness training and physical training. Rigorous training is never easy. Thoughts and emotions can easily sabotage our best intentions. That is where discipline, drive and consistency come in.

From the time she was in high school, Deborah Gruen, whose story we told in Chapter 2 on optimism, routinely got up at 5 a.m. for pre-dawn swimming workouts. Did she enjoy the jarring ring of her alarm clock, or dragging herself out of bed, or walking with the assistance of her two canes through the snow to the school gym, or jumping into the chilly water to swim 150 lengths of the pool before breakfast? "Of course not! There are some days that I just want to stay in bed," she said at the time.

Then why did she do it? Why did she get out of bed and make it to practice on time every day?

> Because the clock never lies. If my lap times are slow, there is a very good reason. Here's an example: your heart rate, you take it and you immediately know if you're not working hard. . . If I didn't study, I know I didn't study. The truth is, I always know because of my conscience. It is always there, it doesn't go away. At the end of the season, if you're not where you hoped, you know why. It's because I didn't get in the water on time and I didn't get to practice on time. You can't get around it. If you added a minute to your time, there is a very good explanation for it. But people are like, "Oh, it's because of the coach." I don't think so. Or, like, "I failed the class because of the teacher." Well, that doesn't go so well when the medical school you applied to is looking at your grades. "Oh, you didn't like your teacher, well that explains everything. That explains why you failed. No problem." I don't think so.

While Deborah certainly has a winning attitude, she has encountered her share of losses. And as Deborah's father, Jeff Gruen, realized from observing his daughters, it is not necessary to win to be happy; instead, what matters is knowing that you did your best. Even better is the ability to use every loss or failure to your advantage. In the book *Mental Toughness*, Karl Kuehl and colleagues point out that ". . .failure is an education. It educates you by telling you that something is not working, that it is time to try something new, time to make an adjustment" (Kuehl *et al.*, 2005, p. 196).

# Training Requires Precision

The most successful training involves what K. Anders Ericsson, author of the *Cambridge Handbook of Expertise and Expert Performance* (Ericsson, 2006; Ericsson & Pool, 2017), refers to as deliberate practice, or "engaging in a practice activity (typically designed by teachers) with full concentration on improving some aspect of their performance."

The late Russian tennis coach Larisa Preobrazhenskaya was famous for turning out champions at the Spartak Tennis Club in Moscow (Zarakhovich, 2003; Nowak, 2007; *Russia Today*, 2009;). In fact, half of the top ten players in the Women's Tennis Association Tours in 2007 trained with her. How did she do it? Working with several groups of up to eight children aged 4–16, six times a week, Preobrazhenskaya would "insist (without concession) that her students are bio-mechanically efficient before they are allowed to compete" (Gonzalez, 2007). Typically, this technical training would last three years – something that American parents might find unacceptable, as they would be unwilling to wait that long to see their children compete and win! But that was not Preobrazhenskaya's way. A *New York Times* reporter noted that she slammed her fist for emphasis when she told him, "If you begin playing without technique, it is big mistake. Big, big mistake!" (Coyle, 2007).

But why the need to practice skills precisely, over and over again for years, before engaging in competition? The answer lies in the structure of our nervous system. A fatty material called myelin coats a portion of many neurons and speeds the transmission of impulses. When we repetitively practice a behavior, we are building myelin. Myelin wraps around and insulates the nerve so that electrical pulses do not diffuse out. When a nerve is stimulated over and over, myelin grows thicker, and the thicker the myelin, the faster the electrical signal travels down the nerve. Increased speed and accuracy of nerve signals means improved control of cognitions and movements. George Bartzokis, a professor of neurology at the University of California, Los Angeles, explained it to a *New York Times* reporter this way: "What do good athletes do when they train? ...They send precise impulses along wires that give the signal to myelinate that wire. They end up, after all the training, with a super-duper wire – lots of bandwidth, high-speed T1 line. That's what makes them different from the rest of us" (Coyle, 2007).

For any training, whether physical, cognitive or emotional, it is important to be disciplined and systematic in planning and executing your training sessions. If you want to improve your physical, cognitive, and emotional skills, you need to strive for perfection. To succeed, you must "target" your practice by pinpointing what you are doing right and what you are doing wrong. Then correct your mistakes. Precision is critical.

# Make Training as Realistic as Possible

It is generally best to make training as realistic as possible. This is true for cognitive, emotional, and physical training. While books, classroom demonstrations and videos are useful, they cannot substitute for experiential, hands-on learning in realistic settings where the individual repetitively practices skills needed to become cognitively, emotionally, and physically stronger and more resilient (Castro & Adler, 2011).

Scenario-based training is a form of highly realistic training that is known to be very effective. It is based on learning through doing, where trainees are provided with constructive feedback in real time so that they learn to master new information and skills. This approach is widely used in training firefighters, police officers, soldiers, pilots, and others who work in high-stress situations where split-second decisions may save a life. Many of us have seen news photos of "disaster drills" in which a large number of actors portray injured victims with artificial wounds and scripted behaviors that mimic what would happen in an actual earthquake, bomb attack, or other emergency. Scenario-based training is also familiar to anyone who has taken a course in cardiopulmonary resuscitation (CPR).

An extreme example of scenario-based training is the Army's SERE (Survive, Evade, Resist, Escape) course. As we described in Chapter 1, SERE is designed to teach soldiers how to survive in enemy-controlled areas, escape detection, and return unharmed to friendly forces. This training is as much mental and emotional as it is physical.

Special Forces instructor Cliff Welch describes how SERE simulates the horror and chaos of war:

> We try to replicate casualties with moulage kits – fake blood, real blood sometimes – pig blood, things like that. It's better to do it in training if we're having a kid fumbling, you know, all thumbs. Do it in training all you want, so when it comes time for the real deal, he's not all thumbs. He's fluid. He knows what he's doing. His adrenaline's up there, way up there, but he knows what he's doing. And he can pretty much do it without having to think, because it's all almost programmed into him.

Another instructor, Gordon Smith, also describes how SERE mimics the "real deal":

> He might get to the edge of a field, starved, the sun comes up and it's a war-torn area, there might be a dead cow there. It's bloated, you can tell it's been dead two or three days, and they might have a guy who went through SERE school, and he'd say, "When it gets dark again, we're going to just hack off a piece of that because we've got to have some food."
>
> [I tell them,] "We're going to give you the instructional knowledge to survive. We're going to teach you how to do it, then we are going to make you do it. . . We're gonna

make you do things you have never done before, maybe you've never started a fire using nothing but what is out there in the woods and two matches. And so we're going to give you the knowledge verbally, and we're gonna show you and then we are going to make you do it." . . .I say, "Look here guys, we're going to challenge you out there in the woods. . . we're going to give you a road kill. And I've got a choice. I've got a bunny rabbit that got hit last night, still nice and fresh, or I've got a maggot-ridden possum. It's been dead for two days. What do you think I am going to give you?" And they're like, "Yeah, the rabbit."

But anybody can eat an old bunny rabbit. . . "I'm going to challenge you so that you can find out how far you can go. . . and I will make you do it under a controlled environment, which this is, a school. Now if you get sick, you get in trouble, we can fix it now, because it's a learning environment. It's not a learning environment once you're out in the real world. . . I'm going to teach you how to cook and eat this disgusting animal now. . . We want you to be out in the world and be able to see that and say, 'Hey, that's a source of food.'"

End of conversation.

The SERE course is harsh because it needs to be as realistic as possible in portraying the harsh conditions of actual combat. Former POWs frequently describe this type of training as invaluable when they were called upon to endure the real thing.

# Taking Responsibility for Your Own Brain Fitness: Practical Applications

Change requires mental and/or physical activity. One cannot become physically stronger simply by wishing for larger muscles. Similarly, one cannot develop or enhance mental skills by allowing the mind to wander randomly from one thought to the next. Instead, change requires focus as well as systematic and disciplined activity. The principles are simple, but the execution demanding. To change in a desired direction, one must identify what needs to be changed, develop a rigorous but realistic training schedule and then follow that schedule. Becoming more resilient may require training in multiple areas, such as mindfulness and meditation, physical strengthening and endurance. It may require adopting new styles of thinking in order to view hardship and failure as opportunities. The process of systematic self-initiated change, while challenging and often difficult, is highly rewarding and can foster a powerful sense of mastery.

In a brief book titled *Keep Your Brain Alive: 83 Neurobic Exercises*, Duke University neurobiologist Lawrence C. Katz and Manning Rubin (2014) describes simple, everyday ways to build and maintain brain fitness, such as writing or brushing your teeth with your non-dominant hand, or getting dressed with your eyes closed. The authors also recommend some more challenging exercises, such as teaching oneself to read Braille well enough to use an elevator with your eyes closed. These activities activate new pathways in your brain. Other researchers, including Gary Small, Professor of Psychiatry and Aging at the UCLA Institute for Neuroscience and Human Behavior, also recommend specific exercises for enhancing cognitive function (Small & Vorgen, 2016).

By placing ourselves in environments that are conducive to learning, by surrounding ourselves with people who stimulate our personal growth and by systematically practicing specific desired skills, we have the capacity to influence the structure and function of our brain and acquire new skills. For Sergeant Bruce Norwood, there is no substitute for training. Like other SF soldiers, he has been trained to deal with stress in a staggering array of circumstances. During his career as a soldier, Norwood has completed dozens of challenging courses that included day and night parachute schools, training in jungle and, desert survival, mountain climbing school, six or seven weapons proficiency courses, hand-to-hand combat instruction, two foreign language schools, bodyguard school, lock-picking courses, numerous counter-terrorist courses, learning to drive motorcycles, Jeeps and large trucks, surveillance detection schools, numerous computer courses, horseback riding instruction, and more.

When asked how training has affected his life, Norwood replied:

I've tried to explain it to my family. I would have no qualms if they came into my house in the middle of the night, took me out of my bed naked, put a blindfold on me, threw me in an airplane, and flew me anywhere south of Mexico and chucked me out with a parachute and nothing else in the middle of nowhere. In a week I'd be living in a nice place, maybe somebody's house. I'd have a vehicle I could use. I'd be clothed. I'd be eating. And I have total confidence I could do that. Why? Because that's what I've been trained to do.

# References

Atchley, R. A., Strayer, D. L. & Atchley, P. (2012). Creativity in the wild: Improving creative reasoning through immersion in natural settings. *PLOS One*, 7(12), e51474. DOI:10.137/journal.pone.0051474

Barger, L. K., Ayas, N.T., Cade, B.E. *et al.* (2006). Impact of extended-duration shifts on medical errors, adverse events, and attentional failures. *PLoS Medicine*, 3(12), e487.

Baxter, L. R., Schwartz, J. M., Bergman, K. S. *et al.* (1992). Caudate glucose metabolic rate changes with both drug and behavior therapy for obsessive-compulsive disorder. *Archives of General Psychiatry*, 49(9), 681–689.

Bezzola, L., Merillat, S., Gaser, C. & Jancke, L. (2011). Training-induced neural plasticity in golf novices. *Journal of Neuroscience*, 31(35), 12444–12448.

Burkeman, O. (2016). Too busy to focus? Try this. *The Guardian*, January 29.

Caria, A., Veit, R., Sitaram, R. *et al.* (2007). Regulation of anterior insular cortex activity using real-time fMRI. *NeuroImage*, 35(3), 1238–1246.

Castro, C. A. & Adher, A. B. (2011). Military mental health training: building resilience. In S. Southwick, B. Litz, D. Charney & M. Friedman (eds.), *Resilience and Mental Health: Challenges Across the Life Span*. Cambridge: Cambridge University Press.

Choi, U. S., Sung, Y. W., Hong, S., Chung, J. Y. & Ogawa, S. (2015). Structural and functional plasticity specific to musical training with wind instruments. *Frontiers in Human Neuroscience*, 9, 597.

Cohn, N. (2008). Concentration camp music. *OzArts Review*, June 3. Available online at http://ozartsreview.hostingsuccess.com/tag/japanese-internment-camp/

Contie, V. (2007). Lack of sleep disrupts brain's emotional controls. *National Institutes of Health, Research Matters*, November 5. Retrieved from www.sleepe ducation.com/Article.aspx?id=637

Coyle, D. (2007). How to grow a super-athlete. *New York Times*, March 5. Retrieved from http://www.nytimes.com/2007/03/05/sports/05iht-web.0305prod igy.4805563.html

Creswell, J. D., Way, B. M., Eisenberger, N. I. & Lieberman, M. D. (2007). Neural correlates of dispositional mindfulness during affect labeling. *Psychosomatic Medicine*, 69(6), 560–565.

Doré, B. P., Boccagno, C., Burr, D. *et al.* (2017a). Finding positive meaning in negative experiences engages ventral striatal and ventromedial prefrontal regions associated with reward valuation. *Journal of Cognitive Neuroscience*, 29(2), 235–244.

Doré, B. P., Weber, J. & Ochsner, K. N. (2017b). Neural predictors of decisions to cognitively control emotion. *Journal of Neuroscience*, 37(10), 2580–2588.

Elbert, T., Pantev, C., Wienbruch, C., Rockstroh, B. & Taub, E. (1995). Increased cortical representation of the fingers of the left hand in string players. *Science*, 270(5234), 305–307.

Ericsson, K. A. (2006). *The Cambridge Handbook of Expertise and Expert Performance*. New York, NY: Cambridge University Press.

Ericsson, K. A. & Pool, R. (2016). *Peak: Secrets from the New Science of Expertise*. New York, NY: Houghton Mifflin Harcourt.

Fackelmann, K. (2006). Study: Long hospital shifts, sleep deprivation can kill. *USA Today*, December 11. Available at: www.usatoday.com/news/health/2006–12-ll-sleep-study_x.htm

Federal Trade Commission (2016). Lumosity to pay $2 million to settle FTC deceptive advertising charges for its "brain training" program. Press release, January 5. Retrieved from https://www.ftc.gov/news-events/press-releases/2016/01/lumosity-pay-2-million-settle-ftc-deceptive-advertising-charges

Fernandez, A. (2008). ABC reporter Bob Woodruff's incredible recovery from traumatic brain injury. *Huffington Post*, September 15. Available at: www.huf fingtonpost.com/alvaro-fernandez/abc-reporter-bob-woodruff_b_125863.html

Gerin, M. I., Fichtenholtz, H., Roy, A. *et al.* (2016). Real-time fMRI neurofeedback with war veterans with chronic PTSD: A feasibility study. *Frontiers in Psychiatry*, 7, 111.

Goleman, D. (2013). *Focus: The Hidden Driver of Excellence.* New York, NY: HarperCollins.

Gonzalez, A. C. (2007). Prepvolleyball.com. Retrieved from http://prepvolleyball.com

Grant, J. A., Courtemanche, J., Duerden, E. G., Duncan, G. H. & Rainville, P. (2010). Cortical thickness and pain sensitivity in Zen meditators. *Emotion*, 10(1), 43–53.

Grossman, P., Niemann, L., Schmidt, S. & Walach, H. (2004). Mindfulness-based stress reduction and health benefits. A meta-analysis. *Journal of Psychosomatic Research*, 57(1), 35–43.

Hambrick, D. Z. (2014). Brain training doesn't make you smarter: Scientists doubt claims from brain training companies. *Scientific American*, December 2. Retrieved online from https://www.scientificamerican.com/article/brain-training-doesn-t-make-you-smarter/

Hamilton, J. (2009). Music News: Say what?! Musicians hear better. National Public Radio, October 19. Available at: www.npr.org/templates/story/story.php?storyId=113938566

Hamilton, J. P., Glover, G. H., Hsu, J. J. & Gotlib, I. H. (2011). Modulation of subgenual anterior cingulate cortex activity with real-time neurofeedback. *Human Brain Mapping*, 32(1), 22–31.

Hammond, C. (2004). Impacts of lifelong learning upon emotional resilience, psychological and mental health: Fieldwork evidence. *Oxford Review of Education*, 30(4), 551–568.

Holzel, B. K., Carmody, J., Vangel, M. *et al.* (2011). Mindfulness practice leads to increases in regional brain gray matter density. *Psychiatry Research*, 191(1), 36–43.

Iacoviello, B. M. & Charney, D. S. (2014). Developing cognitive-emotional training exercises as interventions for mood and anxiety disorders. *European Psychiatry*, 30, 75–81.

Iacoviello, B. M., Wu, G., Alvarez, E. *et al.* (2014). Cognitive-emotional training as an intervention ofr major depressive disorder. *Depression and Anxiety*, 31, 699–706.

Jaeggi, S. M., Buschkuehl, M., Jonides, J. & Perrig, W. J. (2008). Improving fluid intelligence with training on working memory. *Proceedings of the National Academy of Sciences USA*. DOI:10.1073/pnas.0801268105

Johnson. D. C., Thom, N. J., Stanley, E. A. *et al.* (2014). Modifying resilience mechanisms in at-risk individuals: A controlled study of mindfulness training in Marines preparing for deployment. *American Journal of Psychiatry*, 171(8), 844–853.

Johnston, S. J., Boehm, S. G., Healy, D., Goebel, R. & Linden, D. E. J. (2009). Neurofeedback: A promising tool for the self-regulation of emotion networks, *Neurolmage*, 49, 1066–1072.

Kabat-Zinn, J. (1990). *Full Catastrophe Living: Using the Wisdom of Your Body and Mind to Face Stress, Pain, and Illness.* New York, NY: Delacorte.

Kabat-Zinn, S. (1994). *Wherever You Go, There You Are: Mindfulness Meditation in Everyday Life*. New York, NY: Hyperion.

Kaplan, S. (2001). Meditation, restoration, and the management of mental fatigue. *Environment and Behavior*, 33(4), 480–505. Retrieved from http://eab.sagepub.com/content/33/4/480

Karl, A., Birbaumer, N., Lutzenberger, W., Cohen, L. G. & Flor, H. (2001). Reorganization of motor and somatosensory cortex in upper extremity amputees and phantom limb pain. *The Journal of Neuroscience*, 21(10), 3609–3618.

Katz, L. C. & Rubin, M. (2014). *Keep Your Brain Alive: 83 Neurobic Exercises to Help Prevent Memory Loss and Increase Mental Fitness*. New York, NY: Workman Publishing.

Keller, H. (1903). *The Story of My Life*, Chapter 20. New York, NY: Doubleday.

Kolditz, T. A. (2007). *In Extremis Leadership: Leading as If Your Life Depended on It*. Hoboken, NJ: John Wiley & Sons.

Kuehl, K., Kuehl, J. & Tefertiller, C. (2005). *Mental Toughness: A Champion's State of Mind*. Chicago, IL: Ivan R. Dee.

Lustig, C., Shah, P., Seidler, R. & Reuter-Lorenz, P. A. (2009). Aging, training, and the brain: A review and future directions. *Neuropsychology Reviews*, 19(4), 504–522.

Lutz, A., Greischar, L. L., Rawlings, N. B., Ricard, M. & Davidson, R. J. (2004). Long-term meditators self-induce high-amplitude gamma synchrony during mental practice. *Proceedings of the National Academy of Sciences USA*, 101(46), 16369–16373.

Maas, J. B. (1998). *Power Sleep: The Revolutionary Program That Prepares Your Mind for Peak Performance*. New York, NY: Harper Paperbacks.

Morran, C. (2016). LearningRx to pay $200k for allegedly unproven claims that brain training can improve income, treat autism & ADHD. *Consumerist*, May 18.

Nash, W. P. (2011). US Marine Corps and Navy combat and operational stress continuum model: A tool for leaders. In E. C. Ritchie (ed.), *Operational Behavioral Health*, pp. 193–204. Washington, DC: Borden Institute.

Newberg, A. B. (2011). Spirituality and the aging brain. *Generations*, 35(2), 83–91.

New York Times (2009). Times Topics: US Airways Flight 1549. *New York Times*, June 9. Available at: http://topics.nytimes.com/top/reference/timestopics/subjects/a/airplane_accidents_and_incidents/us_airways_flight_1549/index.html?scp=2&sq=Sullenberger&st=cse

Nowak, D. (2007). Mother of Russian Tennis. *The Moscow Times*, November 12. Available at: www.themoscowtimes.com/sitemap/paid/2007/11/article/mother-of-russian-tennis/193046.html

Ochsner, K. N. & Gross, J. J. (2005). The cognitive control of emotion. *Trends in Cognitive Sciences*, 9(5), 242–249.

Parbery-Clark, A., Skoe, E. & Kraus, N. (2009). Biological Bases for the Musician Advantage for Speech-In-Noise. Poster session presented at the annual meeting of the Society for Neuroscience, Neuroscience, October 2009, Chicago.

Pascual-Leone, A. (2001). The brain that plays music and is changed by it. *Annals of New York Academy of Sciences*, 930 (June), 315–329.

Plumb, J. C. (1973). *I'm No Hero: A POW Story as Told to Glen Dewerff.* Calabasas, CA.

Posit Science (n.d.). Brain training program design. Accessed October 22, 2010 at www.positscience.com/science/teams-and-approach/design-approach

Ricard, M., Lutz, A. & Davidson, R. J. (2014). Mind of the mediator: Contemplative practices that extent back thousands of years show a multitude of benefits for both body and mind. *Scientific American*, 3(11), 39–45.

*Russia Today* (2009). All-Russian tennis final: Recipe for success. June 6. Available at: http://rt.com/Sport/2009–06–06/All-Russian_tennis_final__recipe_for_success.html

Rochman, B. (2010). Workouts for your brain. *Time* magazine, January 18. Accessed July 2, 2010 at www.positscience.com/news/workouts-your-brain.

Scholz, J., Klein, M. C., Behrens, T. E. & Johansen-Berg, H. (2009). Training induces changes in white-matter architecture. *Nature Neuroscience*, 12(11), 1370–1371.

Schwartz, J. M. & Begley, S. (2002). *The Mind and the Brain: Neuroplasticity and the Power of Mental Force.* New York, NY: Harper.

Science 2.0 News Staff (2007). Sleep deprivation and the brain's emotional "disconnect". [Web log post, October 22]. Retrieved from www.science20.com/news_account/sleep_deprivation_and_the_brains_emotional_disconnect

Simons, D. J., Boot, W. R., Charness, N. *et al.* (2016). Do "brain-training" programs work? *Psychological Science in the Public Interest*, 17, 103–186.

Singer, T., Seymour, B., O'Doherty, J. *et al.* (2004). Empathy for pain involves the affective but not sensory components of pain. *Science*, 303(5661), 1157–1162.

Small, G. & Vorgen, G. (2016). *2 Weeks to a Younger Brain: An Innovative Program for a Better Memory and Sharper Mind.* West Palm Beach, FL: Humanix Books.

Smith, G. E., Housen, P., Yaffe, K. *et al.* (2009). A cognitive training program based on principles of brain plasticity: Results from the Improvement in Memory with Plasticity-based Adaptive Cognitive Training (IMPACT) study. *Journal of the American Geriatric Society*, 57(4), 594–603.

Song, J., Skoe, E., Banai, K. & Kraus, N. (2009). *Enhancement of Brainstem Encoding of the Fundamental Frequency in Listeners with Good Speech Perception in Noise.* Poster session presented at the annual meeting of the Society for Neuroscience, Neuroscience, October 2009, Chicago.

Southern Methodist University (2008). Turner Construction Student Forum: Roadside bomb explosion changed their lives. News and communications, March 5. Available at: http://smu.edu/newsinfo/stories/bob-woodruff-4march2008.asp

Stelter, B. (2009). TV journalist wounded in Iraq returns to the war. *New York Times*, July 13. Available at: www.nytimes.com/2009/07/14/arts/television/14woodruff.html

Strait, D. L., Kraus, N. & Ashley, R. (2009). Musical Experience Shapes Top-down Auditory Mechanisms: Evidence from Masking and Auditory Attention Performance. Poster session presented at the annual meeting of the Society for Neuroscience, Neuroscience, October 2009, Chicago.

Sullenberger, C. B. III, with Zaslow, J. (2009). *Highest Duty: My Search for What Really Matters.* New York, NY: HarperCollins.

Tang, Y. Y., Hölzel, B. K. & Posner, M. I. (2015). The neuroscience of mindfulness meditation. *Nature Reviews: Neuroscience*, 16(4), 213–225.

University of Southern California (2009). Computer exercises improve memory and attention, study suggests. *Science Daily*, February 11. Retrieved July 2, 2010, from www.sciencedaily.com/releases/2009/02/090211161932.htm.

Urry, H. L., Nitschke, J. B., Dolski, I. *et al.* (2004). Making a life worth living: Neural correlates of well-being. *Psychological Science*, 15(6), 367–372.

Willis, S. L., Tennstedt, S. L., Marsiske, M. *et al.* (2006). Long-term effects of cognitive training on everyday functional outcomes in older adults. *Journal of the American Medical Association*, 296(23), 2805–2814.

Wittenburg, G. F. (2010). Experience, cortical remapping, and recovery in brain disease. *Neurobiology of Disease*, 37(2), 252–258.

Woodruff, B. (2009). Why I've gone back to Iraq. [Web log post at *The World Newser: World News' Daily Blog*, July 13, 8:40 AM]. Accessed June 22, 2010 at http://blogs.abcnews.com/theworldnewser/2009/07/bob-woodruff-why-ive-gone-back-to-iraq.html

Yoo, S., Gujar, N., Hu, P., Jolesz, F. A. & Walker, M. P. (2007). The human emotional brain without sleep – a prefrontal amygdala disconnect. *Current Biology*, 17(20), R877–R878.

Zarakhovich, Y (2003). Tennis, everyone? *Time* magazine, August 24. Available at: www.time.com/time/magazine/article/0,9171,901030901-477901-3,00.html#ixzz0YeVMDwUR

# CHAPTER 10

# Cognitive and Emotional Flexibility

People who are resilient tend to be flexible – flexible in the way they think about challenges and flexible in the way they react emotionally to stress. They are not wedded to a specific style of coping. Instead, they shift from one coping strategy to another depending on the circumstances. Many are able to accept what they cannot change; to learn from failure; to use emotions like grief and anger to fuel compassion and courage; and to search for opportunity and meaning in adversity.

As entrepreneur and motivational speaker Pete Koerner (2010) observes, "Life = change. If you're changing anyway, why not change for the better? Better or worse are your only choices; you can't stay where you are forever."

## When Life Blows Up

As a young man, Jerry White attended Brown University, where he majored in Judaic Studies. Jerry was raised in the Catholic Church and was particularly interested in the teachings of Jesus Christ. He wanted to walk in the footsteps of the prophets, so during his junior year at Brown he chose to study in Israel.

When school in Israel closed for Passover, Jerry and his friends Fritz and David went camping and hiking in the Golan Heights.

> We wanted to get away from people, off the beaten track. We found a primo camping spot, where we could see the valleys of Syria and Jordan. An old bunker from the Six Day War seemed like the perfect shelter. It was a beautiful sunny day, April 12, 1984. I was walking out ahead of my friends, with a song in my heart. I like being the leader, the one out in front. Then, BOOM! A huge explosion. The whole earth seemed to be exploding under me. I thought we were under terrorist attack. I thought someone was shooting at us.

The explosion knocked Jerry off his feet. Stunned and lying face down, he screamed for help. When he tried to crawl, he immediately collapsed. Within seconds, David knew that Jerry had stepped on a landmine. David jumped to safety onto the nearest rock and commanded Fritz to do the same. But as Jerry lay immobile, pleading for help, his friends stepped off their rocks and came to his aid.

Blood poured from Jerry's leg, the skin was shredded and charred, and splinters of bone were covered with dirt and blood. Small toe bones, as if shot from an arrow, impaled his calf.

"I have no foot! I have no foot!" Jerry screamed, again and again. Slipping in and out of consciousness, imagining the fluids draining out his body, Jerry yearned for a cool jug of water. And then, as David and Fritz flipped him onto his back, Jerry was touched by a profound presence.

> I felt something touch me, like God's hand, telling me to shut up. Later I asked my friends if they told me to shut up and they didn't. It seemed like something forceful saying, "Quiet, listen." I stopped screaming... And then I focused and felt a sense of peace and purpose. I knew I didn't die. This is not how the story ends. I don't die here. And there's a purpose in the Middle East. This focused my brain, like someone gave me a pill that said, "Focus, and be calm."

As Jerry lay in a state of surreal calm, David removed his own shirt, wrapped it over Jerry's stump, and tied a makeshift tourniquet around the injured leg. Fritz searched for Jerry's foot and found the boot but not the foot. ("They never did find my foot, but the boot was intact. It was in good shape. This is what I would call a very good advertisement for Timberland," Jerry would later joke.)

Once the tourniquet began to slow the bleeding, David and Fritz took a hard look at the situation. Their good friend Jerry was bleeding to death, they were many miles from a hospital, and they were standing in the middle of a minefield.

Jerry was 6′ 3″ and weighed 200 pounds. As David and Fritz maneuvered their way through the minefield, Jerry's body became entangled in the thick underbrush and briar patches. They dropped him three times, and each time Jerry hit the ground, he flashed back to the explosion, waited for another blast, and imagined he would die. It took them an hour to reach the edge of the minefield, which was enclosed by a fence with a sign reading *Muqshim* – mines. (They were Soviet mines laid by the Syrians in the 1960s.) An Israeli from a nearby Kibbutz had heard the explosion and was standing on the other side of the fence, waiting to see what had happened. As David and Fritz approached carrying Jerry, the Israeli began to cut through the wire fence to come to their aid.

This was Jerry's first serious physical injury. Growing up, he had never been forced to deal with substantial physical pain: he had been in good health; had never broken a bone; had never even gotten stitches. This was different. This was far beyond anything he had ever imagined. For seven days, he stayed in a small hospital in Safed, where an Arab surgeon saved as much of the leg as he could. The surgeon performed a relatively risky operation, called the Symes Procedure. Unfortunately, gangrene set in several weeks later, forcing Jerry to undergo a second surgery in which more of the leg was amputated. For several months after the accident, Jerry was unable to walk because his good leg had also been blown open. Bones and shrapnel had to be plucked out, and skin from his back grafted to his legs.

Once stable, Jerry faced a critical decision: whether to return home for further surgery and rehabilitation or to remain in Israel for treatment. Jerry's father was the president of a hospital in the Boston area. If Jerry returned home, he would be treated as a VIP in one of the world's best hospitals by some of the world's best doctors, and he would be surrounded by his loving family and friends. Jerry chose to stay in Israel. There, he thought, "the fellowship of suffering was normal," and Israeli doctors were experts in treating traumatic amputations. If he stayed in Israel, he could spare his family from feeling his pain, sensing his anger, or seeing him cry. Israel was also the place where he felt he could best address the question, "Where is God?"

And so Jerry was transferred to the Tel Hashomer rehabilitation hospital outside Tel Aviv. Even though many friends visited him, Jerry felt afraid, isolated, and self-conscious. "I was alone in this hospital. Like, here's your room, here are your roommates: Israelis my age who were doing physical therapy. And everybody is looking at you. Suddenly you're like a freak. 'Oh, here's the American, the dumb tourist, who got blown up camping in Northern Israel.'"

One of his roommates, a soldier who had lost both legs and wanted to die, slept the day away and stashed pills, perhaps intending to kill himself.

> It felt like *One Flew Over the Cuckoo's Nest,* and I suddenly felt sad and alone. I thought that I might be crazy. People were trying to introduce themselves, but they were all missing arms, legs, eyes, or they were burn victims. I felt sick and afraid, and all of these people were like ghosts. And I remember this older guy who was doing rehab and he had this new above-the-knee prosthesis and he said, "You're gonna get one of these, too," and he took it off and I saw his stump and his leg, and he was making light of it. And I remember feeling that I hated him, that I hated his stump, that I hated his prosthesis. I hated that he was talking to me, and I felt sick, and all I wanted to do was vomit the baba ganoush that I had just eaten.

When Jerry did go home to Boston, he worried about his friends. Would they feel uncomfortable around him? Would they treat him differently? Would they avoid him? Could they fully accept him as the same old Jerry?

> Some of my closest friends drove up to see me, and I remember how afraid they were. I had been living with this for six months but no one else had; they had only heard the awful news. Was I changed? Was I the same Jerry? How should they act? Should they look really glum and sad? Should they just hug, you know, an extra beat too long?

> I probably overcompensated by trying to make people feel comfortable. Like asking them if they wanted to see my stump or making fun of it and treating my stump like a puppet and making it bark. I even had a pet name for it – Dino.

Jerry White went back to college and completed his studies, then moved to Washington, DC to look for a job in international affairs. While job hunting, he worked as a substitute teacher and, perhaps surprisingly for someone with an artificial leg, he also worked as a home builder. White's career took a new turn when the Brookings Institution hired him as a research assistant in its Middle East Policy section. This experience led him to a position as Assistant Director of the Wisconsin Project on Nuclear Arms Control, an affiliate of the University of Wisconsin Law School. Jerry had grown accustomed to his disability and learned to compensate for the inconvenience. He had married, reaffirmed his Catholic faith, and found a job serving society. He believed that he had fully accepted his disability. He had moved on.

Then in 1995, White got a phone call from a stranger named Ken Rutherford, who had met one of White's college friends at a party, and the friend recommended that Ken call Jerry. Although Rutherford knew that White was an amputee, he did not know how much the two of them had in common. White recalls:

> He thought that he was perhaps the only American civilian amputee who had lost a leg to a landmine. Actually, he lost both of his legs in Somalia. And he was like, "I can't believe it, a landmine survivor, and with your work! Don't you know that landmines are called weapons of mass destruction in slow motion? They've killed more people than nuclear chemicals and biological weapons combined. So with your work experience in nonproliferation and weapons of mass destruction and your personal experience losing a leg to a landmine, you could really be effective. Do you know about the emerging campaign to ban landmines?"

White had read several articles about landmines in arms control magazines but had never made the conscious connection between the two types of weapons. Once he did, he was hooked. Three months later, he and Rutherford attended the UN-sponsored First International Conference on Landmines in Vienna. There, each man told his story, for the first time in public, and bore witness before a UN panel, an opportunity that ignited Jerry White's imagination.

> I saw immediately how this could tap into my passion for a cause and also how powerful the voices of survivors were in this movement. They were living evidence – the lifeblood of the campaign to end landmines. Vienna was a turning point for me, a philosophical turning point that set me on fire for the advocacy issue.

By working for nuclear nonproliferation, he had already prepared for similar activism. Yet it took years for him to find his way to this new mission.

At first, White's boss allowed him to fundraise for landmine survivors by creating a subdivision of the Wisconsin Project on Nuclear Arms Control. But by 1996, Jerry had become consumed by his new passion, and his boss knew that he would eventually lose his valued colleague. Despite his considerable family responsibilities – by now he and his wife had four children under age six – White left his job, cashed out his retirement plan, and set up an office in his basement. It was a risky move, to put it mildly. But he was committed to the cause. He spent day and night fundraising. Even after the group had achieved a great deal, Jerry was willing to acknowledge that he might not succeed.

> All along I felt that, even if it doesn't work, even if I fail, it's not failure because, look, we will have helped change the world, drafted a treaty to ban landmines, saved millions of lives, helped thousands of survivors. So, if I fail as a director of a nonprofit organization because I'm not a good enough fundraiser or I don't know how to build properly as an entrepreneur, then I still succeeded. The failure would still be glorious.

Twenty years after losing his foot in Israel, Jerry White, along with his friend and colleague Ken Rutherford, accepted the Nobel Peace Prize, which honored the work of International Landmine Survivors Network (the group has since been renamed Survivor Corps).

How did White evolve from feeling sad, alone, and sick about the loss of his leg to feeling joyous, passionate, and committed to the welfare of other landmine survivors? How did he progress from victim to survivor – then to what he calls "super-survivor"? White answers these questions in his book *I Will Not Be Broken*, which outlines five steps to overcoming a life crisis (White, 2008):

- Face facts: accept what has happened.
- Choose life: live for the future, not in the past.
- Reach out: connect with other survivors.
- Get moving: set goals and take action.
- Give back: service and acts of kindness empower the survivor to be an asset rather than a victim.

Jerry White's story is an example of what numerous researchers have found. As Donald Campbell and colleagues from the Department of Behavioral Science and Leadership, US Military Academy, West Point, write "Rather than seeing themselves as victims of a terrible and mindless fate, resilient people and groups devise ways to frame their misfortune in a more personally understandable way, and this serves to protect them from being overwhelmed by difficulties in the present" (Campbell, Campbell & Ness, 2008, p. 63). This concept appears over and over again in the literature on resilience (Coutu, 2002).

## Acceptance

An important component of cognitive flexibility is accepting the reality of our situation, even if that situation is frightening or painful. To remain effectively engaged in problem-oriented and goal-directed coping, we must keep our eyes "wide open," and acknowledge, rather than ignore, potential roadblocks. Avoidance and denial are generally counterproductive mechanisms that may help people cope for a while, but that ultimately stand in the way of growth, interfering with the ability to actively solve problems.

Sometimes acceptance involves not only acknowledging the reality of one's situation, but also assessing what can and cannot be changed, abandoning goals that no longer seem feasible, and intentionally re-directing efforts toward that which can be changed. Thus, acceptance is not the same as resignation and does not involve giving up or quitting. Instead, acceptance is based on realistic appraisal and active decision-making.

For White, as for many trauma survivors, fully accepting his loss took a very long time. It was not until many years after his accident, when he was invited to a conference on landmine survivors in Cambodia, that he experienced what he calls an "emotional turning point." It was August, the temperature was well over 100 degrees with nearly 100 percent humidity, the streets smelled of putrefied food, and White was drenched with sweat. As he stopped to change the dressing on his stump, a young, one-legged beggar, with a crutch under her arm, approached him and said, "You're one of us."

> First, I was repulsed by her. I thought, "I'm not a Cambodian beggar. I'm not like you. You've lost a leg, but you're begging in the streets. That's not me." Then I was repulsed by myself. She was right. How dare I separate myself and turn my back on her? How could I turn my back and leave if there was something I could do? She showed me that I was a jerk. What I didn't know, at the time, was that I was part of a family, the family of landmine survivors.

In seeing himself as belonging to that family, White took another step toward acceptance, a step that allowed him to more fully embrace his status as a survivor.

Many of the other resilient individuals we interviewed also cited acceptance as critical in their ability to thrive under conditions of high stress and trauma. Somehow, they learned how to focus their attention and energies on problems that they believed they could solve, and they rarely wasted time and energy "banging their head against the wall," fighting battles that they could not win. In other words, they were realistic and pragmatic.

Colonel William Spencer, another former Vietnam POW, recalls an experience from his survival school training that taught him an important lesson about acceptance.

> One of the things that they did was put us in a little box. And the box was made to shrink. If you moved, the box would constrict. It was bad. I could hear other guys scream and then they [the instructors] would let them out... When I went in, I tried to push against it, and that panicked me. I realized that's not the thing to do. So then I just relaxed and I tried to [mentally] play golf and occupy my mind with other things...

> Because when I fought it, I was losing. I stopped fighting it when I realized I couldn't change it and pushing made it worse... The same thing that protected me in that box, I think helped me in the environment [prison camp] that I was in later.

Perhaps our most graphic example of acceptance involved another Vietnam POW who, after 15 months in solitary confinement, sensed that he was about to "lose his mind." Each day he struggled to understand how and why his life had taken such a dramatic turn. Less than two years earlier, as a Navy aircraft carrier pilot, he had reached the top of his game. He was highly respected, had the "best job in the world," and was happily married with two children. Now, starved and emaciated, he lay shackled in a rat- and mosquito-infested windowless concrete prison cell, refusing to believe or accept that his life had been reduced to mere survival.

And then, one morning, he heard a loud and distinct voice that startled him.

> "This is your life."

And it was true. This was his life, not a dream, not his imagination. There was no denying it, no wishing it away. This was real.

> When I heard that voice, things changed. I don't know where it came from. It was pretty loud. I'm sure I heard it. I know it sounds weird but it wasn't my voice. It's almost like it lifted this weight off my shoulders, 'cause the voice was right. I was in this cell and I wasn't going anywhere. So I guess when I really admitted it to myself, I just kind of stopped fighting and things got a lot better. I mean, I always knew I was in prison, but after that voice, it just changed. I just wasn't as miserable anymore, and I started to take care of business, you know. I started to exercise as much as I could, and I tried to stay in touch with some of the guys... After that voice, I felt a lot better.

These experiences echo the essence of the well-known Serenity Prayer: "God grant me the serenity to accept the things I cannot change, the courage to change the things I can, and the wisdom to know the difference."

# The Science of Acceptance

In the scientific literature, acceptance has been cited as a key ingredient in the ability to tolerate highly stressful situations. This has been true both among survivors of extreme environmental hardship and threats to life (Siebert, 1996), among highly successful learning-disabled adults (Gerber & Ginsberg, 1990) and among individuals with a variety of medical and mental disorders (Sirois & Hirsh, 2017; Casier *et al.*, 2011; Huston *et al.*, 2016; Thompson *et al.*, 2011). Acceptance has also been associated with better psychological and physical health in many different groups of people. In a nationwide survey of individuals shortly after the terrorist attacks of September 11, 2001, researchers found reduced levels of posttraumatic stress symptoms in those who accepted the situation (Silver *et al.*, 2002). In a study of mothers whose children had life-threatening cancer diagnoses and were undergoing bone transplants – a painful and highly invasive procedure – Sharon Manne and colleagues (2002) found that those who accepted their situation reported fewer symptoms of depression. Acceptance has also been recommended as a coping mechanism for families of children with cancer (Kazak *et al.*, 1999) and for family members of adults with serious mental illness (Zauszniewski *et al.*, 2015). Further, the most commonly used scale to measure resilience, the Connor–Davidson Resilience Scale, includes a question about positive acceptance of change.

Elsewhere in this book, we have mentioned cognitive behavioral therapy as a means to develop a more positive explanatory style, and as a means to observe the world more realistically. A related therapy called acceptance and commitment therapy uses acceptance as a starting point for taking action to address problems. The American Psychological Association describes it this way:

> The goal of acceptance and commitment therapy (ACT) is to increase psychological flexibility, or the ability to enter the present moment more fully and either change or persist in behavior when doing so serves valued ends. Therapists and clients work to establish psychological flexibility through six core ACT processes, including acceptance, the opposite of experiential avoidance; cognitive defusion, in which negative thoughts are observed mindfully instead of avoided or reasoned away; chosen values; and committed action. (American Psychological Association, 2008)

Therapists have successfully used ACT to treat problems ranging from chronic pain to smoking cessation to eating disorders. Research also suggests that it may be useful in treating stress and anxiety disorders (Orsillo *et al.*, 2005; Woidneck *et al.*, 2014).

# Cognitive Reappraisal

Several years ago, while conducting a study on the psychological and neuro-biological consequences of the Holocaust, a colleague asked an elderly Holocaust survivor if she had ever dreamed about her experiences in the camps.

"Oh yes," the woman replied. "I've never stopped dreaming about those times. I just had a dream the other night. Mostly it's the same horrifying one. It wakes me up in the middle of the night. I'm in a panic. I'm sweating, and it's hard to breathe. Yes, I still dream about the camps."

At that point, our colleague replied, "My goodness, it must be horrible to still have those nightmares after all these years."

"Oh no," the woman said. "It's OK. It's OK because when I awaken, I know that I'm here and not there."

Positive reappraisal requires us to find alternative positive meaning for neutral or negative events, situations and/or beliefs. While this remarkable woman suffered profoundly from her Holocaust experiences, she somehow found a way to reappraise her nightmares. Although she was unable to control the nightmares, she was able to view them as powerful reminders that she was lucky to have survived and now had the privilege of waking up each morning to a new day.

Like this woman, pilot Sullenberger narrowly escaped death, as described in Chapter 9, when his plane's engines failed. Although he remained outwardly calm during the emergency, Sullenberger suffered from the experience afterwards. Like many (if not most) trauma victims, he struggled with insomnia, distracted thinking, diminished appetite, flashbacks, and "second-guessing and what-iffing." Soon, however, he was able to reappraise his circumstances and see that his experience could give him power – in his case, to influence aviation policy. In his book *Highest Duty* (2009), Sullenberger explains how he decided to move forward: "I've been asked by colleagues to be a public advocate for the piloting profession and for airline safety... I know I now have the potential for greater influence in aviation issues, and I plan to be judicious in how I wield that influence" (p. 275).

Decades earlier, in his groundbreaking work on crisis intervention and prevention, Norman J. Finkel coined the term "strens" to describe life events that were health-promoting or growth-enhancing. Although most of these events were positive in nature, a substantial number were clearly traumatic. After years of crisis-oriented research, Finkel (1974) concluded that some people possess the capacity to convert trauma into growth and that they do so through "some cognitive restructuring mechanism." That is, they tend to reframe the negative, search for opportunity in the midst of adversity, and extract positive meaning from trauma and tragedy. Although the term "strens" never gained widespread acceptance, the concept of cognitive reapprasial has been widely recognized.

In the decades since Finkel made his observations, numerous researchers have found that the capacity to positively reframe and extract meaning from adversity is an important component of stress resilience: resilient individuals often find that trauma has forced them to learn something new or to grow as a person (Park *et al.*, 1996; Southwick *et al.*, 2016). The reported potential "benefits" of trauma have been numerous and far-ranging: greater compassion for and acceptance of others; closer ties with family and friends; a greater sense of kinship with humanity; an enhanced sense of community; a heightened appreciation of nature; renewed religious faith; development of more effective coping skills; commitment to a healthier lifestyle; improved self-esteem and self-respect; increased emotional strength; enhanced wisdom and maturity; a shift in values, priorities, and perspective; intensified appreciation of life;

and a new sense of meaning and purpose (Tedeschi, Park & Calhoun, 1998; Anderson & Anderson, 2003).

As human rights worker Sister Dianna Ortiz writes of torture survivors, "From a position of slowly increasing strength, many of us can then begin to redirect our energies to helping other survivors, raising public awareness about the practice of torture, confronting our perpetrators, or simply learning to live life anew with some sense of hope" (Ortiz, 2001, p. 29).

# Gratitude as a Form of Reappraisal

The old advice to "count your blessings" is a time-honored way of promoting a positive view of life. Perhaps surprisingly, even survivors of severe trauma can express a measure of gratitude, feeling that the ordeal has enriched their lives in some way. "First of all, it makes you very humble," says former Air Force pilot Steve Long when describing the effects of more than five years as a POW in Vietnam.

> A lot of the old axioms that you hear – like, "You never really appreciate anything until you take it away" – those axioms exist because they're true. And I think anybody that goes through an experience like this, and even like the World Trade Center, the families that were associated with it, they all come to understand this sooner or later: Life is precious. Appreciate it while you can, while you have it, because it can be taken away very easily.

Since his return from Vietnam, Long has been invited to speak about his war experiences to many audiences, including high school and college students. For some people, talking about past traumas can be painful, reactivating old feelings of fear and sadness. However, for Long, it provides a way to educate others about the importance of moral integrity, perseverance, learning from role models, and facing fear with trusted colleagues and friends. It also reminds him what the experience taught him.

> It keeps things fresh in my mind that I want to remember. I want to remember to appreciate the things that we have, the freedoms that were taken away from me. I want to remember to place my family first. I don't want to fall back into taking things for granted. I swore that when I got home I'd never forget to be thankful for that piece of bacon, because that was one of the things that I thought about a lot. Just simple things in life.

In their 2003 book *Emotional Longevity*, Norman and Elizabeth Anderson point out that a surprisingly high percentage of people who survive a major crisis later describe the crisis as having affected their lives positively, at least in some important ways. In addition, they cite research showing that individuals who reframed a crisis positively were less likely to develop posttraumatic stress symptoms after being exposed to combat or natural disasters, and adjusted better after losing a family member. This was also true for survivors of incest. Even medically, patients who had suffered a heart attack were less likely to suffer a second one if they were able to view the crisis as a wake-up call or inspiration to re-evaluate their lives. In our own research on a large, nationally representative sample of US military veterans, we found that dispositional gratitude was associated with resilience, posttraumatic growth, and reduced risk of suicide (Tsai *et al.*, 2016; Smith *et al.*, 2016; Isaacs *et al.*, 2017).

Gratitude in the form of journal writing or intentional expressions has been used as an adjunct to psychotherapy in treatment for depression and other disorders. Such gratitude interventions show promise in improving well-being and positive affect and in reducing worry. Expressing gratitude may also improve physical health and foster healthy behaviors (Millstein *et al.*, 2016).

In some cases, the cognitive reframing that accompanies trauma can be life-altering. In her innovative work with trauma survivors, Ronnie Janoff-Bulman (1992) proposed that personal psychology and personality can change when survivors experience a shattering of their world view followed by questioning, and then rebuilding basic assumptions.

And indeed, many of the resilient Vietnam POWs whom we interviewed believed that their imprisonment, while it shattered their previous approach to life, eventually proved meaningful and in some cases even positive. Bill Spencer, for example, believes that life is a test and that our mission here on Earth is to learn lessons that lead to growth and maturity, and that many important lessons are the byproducts of adversity:

In my view, life is an experiment, a test. I think our Lord puts us here to learn things about ourselves. And we really grow and mature more during trials than during the good times. When things are really going well, we start getting real sloppy and we get gregarious and we waste our time. The job's great, everything's wonderful! But when things really go bad, if we concentrate, we can learn a lot. It's not fun. It's not what we ordered. The fun times are better. But really we mature more when we're under an intense trial.

Quite apart from his POW experience, Spencer also lived through a family tragedy. He had a son who was physically handicapped and died at a young age, an experience that profoundly affected the family. Spencer remembers:

I lost a son. And as he became more and more ill I realized how valuable he was and all he had taught me, all the lessons I learned from him. I learned more from him than from anyone or from any lesson. But his life was full of trial. He died when he was 24. And he was handicapped.

When I was a kid, I was very athletic and everything came easy to me. So I have a son who can't do anything. It's good for me. Bad for him. He was here, I think, to teach me those lessons, and the rest of our family. I learned a lot from him... You don't necessarily learn that much from a normal child. It sounds funny. . . I didn't volunteer for it. But after it's all over you realize I can write down 18 things that I learned from him, more than any other source. So did a lot of other people: my wife, his sisters, people who cared for him.

When we had his funeral, there were hundreds of people there we'd never seen. And they just came and told their stories about all the things that he had taught them, because he was handicapped. We learn a lot when we care for somebody, when they can't do it for themselves, that's when we really learn a lot.

One morning, he was about three or four and we always said prayers around a little chest that we had gotten in the Philippines. We always knelt. And I had two daughters and a son and wife. And the five of us would kneel and I would say prayers and I would usually lead or call on one of them and then I'd go to work. And on this morning, I was in a hurry. I failed to get up in time and I was rushed for my schedule. Nobody else was rushed, just me. So I said, "Well, we're just going to say our prayers standing up. I'll give the prayer."

I started saying the prayer and I looked down and my three-year-old was on his knees. So without saying anything I knelt and without saying anything more, the rest of the family knelt. He led us. And that's just one example. He taught me how to pray. You don't say prayers hastily. If you're going to say prayers, do it right. He did a lot of things like that. It was just easy for him. He was never in a hurry. So he didn't take shortcuts on important things.

Despite the grief over losing his son, Bill Spencer continues to search for positive lessons embedded in tragedy. And by reframing the tragic, he finds meaning in suffering, thereby enriching his own life and the lives of those around him.

# The Science of Cognitive Reappraisal

In reviewing an extensive scientific literature on cognitive strategies to regulate emotions, researchers Allison Troy and Iris Mauss (2011) propose that positive cognitive reappraisal fosters resilience through its effect on negative emotions. More specifically, reappraising the meaning of a stressful event as less negative or more positive changes emotional reactions to the event and results in a more adaptive and resilient response. Studies have shown that individuals who frequently use positive cognitive reappraisal to change their emotional reactions to stress report greater psychological well-being and more positive outcomes compared to individuals who do not use reappraisal to cope (John & Gross, 2004; Martin & Ochsner, 2016).

We can also take cues from those around us to help us interpret (or reinterpret) our own experiences in a more positive light. For example, in the workplace a manager or supervisor may point out the positive aspects of an adverse situation or event, providing employees with cognitive and emotional tools to view the adversity as a challenge. Similarly, if a husband is upset about something a neighbor has done, his wife might provide an alternative explanation for the neighbor's behavior that allows for a more constructive interpretation (Reeck, Ames & Ochsner, 2016).

Neuroscientists have found that reappraising an event as being more negative or more positive changes activation in brain regions associated with emotions. Columbia University researcher Kevin Ochsner and colleagues (Ochsner *et al.*, 2009; Martin & Ochsner, 2016; McRae *et al.*, 2010) have conducted a series of fMRI studies in which subjects were instructed to reinterpret visual stimuli (e.g., neutral or negative images) while being scanned. In some studies, subjects were asked to pay attention and respond naturally to a set of pictures that depicted various situations, some negative in content. Subjects were then instructed to reinterpret these situations so that they felt less negative about them. Overall, Ochsner's research found that reappraisal of negative situations decreased negative emotions, increased activation in areas of the prefrontal cortex related to cognitive control, and decreased activation of the amygdala.

As described in Chapter 1 and elsewhere, the prefrontal cortex is the "executive" region of the brain, involved in planning, directing, and inhibiting; and the amygdala is the "alarm center," where the brain processes emotion and fear outside of conscious awareness. Ochsner's study suggests that conscious efforts to positively reframe or reappraise an aversive situation activates the brain's executive region (the prefrontal cortex) and inhibits its emotion center (the amygdala). Recent meta-analyses evaluating numerous brain imaging studies examining the effects of cognitive reappraisal on activation of relevant brain regions have supported Ochsner's findings (Etkin, Bücher & Gross, 2015).

## Cognitive Reappraisal of Failure

Resilience demands the emotional stability to handle failure, what Admiral James Stockdale referred to as the "ability to meet personal defeat with neither the defect of emotional paralysis and withdrawal nor the excess lashing out at scapegoats or inventing escapist solutions." In our experience, people who are resilient generally meet failure head-on and use it as an opportunity to learn and to self-correct. Stockdale used his knowledge of history to do that.

> The only way I know how to handle failure is to gain historical perspective, to think about men who have successfully lived with failure in our religious and classical past. When we were in prison we remembered the Book of Ecclesiastes: "I returned and saw that the race is not always to the swift nor the battle to the strong... but time and chance happeneth to them all." ...Failure is not the end of everything, a man can

always pick himself up off the canvas and fight one more round. To handle tragedy may, in fact, be the mark of an educated man, for one of the principal goals of education is to prepare us for failure. (Stockdale, 1984, pp. 56, 73)

There's truth to the cliché, "It's not how many times you fall down that counts – it's how many times you get up." Failure can teach us to adjust, to improve, and to find new ways to overcome difficulties. Thomas Edison provided a classic example of reframing: "If I find 10,000 ways something won't work, I haven't failed," he said, "I am not discouraged, because every wrong attempt discarded is another step forward."

Another popular saying is worth remembering: "Learn from the mistakes of others. You can't possibly live long enough to make them all yourself."

# Humor: Another Form of Cognitive Reappraisal

In his classic book *Man's Search for Meaning,* Viktor Frankl refers to humor as "another of the soul's weapons in the fight for self-preservation. It is well-known that humor, more than anything else in the human makeup, can afford an aloofness and an ability to rise above any situation, even if only for a few seconds" (1963, p. 63). For Frankl, humor provided a healthy means to gain perspective. And with perspective comes the capacity to reappraise and generate alternative approaches and solutions to problems.

Like other positive emotions, humor tends to broaden one's focus of attention and thereby foster exploration, creativity and flexibility in thinking. In so doing, humor may incorporate a number of other resilience coping mechanisms such as cognitive reappraisal, active problem-focused coping, and infusion of positive meaning into ordinary events. As noted by the philosopher André Comte-Acheg:

The best or most profound humor plays on meaning that touches important areas of our lives, drawing us into its wake and shaking up larger fields of significance, our beliefs, values, illusions, in short our seriousness. Sometimes humor seems to bring about an implosion of thought... Humor can zero in on the very meaning of our behavior and reactions, shaking their foundations and calling them into question, scrambling our values, pretensions, and points of reference. (1996, p. 219)

Humor can also serve as a tool to help us face our fears. Humor provides distance and perspective, but does so without denying pain or fear. Humor manages to present the positive and negative wrapped into one package. As the noted Viktor Frankl scholar, Ann Graber, puts it, humor combines "optimism with a realistic look at the tragic." Without Pollyanna-like optimism, humor can actively confront, proactively reframe and at times transform the tragic. Consider screenwriter and director Woody Allen musing on mortality. "I'm not afraid of dying," says Allen. "I just don't want to be there when it happens."

And, "I don't want to achieve immortality through my work. I want to achieve it by not dying."

Of course, we have all known people who use humor as a form of avoidance, making jokes even when circumstances call for seriousness. This is not what we are recommending. However, while it may sometimes appear incongruous, humor can be a creative way to confront and cope with what we fear or find painful.

In this sense, perhaps humor may be viewed as a user-friendly and creative form of exposure. As noted in Chapter 3, on facing fear, exposure therapy is a category of treatment for fears that involves facing the feared object or situation. It allows the patient to extinguish or lessen fear by encountering the fear in a safe environment. Humor tends to be safe because it incorporates the feared stimulus in a palatable form, sometimes even belittling it and thereby gaining some control over it.

Jerry White used humor when he endorsed Timberland boots and gave a nickname to his stump. In addition, he recalls:

> We started to play tricks on other amputees in the hospital, like telling new amputees that part of their treatment would be sex therapy with a beautiful psychologist, but that no one really talked about it. [We said] it was the hospital's way of helping you to feel like a man again.
>
> I have always said that humor is everything in recovery, so I'll gravitate to whoever laughs the most. No matter what it's about, even if it is dark humor, it just sort of helps. Once, when lights were going out and I was making some kind of joke, one guy said, "But look at us. Don't you realize what has happened?" And the room went quiet. I thought to myself, stay away from this man, he's toxic to me. I felt irritated and wanted to say, "Shut up, of course we know, but if laughter and joking is one of the ways to muscle your way through, then why would you want to take that away?" And if you do take it away, look at what you become, as sad and depressed as this guy who is really sinking down and not dealing well with his limb loss.

Most of the POWs we interviewed also cited humor as an essential tool in their ability to survive and resist. For example, when Rod Knutson could no longer withstand another day of brutal torture, he "succumbed" to the demands of the North Vietnamese to provide them with information about his personal life. "I told them my dad had a chicken farm and he raised three chickens. I told them that I went to school at Farm District Number One and the only job I ever had was selling peanuts to basketball players." Another POW, Ken Coskey, remembers the nicknames "Big Ug, Zero, and Rudolf" that he and his fellow prisoners used when referring to their guards. Rudolf was the guard with the large red nose.

Staff Sergeant Bobby Henline was never a POW, but his experience ranks among the most severe traumas survived by military veterans (Ledford, 2008). Henline, now married and a father of three, had enlisted in Operation Desert Storm when he was only 17, then returned to civilian life. After the terrorist attacks of September 11, 2001, he re-enlisted and was sent to Iraq. By 2007, he was serving his third deployment there when his luck ran out. Traveling in a convoy, Henline's vehicle struck a roadside bomb; the four other soldiers in his Humvee were killed. Burned over 50 percent of his body, he lost his left hand and part of the arm. His face and scalp were permanently disfigured; most of his hair, ears, and eyelids are gone.

During the months he spent recovering and undergoing multiple surgeries in Brooke Army Medical Center's burn unit, Henline had such a habit of joking with the staff that they told him, "You've got to go do standup." And he thought, "I can't do that." But a year later, he had a new hobby: performing on open mic night at a comedy club in his Texas hometown of San Antonio. In a 2009 interview with National Public Radio, Henline provided a glimpse of his routine:

> In case you didn't notice, I'm a burn survivor. I've been extinguished for years now. It's actually a rare birth defect. It's a sad story. My mother had to work in the circus as a fire eater while she was pregnant and she thinks she has the right to complain about her acid reflux. Mom, come on! (Gildea, 2009)

# Humor and the Brain

Substantial evidence exists for the effectiveness of humor as a coping mechanism. Studies involving combat veterans (Hendin & Haas, 1984), cancer patients (Carver, 1993), and surgical patients (Culver *et al.*, 2002) have found that using humor to reduce the threatening nature of stressful situations is associated with resilience and the capacity to tolerate stress (Martin, 2003). In patients with depression, humor can sometimes diminish depressive symptoms by reducing tension and psychological discomfort, attracting support from others, and creating a positive perspective on difficult circumstances.

Like positive emotions and optimism, humor has been shown to activate a network of subcortical brain regions that constitute core elements of the dopaminergic reward system. In an fMRI brain imaging study of healthy volunteers, Dean Mobbs and colleagues at Stanford University found that funny cartoons, in comparison to non-funny cartoons, caused activation of the nucleus accumbens and the amygdala. A time series analysis showed that as the intensity of the humor increased activity in the nucleus accumbens increased; the nucleus accumbens has repeatedly been linked to psychologically and pharmacologically mediated rewards. Although the amygdala plays a well-known role in fear and fear-related behaviors, it has also been associated with processing positive emotions, and laughter and magnitude of reward (Mobbs *et al.*, 2003; Moran *et al.*, 2004).

Our response to humor can be divided into a cognitive component (understanding the joke – or "getting it") and an affective component (enjoying the joke – finding it funny). In a study of jokes, Vinod Goel and Raymond

J. Dolan (2001) reported that the two components activated different regions of the brain: the cognitive component of humor was associated with activation of the posterior middle temporal gyrus, the affective component with activation of the ventromedial prefrontal cortex. Like the nucleus accumbens and the amygdala, the ventromedial prefrontal cortex has been implicated in representation and control of reward-related behaviors. Thus, humor is linked with areas of the brain that are involved in cognitive appraisal and with reward and motivation, which both appear to be associated with resilience.

# Applying Cognitive Flexibility in Your Own Life

Recent research on coping has shown that successful adaptation depends less on which specific strategies people adopt, than on whether they apply coping strategies flexibly depending on the nature of the stressor (Cheng, Hui & Lam, 1999; Whealin, Ruzek & Southwick, 2008; Bonanno & Burton, 2013). Sometimes it is wise to accept and tolerate a situation, while at other times it is best to change it. Similarly, emotion theorists argue that expression of emotion is not necessarily better than suppression. What helps people cope is having the flexibility to express or suppress emotions in accordance with the demands of a given situation (Barrett & Gross, 2001).

In her *Harvard Business Review* article on resilience, Diane Coutu evokes the concept of *bricolage,* or tinkering, as proposed by the French anthropologist Claude Lévi-Strauss.

> Bricolage in the modern sense can be defined as a kind of inventiveness, an ability to improvise a solution to a problem without proper or obvious tools or materials. . . When situations unravel, bricoleurs muddle through, imagining possibilities where others are confounded. . . Consider UPS, which empowers its drivers to do whatever it takes to deliver packages on time. Says CEO [Mike] Eskew: "We tell our employees to get the job done. If that means they need to improvise, they improvise. Otherwise we just couldn't do what we do every day. Just think what can go wrong: a busted traffic light, a flat tire, a bridge washed out. If a snowstorm hits Louisville tonight, a group of people will sit together and discuss how to handle the problem. Nobody tells them to do that. They come together because it's our tradition to do so." (Coutu, 2002, pp. 54–55)

This practice has served UPS well even through major disruptions such as hurricanes. Moreover, concludes Coutu, the company's ability to continue making deliveries "gave others a sense of purpose of meaning amid the chaos" (p. 55).

We can summarize the strategies in this chapter as: acceptance, reappraisal, dealing with failure, and generating humor. These all require cognitive and emotional flexibility. Here are some suggestions that may be useful if you wish to further develop your cognitive flexibility.

# Acceptance

The well-known Serenity Prayer, which we mentioned earlier in this chapter, captures the essence of the kind of acceptance that contributes to resilience: an acceptance of those things that we cannot change. This type of acceptance is not passive "giving up," but rather a well-considered decision not to waste effort and energy on a fruitless attempt to change the unchangeable. Mindfulness meditation, and acceptance and commitment therapy, are two modalities that readers may explore to help increase acceptance and cognitive flexibility.

The Serenity Prayer is, in fact, a key element of 12-step programs such as Alcoholics Anonymous. "The Big Book" of Alcoholics Anonymous says this about acceptance:

> . . .acceptance is the answer to ALL my problems. Today. When I am disturbed, it is because I find some person, place, thing or situation – some fact of my life – unacceptable to me, and I can find no serenity until I accept that person, place, thing or situation as being exactly the way it is supposed to be at this moment. (Alcoholics Anonymous, 1976, pp. 449–451)

Once we have accepted that which we cannot change, we can focus our attention on what we can change.

In exploring acceptance from a research perspective, Emily Lindsay and David Creswell (2016) have developed a "monitor and acceptance" theory. This theory relates acceptance to mindfulness in a two-phase model. First comes awareness of the present moment. Second is an attitude of "an objective, non-reactive lens" through which to view the present moment, to see the moment for what it is without judging it.

# Reappraisal

The technique of reappraisal is at the heart of cognitive behavioral therapy, which we have described in various chapters in this book. Whether working with a therapist or practicing self-help, one can always ask, "How else can I think about this? How would someone else think about this? What was it like for the other people involved?" Questions like this help to get us out of our own narrow view of a situation and open up new possibilities for coping and problem solving. In their book *Resilience at Work: How to Succeed No Matter What Life Throws at You,* Salvatore R. Maddi and Deborah M. Khoshaba (2005) outline seven steps for a type of reappraisal they call transformational coping:

- Fully describe the stressful situation.
- How could this situation be worse?
- How could the situation be better?
- Create a story about a worse version.
- Create a story about a better version.
- What can you do to create the better version and decrease likelihood of the worse version?
- Place the situation into perspective.

# Learn from Failure

Regardless of how resourceful we are, there will be times when we simply cannot attain a cherished goal. In such situations, when an endeavor, big or small, does not work out, flexibility can be critical.

In an article titled "Failure is the seed of success," business writer Zach Cutler (2014) summarizes five benefits we can derive from experiencing a failure: It propels us to frame our thoughts and goals in a new way, it builds tough skin, it keeps our ego in check, it creates "Aha!" moments, and it prepares us for the unexpected.

David Levin, co-founder of the KIPP network of charter schools in New York City, whose students are almost all from low-income families, observed the importance of character in student success over the long term (i.e., college graduation rates after the students leave KIPP). It was not the students who were brilliant and easily attained top grades who went on to do well, he found; instead, it was the students who struggled but persevered toward their goals (Tough, 2011). Dominic Randolph, headmaster of the highly competitive Riverdale Country School, an exclusive private prep school, came to similar conclusions. Levin and Randolph worked with psychologists Martin Seligman and Christopher Peterson, authors of *Character Strengths and Virtues: A Handbook and Classification* (2004), and Angela Duckworth, who devised the Grit scale (2007), to develop an evaluation system that assessed the character traits that students would need for long-term success. To succeed, the educators concluded, students must first learn how to fail (Tough, 2011).

In their book *Mental Toughness: A Champion's State of Mind* (2005), Karl Kuehl and his co-authors point out, "The ability to make adjustments begins with attitude, and the first attitude is accepting that failure is an education, then learning from the experience rather than becoming engulfed in frustration..." (p. 198). In her book *Stoic Warriors: The Ancient Philosophy Behind the Military Mind*, Nancy Sherman (2007) writes, "If we fail we can always get up again and try again. To be defeated need not mean we are out of the race. Life gives us new contests and new opportunities in which happiness can prevail" (p. 35).

# Humor

Of all the aspects of resilience, obviously humor is the most fun. Humor's value has been recognized for millennia: Proverbs 17:22 tells us, "a merry heart doeth good like a medicine." In his classic book *Anatomy of an Illness as Perceived by the Patient*, first published in 1979, Norman Cousins describes his recovery from an arthritis-like illness that involved chronic pain. After pain-relieving medications failed to help him, Cousins decided to surround himself with funny movies, books, and other sources of humor. He reported, "I made the joyous discovery that ten minutes of genuine belly laughter had an anesthetic effect and would give me at least two hours of pain-free sleep" (2nd edn, 2001, p. 43). Cousins's work inspired a new form of therapy known as humor therapy or laughter therapy. There are even "laughter workshops" and laughter yoga which some people find helpful. Any of us can imitate these strategies and go out of our way to watch funny movies, read funny books, and choose to hang around with people who have a good sense of humor. In *Toughness Training for Life*, Jim Loehr recommends: "Think nutty, goofy, silly, funny, off-the-wall thoughts. . . In almost every situation, being able to laugh puts you in emotional control" (1993, p. 190).

In sum, people who are resilient tend to be flexible: they know when to accept that which cannot be changed and how to positively reframe life's challenges and failures; they use humor to reframe the tragic and that which is frightening; and they regulate their emotions, sometimes suppressing feelings and at other times expressing them. In many respects, resilience requires creativity and flexibility: the creativity to explore multiple viewpoints and the flexibility to embrace a positive but realistic assessment – or reassessment – of a challenging situation.

# References

Alcoholics Anonymous (1976). *Alcoholics Anonymous Big Book*. New York, NY: Alcoholics Anonymous World Service.

American Psychological Association (2008). Acceptance and commitment therapy (abstract). *Systems of Psychotherapy* Video Series. Accessed July 8, 2010 at www.apa.org/pubs/videos/4310860.aspx

Anderson, N. B. & Anderson, P. E. (2003). *Emotional Longevity: What Really Determines How Long You Live*. New York, NY: Viking Press.

Barrett, L. F. & Gross, J. J. (2001). Emotional intelligence: A process model of emotion representation and regulation. In T. J. Mayne & G. A. Bonanno (eds.), *Emotions: Current Issues and Future Directions*, pp. 286–311. New York, NY: Guilford Press.

Boelen, P. A., Lenferink, L. I. M., Boelen, P. A. & Lenferink, L. I. M. (2017). Experiential acceptance and trait-mindfulness as predictors of analogue post-traumatic stress. *Psychology and Psychotherapy: Theory, Research and Practice*, July 14. DOI:10.1111/papt.12138 [Epub ahead of print]

Bonanno, G. A., Papa, A., O'Neill, K., Westphal, M. & Coifman, K. (2001). The importance of being flexible: The ability to both enhance and suppress emotional expression predicts long-term adjustment. *Psychological Science*, 15(7), 482–487. Available at https://www.psychologicalscience.org/pdf/ps/bonanno.pdf

Bonnano, G. A. & Burton, C. L. (2013). Regulatory flexibility: An individual differences perspective on coping and emotion regulation. *Perspectives on Psychological Science*, 8(6), 591–612.

Campbell, D., Campbell, K. & Ness, J. W (2008). Resilience through leadership. In Lukey, B. J. & Tepe, V. (eds.), *Biobehavioral Resilience to Stress*. New York, NY: Taylor & Francis.

Carver, C. S. (1993). How coping mediates the effect of optimism on distress: a study of women with early stage breast cancer. *Journal of Personality and Social Psychology*, 65, 375–390.

Casier, A., Goubert, L., Theunis, M. *et al.* (2011). Acceptance and well-being in adolescents and young adults with cystic fibrosis: A prospective study. *Journal of Pediatric Psychology*, 36(4), 476–487.

Cheng, C., Hui, W. & Lam, S. (1999). Coping style of individuals with functional dyspepsia. *Psychosomatic Medicine*, 61, 789–795.

Comte-Sponville, A. (1996). *A Small Treatise on the Great Virtues: The Uses of Philosophy in Everyday Life*. New York, NY: Henry Holt & Company.

Cousins, N. (2001). *Anatomy of an Illness as Perceived by the Patient: Reflections on Healing and Regeneration*, 2nd edn. New York, NY: W. W. Norton.

Coutu, D. (2002). How resilience works. *Harvard Business Review*, May, 46–55.

Culver, J. L., Arena, P. L., Antoni, M. H. & Carver, C. S. (2002). Coping and distress among women under treatment for early stage breast cancer: Comparing African Americans, Hispanics and non-Hispanic whites. *Psychooncology*, 11, 495–504.

Cutler, Z. (2014, November 6). Failure is the seed of growth and success. *Entrepreneur.* Retrieved from https://www.entrepreneur.com/article/239360#

Dore, B. P., Boccagno, C., Burr, D. *et al.* (2017). Finding positive meaning in negative experiences engages ventral striatal and ventromedial prefrontal regions associated with reward valuation. *Journal of Cognitive Neuroscience*, 29(2), 235–244.

Duckworth, A. L., Peterson, C., Matthews, M. D. & Kelly, D. R. (2007). Grit: Perseverance and passion for long-term goals. *Journal of Personality and Social Psychology*, 92(6), 1087–1101.

Etkin, A., Bücher, C. & Gross, J. J. (2015). The neural bases of emotion regulation. *Nature Reviews Neuroscience*, 16, 693–700.

Finkel, N. J. (1974). Strens and traumas: An attempt at categorization. *American Journal of Community Psychology*, 2(3), 265–273.

Frankl, V. E. (1963). *Man's Search for Meaning: An Introduction to Logotherapy.* A newly revised and enlarged edn of *From Death-Camp to Existentialism.* Translated by Ilse Lasch. Preface by Gordon W. Allport. Boston, MA: Beacon Press.

Gerber, P. J. & Ginsberg, R. J. (1990). *Identifying Alterable Patterns of Success in Highly Successful Adults with Learning Disabilities.* Washington, DC: United States Department of Education Office of Special Education and Rehabilitative Services. Accessed January 15, 2010 at www.eric.ed.gov/ERICDocs/data/eric docs2sql/content_storage_01/0000019b/80/23/d2/bf.pdf

Gildea, T. (2009). Wounded vet takes pain of war to comedy club. Texas Public Radio, December 26. Accessed January 15, 2010 at www.npr.org/templates/ story/storyphp?storyId=121767614

Goel, V. & Dolan, R. J. (2001). The functional anatomy of humor: Segregating cognitive and affective components. *Nature Neuroscience,* 4, 237–238.

Hendin, H. & Haas, A.P. (1984). *Wounds of War: The Psychological Aftermath of Combat in Vietnam.* New York, NY: Basic Books.

Huston, S. A., Blount, R. L., Heidesch, T. & Southwood, R. (2016). Resilience, emotion processing and emotion expression among youth with type 1 diabetes. *Pediatric Diabetes,* 17(8), 623–631.

Isaacs, K., Tsai, J., Harpaz-Rotem, I. *et al.* (2017). Psychological resilience in U.S. military veterans: A 2-year, nationally representative prospective cohort study. *Journal of Psychiatric Research,* 84, 301–309.

Iidaka, T. (2017). Humor appreciation involves parametric and synchronized activity in the medial prefrontal cortex and hippocampus. *Cerebral Cortex,* 27(12), 5379–5391.

Janoff-Bulman, R. (1992). *Shattered Assumptions: Towards a New Psychology of Trauma.* New York, NY: The Free Press.

John, O. P. & Gross, J. J. (2004). Healthy and unhealthy emotion regulation: Personality processes, individual differences, and life span development. *Journal of Personality,* 72(6), 1301–1333.

Kazak, A. E., Simms, S., Barakat, L. *et al.* (1999). Surviving cancer competently intervention program (SCCIP): A cognitive-behavioral and family therapy intervention for adolescent survivors of childhood cancer and their families. *Family Process,* 38(2), 175–191.

Koerner, P. (2010). Innovation – There's got to be a better way. [eZine article] Accessed July 2, 2010 at http://ezinearticles.com/?Innovation–Theres-Got-to-Be-a-Better-Way &id=1384677. Note: Pete Koerner is the author of *The Belief Formula: The Secret to Unlocking the Power of Prayer* (2007) (St. Marys, GA: Bell Rock Press).

Kuehl, K., Kuehl, J. & Tefertiller, C. (2005). *Mental Toughness: A Champion's State of Mind.* Chicago, IL: Ivan R. Dee.

Ledford, T. (2008). Nonprofit helps wounded vet start over: Home for a hero. OperationHomeFrontOnline, August 4. Accessed January 15, 2010 at www.homefrontonline.com/article.asp?articleid=1296

Lindsay, E. K. & Creswell, J. D. (2016). Mechanisms of mindfulness training: Monitor and acceptance theory (MAT). *Clinical Psychology Review*, 51, 48–59.

Loehr, J. (1993). *Toughness Training for Life*. New York, NY: Dutton.

Maddi, S. R. & Khoshaba, D. M. (2005). *Resilience at Work: How to Succeed No Matter What Life Throws at You*. New York, NY: AMACOM, a division of the American Management Association.

Manne, S., DuHamel, K., Nereo, N. *et al.* (2002). Predictors of PTSD in mothers of children undergoing bone marrow transplantation: The role of cognitive and social processes. *Journal of Pediatric Psychology*, 27(7), 607–617.

Martin, R. (2003). Sense of humor. In Lopez, S. J. & Snyder, C. R. (eds.) *Positive Psychological Assessment: A Handbook of Models and Measures*, pp. 313–326. Washington, DC: American Psychological Association.

Martin, R. E. & Ochsner, K. N. (2016). The neuroscience of emotion regulation development: Implications for education. *Current Opinions in Behavioral Science*, 10, 142–148.

McRae, K., Hughes, B., Chopra, S. *et al.* (2010). The neural bases of distraction and reappraisal. *Journal of Cognitive Neuroscience*, 22(2), 248–262.

Millstein, R. A., Celano, C. M., Beale, E. E. *et al.* (2016). The effects of optimism and gratitude on adherence, functioning and mental health following an acute coronary syndrome. *General Hospital Psychiatry*, 43, 17–22.

Mobbs, D., Greicius, M. D., Abdel-Azim, E. & Menon, V. (2003). Humor modulates the mesolimbic reward centers. *Neuron*, 40, 1041–1048.

Moran, J. M., Wig, G. S., Adams, R. B. Jr., Janata, P. & Kelley, W. M. (2004). Neural correlates of humor detection and appreciation. *Neuroimage*, 21, 1055–1060.

Ochsner, K. N., Bunge, S. A., Gross, J. J. & Gabrieli, J. D. E. (2002). Rethinking feelings: An fMRI study of the cognitive regulation of emotion. *Journal of Cognitive Neuroscience*, 14, 1215–1229.

Ochsner, K. N., Ray, R. R., Hughes, B. *et al.* (2009). Bottom-up and top-down processes in emotion generation: Common and distinct neural mechanisms. *Psychological Science*, 20(11), 1322–1331.

Ochsner, K. N., Silvers, J. A. & Buhle, J. T. (2012). Functional imaging studies of emotion regulation: a synthetic review and evolving model of the cognitive control of emotion. *Annals of the New York Academy of Sciences*, 1251, E1–E24.

Orsillo, S. M., Roemer, L. & Holowka, D. (2005). Acceptance-based behavioral therapies for for anxiety: Using acceptance and mindfulness to enhance traditional cognitive-behavioral approaches. In S. M. Orsillo & L. Roemer (eds.), *Acceptance-and Mindfulness-Based Approaches to Anxiety: Conceptualization and Treatment*. New York, NY: Springer.

Ortiz, D. (2001). The survivor's perspective: Voices from the center. In Gerrity, E., Keane, T. M. & Tuma, F. (eds.), *The Mental Health Consequences of Torture*. New York, NY: Kluwer Academic/Plenum Publishers.

Park, C., Cohen, L. & Murch, R. (1996). Assessment and prediction of stress-related growth. *Journal of Personality*, 64, 71–105.

Reeck, C., Ames, D. R. & Ochsner, K. N. (2016). The social regulation of emotion: An integrative, cross-disciplinary model. *Trends in Cognitive Sciences*, 20(1), 47–63.

Seligman, M. & Peterson, C. (2004). *Character Strengths and Virtues: A Handbook and Classification*. Washington, DC/New York, NY: American Psychological Association/Oxford University Press.

Sherman, N. (2007). *Stoic Warriors: The Ancient Philosophy Behind the Military Mind*. New York, NY: Oxford University Press.

Shibata, M., Terasawa, Y., Ito, Y. *et al.* (2017). Time course and localization of brain activity in humor comprehension: An ERP/sLORETA study. *Brain Research*, 1657, 215–222.

Siebert, A. (1996). *The Survivor Personality*. New York, NY: Pedigree Books.

Silver, R. C., Holman, E. A., McIntosh, D. N., Poulin, M. & Gil-Rivas, V. (2002). Nationwide longitudinal study of psychological responses to September 11. *Journal of the American Medical Association*, 288, 1235–1244.

Sirois, F. M. & Hirsch, J. K. (2017). A longitudinal study of the profiles of psychological thriving, resilience, and loss in people with inflammatory bowel disease. *British Journal of Health Psychology*, 22(4), 920–939.

Smith, N. B., Mota, N., Tsai, J. *et al.* (2016). Nature and determinants of suicidal ideation among U.S. veterans: Results from the national health and resilience in veterans study. *Journal of Affective Disorders*, 197, 66–73.

Stockdale, J. B. (1984). *A Vietnam Experience*. Stanford, CA: The Hoover Institution.

Sullenberger, C. B. III, with Zaslow, J. (2009). *Highest Duty: My Search For What Really Matters*. New York, NY: HarperCollins.

Tedeschi, R. G., Park, C. L. & Calhoun, L. G. (eds.) (1998). *Posttraumatic Growth: Positive Changes in the Aftermath of Crisis*. Mahwah, NJ: Lawrence Erlbaum Associates.

Thompson, R. W., Arnkoff, D. B. & Glass, C. R. (2011). Conceptualizing mindfulness and acceptance as components of psychological resilience to trauma. *Trauma Violence Abuse*, 12(4), 220–235.

Tough, P. (2011). What if the secret to success is failure? *New York Times Magazine*, September 14. Retrieved from www.nytimes.com/2011/09/18/magazine/what-if-the-secret-to-success-is-failure.html

Troy, A. S. & Mauss, I. B. (2011). Resilience in the face of stress: Emotion regulation as a protective factor. In S. M. Southwick, B. T. Litz & D. Charney *et al.* (eds.) *Resilience and Mental Health: Challenges across the Lifespan*, pp. 30–44. Cambridge, UK: Cambridge University Press.

Tsai, J., Tsai, J., Sippel, L. M. *et al.* (2016). Longitudinal course of posttraumatic growth among U.S. military veterans: Results from the national health and resilience in veterans study. *Depression and Anxiety*, 33, 1, 9–18.

Whealin, J.M., Ruzek, J.I. & Southwick, S. (2008). Cognitive behavioral theory and preparation for professionals at risk for trauma exposure. *Trauma, Violence, and Abuse*, 9, 100–113.

White, J. (2008). *I Will Not Be Broken: Five Steps to Overcoming a Life Crisis.* New York, NY: St. Martin's Press.

Woidneck, M. R., Morrison, K. L. & Twohig, M. P. (2014). Acceptance and commitment therapy for the treatment of posttraumatic stress among adolescents. *Behavior Modification*, 38(4), 451–476.

Zauszniewski, J. A., Bekhet, A. K. & Suresky, M. J. (2015). Indicators of resilience in family members of adults with serious mental illness. *Psychiatric Clinics of North America*, 38(1), 131–146.

# CHAPTER 11

# Meaning, Purpose, and Growth

When philosopher Friedrich Nietzsche wrote, "He who has a why can endure almost any how," he was referring to the power of meaning. Other renowned thinkers have also recognized the powerful effects of meaning – of having a worthy goal or mission in life. As Carl Jung wrote in his classic *Man and His Symbols*, "[Man] can stand the most incredible hardships when he is convinced they make sense" (1968, p. 76). South African dissident Nelson Mandela stands as an inspiring example: Mandela was able to tolerate 30 years of imprisonment with grace and dignity because his imprisonment symbolized the struggle for equality. Meaning can give us strength and meaning can give us courage. During your own life, when called upon to defend a cherished idea, stand up for a worthy cause, or protect a loved one, perhaps you have been surprised by the reservoir of strength and resilience that lies within.

Undoubtedly the best-known and most influential advocate for finding meaning is Holocaust survivor Viktor Frankl, who wrote:

> Deep down, in my opinion, man is dominated neither by the will-to-pleasure [as proposed by Sigmund Freud] nor by the will-to-power [Alfred Adler], but by what I like to call man's will to meaning; that is to say, his deep-seated striving and struggling for a higher and ultimate meaning to his existence. (1958, p. 20)

In psychological research, studies have found that having a clear and valued purpose, and committing fully to a mission, can markedly strengthen one's resilience. University of Missouri psychologist Laura A. King and her colleagues (King, Heintzelman & Ward, 2016) proposed methods for defining and measuring feelings of meaning and the degree to which individuals experience their lives as meaningful. They argue that far from being "the icing on the cake of psychological well-being" (p. 211), living a meaningful life is a basic human need, without which we can easily fall into despair, alienation, or even violent acts against others or ourselves

Yale School of Management professor Amy Wrzesniewski studied how people view the meaning of their work – something that occupies half of many people's waking hours, week after week. She found that "most people see their work as either a Job (focus on financial rewards and necessity rather than pleasure or fulfillment; not a major positive part of life), a Career (focus on advancement), or a Calling (focus on enjoyment of fulfilling, socially useful work)" (Wrzesniewski *et al.*, 1997, p. 21). In keeping with Frankl's conception of service as a pillar of meaning, the ability to see one's work as a calling may enhance resilience. This holds true even for people performing "dirty work" jobs (e.g., hospital cleaners) and for people who have been prevented from pursuing their chosen career.

Donald Campbell and colleagues in the Department of Behavioral Sciences and Leadership at West Point teach future military commanders that it is critical for their soldiers to understand and embrace the significance of their duty, service, and sacrifice. Campbell has found that soldiers who believe in the importance of their mission, even if it is dangerous, derive greater benefits from their work than do soldiers who do not believe in the mission. This was borne out by researchers Thomas Britt, Amy Adler, and Paul Bartone (2001) in a prospective study of 161 US soldiers participating in a stressful peacekeeping mission in Bosnia. The researchers found that soldiers who considered this work to be meaningful later reported greater benefits from the mission compared to soldiers who found it less meaningful.

Civilian workers who feel a sense of purpose in their work also exhibit strength in the face of work-related stress. In a study of city bus drivers, Paul Bartone (1989) found that those who were high in hardiness (a construct related to resilience) were generally proud of their work and found it to be meaningful. When faced with work-related stressors, these individuals fared better than those for whom driving a bus was "just a job." Similarly, in a 12-year longitudinal study of employees at Illinois Bell Telephone, Salvatore Maddi (1987) found that workers who reported a purposeful direction in their community, school, and work activities were more resilient during an organizational crisis than were workers who lacked such direction.

In our own clinical work and research, we have looked for ways to help patients derive strength in the wake of their traumatic experiences. Twenty years ago, at the Yale University-affiliated division of the Veterans Administration National Center for PTSD, McDonough, Gilmartin, Morrissey and Southwick (2006) developed a treatment program for combat veterans with chronic PTSD that was based on logotherapy, an intervention created by Frankl and several of his students. The literal meaning of logotherapy is "healing through meaning." For years we had worked with veterans who expressed doubts about the meaning of their lives. Many of them had experienced the darkest side of human nature and were plagued by painful memories and feelings of aimlessness and sometime guilt.

These feelings affected their work, family relations, and spirituality. Many had little desire to fully engage in life.

In a 2006 article that described this treatment program, we wrote that logotherapy directly addresses

> the dialectic of fate and freedom that may be expressed as follows: Even though we as human beings cannot often control the circumstances in our lives (fate), we usually can control our attitudes and responses to those circumstances. As one protégé of Frankl put it, "[T]he meaning of fate lies in our response to it. . . Chance decides what happens, but we decide how to take it." (Southwick *et al.*, 2006, p. 162; quote from Lukas, 2000)

In this article, we described how community service was an integral part of the treatment plan for these veterans. Through community service, patients often discover a sense of purpose by giving to others.

> During orientation to community service, veterans are reminded that they are already experts in many respects: They are experts in fear and psychological trauma, experts in personal and spiritual pain, experts in loss and failure, experts in hopelessness and emptiness, experts in coping with a society that rejects its injured members, and experts in survival and resilience. We next pose the question, "What can you do and what will you do with your expertise?" (Southwick *et al.*, 2006, p. 166)

Each veteran was assigned to a community service site that tapped into his or her special expertise. For example, if a veteran had been homeless, we recommended volunteering for Habitat for the Humanity. Another veteran, who had spent years living alone, volunteered with Meals on Wheels, which delivers meals to elderly shut-ins. Like the veteran, the recipient of meals may have felt socially isolated and afraid. Or veterans might tutor underprivileged school children, many of whom have been exposed to violence in their inner-city neighborhoods. As a group, the veterans also initiated their own projects.

> For example, the first project – a toy drive and holiday party for children in the foster care system – was meaningful to one veteran who had been abused as a child and wanted "the kids to know someone cares." For another group member, anguished over his inability as a soldier to help children orphaned by war, this work enabled him to effectively help children harmed by their circumstances. And, for a third veteran, the project provided a means for him to confront his regrets of not connecting with his own children, due to longstanding trauma-related emotional numbing, and to work towards connection with his grandchildren. (Southwick *et al.*, 2006, p. 167)

Much of the impetus for the service work was fueled by personal experiences of suffering, guilt, and loss in war.

> One group member, acting on his own, decided to devote a portion of his service-connected disability benefits to fund a partial scholarship in the name of his friend who died in Vietnam. This veteran, who has struggled with survivor guilt over the years,

found a meaningful way to honor his friend, who had planned to return to college after Vietnam. (Southwick *et al.*, 2006, p. 168)

The veterans' role in choosing and originating projects aligns with the idea that "chance decides what happens but we decide how to take it" (Lukas, 2000). Similarly, most of the people we interviewed for this book found ways to exercise whatever freedom they had as they searched for meaning in the aftermath of trauma. Elizabeth Ebaugh, the social worker who was abducted and raped, eloquently describes her search.

> I go inside and ask what this is trying to show me about my own life. What is this trying to teach me? The overarching philosophy that's guiding me is in the way I handle it. There's room for getting really angry that I got raped. What's important is where you stay. If I were to stay in that place of anger and "why me?" and "why did this happen?" then I'm only going to be like a hamster in a cage. So... I take it to a more transcendent place, where I think, how can I use this in my spiritual journey? Maybe this didn't have to happen, maybe there is no reason, but if I give it a reason, if I find a reason for how it can better my life, then that makes it a golden nugget in my life, rather than something horrible.

Although Ebaugh could not control her fate on the night of the horrific incident, she could and did, to a large degree, determine how she responded. Over time, she chose to find value in her trauma, to be strengthened by it, and to use it as a motivation for her own emotional and spiritual growth.

Like Ebaugh, Jerry White chose to find meaning in trauma – in his case, losing his leg to a landmine.

> There are three types of trauma victims: Those people who say why me, and the pity piece that goes with that. Then there's the other Christian martyr thing, why *not* me – with suffering all around, why do I deserve *not* to be in a wheelchair or maimed or burned or whatever? And the third type simply asks, "Why?" This is a healthy question. This question is a search for meaning. For years I never asked the "why" questions, like "Why did I step on that landmine?" Or, "Why were those minefields there in the first place? Who put them there? Why are minefields blowing up people during wars and even years after wars are over?" Now, 20 years later, with perspective and enough living, I understand that the better question is "Why?"
>
> We each have a choice not to be a victim. If someone wants help from me or from the Landmine Survivors Network, they have to make movement toward us because we're not hanging around with the victim club. It's a radical stance. You have to choose to get up, choose life not death. The word "survivor" means to live through it, to refuse to accept defeat. It is a romantic idea and I am still striving to fully achieve it. I won't be defeated.
>
> There is a rescue side to the work, a life-saving side. And that's related to understanding that people get stuck on their victim platforms and that we want to help them get unstuck, and we want to prod them forward.

But White asks survivors to do more than to quit "the victim club."

> It's not just moving people from death to life or from victim to survivor, it's an expectation of survivor citizenship, where people move on and become givers to the community. They could become community leaders, change agents, future peer supporters, whatever, but our expectation, all along, for the Landmine Survivors Network was that it be a movement forward that blessed the community, that took shattered lives, offered some tools to overcome, and then encouraged individual survivors to come back and serve as a role model for others, a living example of survivorship.

Jerry White uses the term "super-survivor" to describe the person who moves from victim to survivor and then takes it a step further. Super-survivors recognize the healing and strengthening value of "paying forward," giving to others and to the community.

One person who has "paid it forward" for most of his adult life is W. Aubrey Webson, a native of the Caribbean country of Antigua and Barbuda who has been blind from early childhood. Webson recalls the general attitude in his rural community: a blind child would either not survive to adulthood or, if he did survive, would be a burden on the family. Nevertheless, he says, his parents "were never ashamed of me and of the fact that I am blind... I always had people who believed in me" (Fleck, 2016, p. 84). He was sent abroad to school in Trinidad because there was no school for blind children on his home island (Robison, 2016). Throughout his career, Webson has been a proponent of blind people and others with disabilities. He has served with the Caribbean Council for the Blind, Sight Savers International, Helen Keller International, and other non-governmental organizations in the United States and elsewhere. For more than 20 years he was a top administrator at Perkins International School for the Blind in Watertown, Massachusetts – and for three of those years he commuted to Cleveland, Ohio, to earn a Doctor of Management degree from Case Western Reserve University. In 2014, he was named Ambassador to the United Nations representing Antigua and Barbuda, and he has used that post to advocate not only for persons with disabilities but also for measures to limit global climate change, an urgent concern for a small Caribbean nation situated on low-lying islands (Robison, 2016). Webson is determined to help others have greater opportunities than those that were available to him in his formative years: "Persons with disabilities should not have to work harder than others to make their contribution, but very often we have to because there are so many cultural and attitudinal barriers to break down" (Fleck, 2016, p. 85).

Judith Herman, a well-known trauma researcher, refers to transformations such as White's and Webson's as a "survivor mission." Trauma survivors who find such a mission recognize "a political or religious dimension in their misfortune and discover that they can transform the meaning of their personal tragedy by making it a basis for social action. While there is no way to compensate for an atrocity, there is a way to transcend it by making it a gift to others" (Herman, 1997, p. 201). That is, these individuals have used their adversity as a catalyst for reaching out to others. In doing so, they try to make life better for their families, their communities, and even for people in societies far beyond their own personal experiences and day-to-day lives. They create foundations and advocacy groups, become tireless volunteers, assume difficult leadership responsibilities, and mentor others.

# Survivor Mission: Shining a Light on the Sudan Genocide

If the word "survivor" can be applied to anyone, it is to Valentino Achak Deng and the thousands of young men and women like him who endured one of the most horrific – yet little-known – humanitarian crises of the twentieth century.[1] Valentino was born in southern Sudan, a region of rivers, grasslands, and tropical forests where for generations his ancestors, the Dinka people, have herded cattle and raised millet, sorghum, and other crops. Many Americans have seen headlines about genocide in western Sudan's Darfur provinces, but the outside world is less aware of similar atrocities within the southern half of the country, beginning in the late 1970s when oil was discovered there.

Valentino was six or seven years old in 1988 when he was one of tens of thousands of children who fled when their homes were attacked by militias from the north. They had seen their parents killed, entire villages burned, wells contaminated, and cattle and crops laid waste. Hiding among the grasses, roots of trees, and in riverbank swamps, these "lost boys" (girls were more likely to have been killed with the adults or carried off as slaves) eventually made their way across the conflict-ridden region, where raiding militias had destroyed sources of food across the Ethiopian border. Along the way, many boys died of disease and dehydration; others were killed by wild animals or by gunfire from the militia groups, against which they were constantly on alert. Valentino had walked more than 500 miles from his village when he and the other survivors reached the relative safety of a United Nations refugee camp.

Life in the camp was comfortable by comparison; the refugees built shelters of sisal bags supported by sticks, and they received regular rations of dried corn and beans, which they cooked in water drawn from the nearby river. Many young boys, Valentino among them, were soon assigned to carry the dead from the hospital tent to the camp's burial area and to dig graves for them. Weeks, months, and years passed as the displaced Sudanese in the camp, now

---

[1] Information about Valentino Achak Deng is drawn from http://www.valentinoachak deng.org/ and Eggers, D. (2006).

numbering over 40,000, awaited word that they could safely return home. Then, in 1991, the overthrow of the Ethiopian government forced them to flee again. This time they went to Kenya, where first one and then another United Nations refugee camp served as home for Valentino.

More than a decade after he had run away from his village, Valentino Achak Deng was accepted as a refugee by the United States. A nonprofit organization called the Lost Boys Foundation helped him to settle in Atlanta, where he supported himself with low-wage jobs and enrolled in college. Ironically, in the United States he experienced not only the pre-judice of white people against black people, but also of African Americans against African newcomers, and of different Sudanese groups against one another.

He witnessed how alcohol, drugs, compulsive gambling, and violent crime harmed some of his fellow Sudanese immigrants. It would be understandable if he and others like him chose to become hostile, or fearful, or simply alienated from the world. But instead, here are Valentino Achak Deng's thoughts as recorded by the American writer Dave Eggers:

> I will reach upward. I will attempt to do better. I will not be a burden... I will always be grateful for what pleasures I have enjoyed, what joys I have yet to experience... I will live as a good child of God, and will forgive him each time he claims another of the people I love. I will forgive and attempt to understand his plans for me, and I will not pity myself. (Eggers, 2006, p. 533)

Valentino Deng had been in the United States for only a short time when the Lost Boys Foundation put him in touch with Eggers, who chronicled his story in the novel *What Is the What* (2006). Valentino's purpose from the beginning of the book project was to draw public attention to the continued suffering in southern Sudan and the political complexities of the fragile peace achieved there in 2005. Eggers channels profits from the book into the Valentino Achak Deng Foundation. Like other humanitarian groups such as Sudan Sunrise, this foundation builds schools, libraries, and teacher-training facilities in southern Sudan, now the nation of South Sudan. In 2009, the foundation opened an educational complex with 15 buildings in Valentino's home village, Marial Bai, and in 2015 he became the education minister for one of the ten states in South Sudan and is now the vice president of corporate social responsibility at an international investment firm. As he wrote in the preface to *What Is the What*,

> My desire to have this book written was born out of my faith and beliefs in humanity; I wanted to reach out to others to help them understand Sudan's place in our global community...
>
> I am blessed to have lived to inform you that even when my hours were darkest, I believed that some day I could share my experiences with others. This book is a form of struggle, and it keeps my spirit alive to struggle. To struggle is to strengthen my faith,

my hope and my belief in humanity. Since you and I exist, together we can make a difference! (Eggers, 2006, pp. xiv–xv)

There are countless other examples of "super-survivors", individuals who have turned their misfortune into a survivor mission; they include, to name just a few:

- Carolyn McCarthy, who was elected to the US Congress on a gun control platform after her husband was killed in a random shooting on the Long Island Railroad;
- Candy Lightner, Cindy Lamb, and the other women who founded Mothers Against Drunk Driving after their children were injured or killed by drunk drivers;
- Terry Fox, the young cancer patient who founded the Marathon of Hope, an annual run across Canada that has since raised nearly $300 million for cancer research;
- Jim Muller, Charles Kenney, Peggie Thorp, and other Roman Catholics who founded Voice of the Faithful in response to sexual abuse by priests; its goal is to "keep the faith, change the church";
- Eddie Canales and Mike Kipp, who founded Gridiron Heroes Spinal Cord Injury Foundation to help injured high school football players after Canales' son became paralyzed from a football injury;
- John Walsh, host of the TV show *America's Most Wanted*, who began his crusade to bring criminals to justice and to help find missing and exploited children after the 1981 abduction and murder of his 6-year-old son.

# Making a "Small" Difference Is Better Than Doing Nothing

One of Viktor Frankl's observations is that meaning may be found even in the most ominous circumstances.

> We must never forget that we may also find meaning in life even when confronted with a hopeless situation, when facing a fate that cannot be changed. For what then matters is to bear witness to the uniquely human potential at its best, which is to transform a personal tragedy into a triumph, to turn one's predicament into a human achievement. When we are no longer able to change a situation – just think of an incurable disease such as inoperable cancer: We are challenged to change ourselves. (Frankl, 1963, p. 116)

Frankl referred to the capacity for finding meaning in adversity as "tragic optimism," optimism in the face of human suffering, guilt, and even certain death. Tragic optimism encompasses the human potential to transform suffering into human achievement and guilt into meaningful action.

Col. Paul Morrissey is a psychiatrist with an emergency medicine background. For several years he directed the mental health program for the

US Military Academy at West Point. Before that, Morrissey served in Iraq, where his mission was to provide combat stress control services to US soldiers stationed south of Baghdad at Forward Operating Base Scania. Adjacent to the base, there was a makeshift burn clinic for Iraqi children.

> We had an Iraqi doctor who served as a translator officially, but he was the main person taking care of the kids, and some of our medics would help out, too. One thing I push out of my mind is that the "clinic" was a Conex, a shipping container with lights, a primitive table, that's it. These kids would come in after being bounced and tossed over rough roads for hours, and their wounds would be covered with yellow, gooey pus, and flies; kids would be sitting there with flies buzzing all around them. It was a horrific thing to see. Some of the kids would come in on stretchers because they were so malnourished they couldn't walk. We would do what we could to fix them up, and send them out looking good with antibiotics and fresh bandages, and they always left with a few Jolly Rancher candies. We were able to provide at least some comfort which seemed to make a little difference, and increased the odds that they would live another week.
>
> One thing that really got to me was the day two burned Iraqi boys came in, one in the morning and a second in the afternoon. The first was a beautiful 15-month-old boy. . . He was turning blue and had no palpable pulses because of low blood pressure, in shock caused by a bacterial infection from the burns. We resuscitated him and were so happy to have saved his life. It was the greatest feeling to win one, and we were all proud and elated. But then the 18-month-old showed up with almost the exact same problem, and quickly coded and died. It was devastating to lose him and we were all despondent, both from seeing this dead kid in front of us, hearing his father's wailing sobs, and knowing that many other Iraqi kids were dying because they weren't getting adequate medical care.
>
> That's combat stress for doctors, watching little kids die of treatable illnesses. There's a sense of powerlessness when you don't have nurses and staff and millions of dollars' worth of equipment supporting you. There you are with 50 Iraqi kids in a shipping container, it's just – whoa – like holy crap, what can we do? When you're here in the US, there's always someone to ask, always someone to help out. There, it's you and a kid – you and your little bag, and someone in deep trouble. It helped us to understand what it was like to be a general practice doctor 100 years ago.

Morrissey explains that most of the children's burns were not related to combat, but occurred instead from open-flame heating in the home, and, in some cases, from abuse. And in addition to burn victims, some children came in with cancer, congenital heart defects, and other life-threatening conditions. For example, one teenage boy arrived with a softball-sized tumor in his neck that impaired his breathing. The diagnosis turned out to be Hodgkins lymphoma – for which, according to Morrissey, the chances of survival in Iraq are slim. One thing most of the patients had in common was that Iraqi doctors had already done all they could for them.

> The families had been told, "Your fate is in Allah's hands. Now go home," because the care of burns is too labor-intensive and the Iraqi hospitals lacked basic supplies. But some parents still decided to travel four or five hours to reach the American base, which is a very dangerous thing to do in Iraq.
>
> There was a five-year-old boy with about half of the skin on his scalp and face burned off. Somebody in Iraq at some point had tried skin grafts, but it didn't work very well, and half of his head was an open oozing wound. Over the course of a few months he was coming in two or three times a week for dressing changes, which was very painful, and he would try to be tough and not cry, but often he couldn't help it. We were all frustrated because we were supposedly "helping" this kid, but what we were actually doing was torturing him. We would give him pain medication, but that made him dizzy for a few hours, so eventually he didn't want any pain medication. I was amazed at his strength and stoicism and courage, but I knew that he needed much more than we could give him in Iraq.

Soon Morrissey was talking with military chaplains and US embassy staff to unravel the bureaucratic logistics of securing passports and visas for the young boy and his father to leave Iraq, raising money for his travel expenses, and finding a US hospital willing to donate care. Many enlisted soldiers at Forward Operating Base Scania made donations, small and large, out of their modest earnings. This was the beginning of the Iraqi Children's Project, a not-for-profit corporation that partners with Boston Shriners Hospital and various other hospitals in the United States, including Massachusetts General Hospital, Jefferson Medical College in Philadelphia, SUNY Upstate Medical University in Syracuse, and others – to bring critically ill and injured Iraqi children and their parents and guardians to the United States to provide advanced medical care.

In organizing the Iraqi Children's Project, Morrissey took meaningful action in the midst of a seemingly impossible situation. Despite the "whoa," the seemingly hopeless circumstances, Morrissey created meaning. This reminds us of the Jewish proverb, "It is better to light one small candle than to curse the darkness." Morrissey has what we referred to earlier as tragic optimism, optimism in the face of human suffering. He and the partners of the Iraqi Children's Project have been doing what they can, rather than cursing the darkness.

Morrissey's work illustrates the concept we described in Chapter 4 on moral compass: that we are responsible for what we can control, and not responsible for what is beyond our control. This distinction, central to Stoic philosophy, was also described by World Trade Center survivor Jimmy Dunne, whom we introduced in Chapter 1. Speaking to a business audience in 2004, Dunne distinguished between "the infinite things," which an individual person cannot control such as, the horror of an airplane smashing into a building – and "the finite things" that we can control: attitude, effort, conduct.

In choosing to turn misfortune into a springboard for helping others, survivors of trauma often discover in themselves unexpected tenacity and strength, and these qualities become of the foundation for purposeful living.

It is important to acknowledge that in some cases becoming a "super-survivor" is not an option. For example, a terminally ill patient may be incapacitated to the point of depending upon others even for basic daily activities like eating and bathing. Sometimes the best one can do is to accept and find meaning of a personal nature while living through the last stages of an illness. Accepting one's own imminent death, or that of a loved one, may be one of the most difficult tasks that we face as humans. In his book *Hand to Hand: From Combat to Healing*, former British Royal Marine and PTSD sufferer Nigel Mumford (2000) points out that "cure" is a medical term, and that not everyone can experience cure. However, healing can be spiritual and emotional, and, unlike cure, healing may be available to those who have the capacity to choose it. In her book on death and dying, *The Journey Home*, Ann Graber writes,

> As a first step when hospice is invited into the treatment team, the illusion that recovery will be forthcoming has to be given up. Denial of approaching death can no longer be sustained; neither by the patient, nor by the family. Those who can accept this inevitability, in spite of the anguish it may cause, are preparing for a harmonious parting of ways on their journey home... The transformative process – inherent in unavoidable suffering – makes us realize that tragedy often contains the seeds of grace: We can become more than we were before, by facing the challenges life presents to us. (2009, pp. 31–32)

## Posttraumatic Growth

To understand how some trauma survivors create new meaning and purpose out of what may seem to be a cruel and meaningless world, Ronnie Janoff-Bulman (1992) from the University of Massachusetts has described two types of meaning: meaning as comprehensibility, and meaning as significance. In the immediate aftermath of a trauma, survivors struggle to comprehend what has happened. They may have trouble believing and accepting that a loved one is gone forever or that they have lost all of their possessions. Their longstanding assumption that the world is safe and predictable may be shaken, leaving them feeling vulnerable and lost, and they may repeatedly experience intrusive thoughts about the trauma. However, over time, many survivors find that their attempts to comprehend the trauma gradually shift; their new focus is then to create meaning out of the trauma.

To assess posttraumatic growth, Richard Tedeschi and Lawrence Calhoun developed the Posttraumatic Growth Inventory (1996), which includes three general domains: changes in the perception of self, changes in the experience of relationships with others, and changes in one's philosophy of life. Changed perception of self can be summarized by the statements, "I've been through the absolute worst that I know. And no matter what happens, I'll be able to deal with it," and "I am more vulnerable than I thought, but much stronger than I ever imagined." Changes in the experience of relationships with others include feeling a stronger connection with other people and greater compassion for those who suffer. Changes in philosophy often grow out of existential questions about the meaning of life and one's purpose in a world replete with inexplicable suffering. Recognizing that the trauma has engendered growth may give purpose to the trauma.

We have used Tedeschi and Calhoun's Posttraumatic Growth Inventory in our own research with veterans of Operation Enduring Freedom (Afghanistan) and Operation Iraqi Freedom, as well as with former Vietnam POWs. In a study of nearly 300 Iraq and Afghanistan veterans (Pietrzak *et al.*, 2010), our colleague Robb Pietrzak found that 72 percent reported growth in at least one of the assessed areas as a result of their service. The most common areas of growth were changing priorities about what is important in life (52.2 percent) and greater perception of ability to handle difficulties (48.5 percent). In a more recent study of 3,157 US veterans (Tsai *et al.*, 2015) approximately 50 percent of all veterans – and 70 percent of those diagnosed with PTSD – reported at least moderate posttraumatic growth in relation to their worst traumatic event. Posttraumatic growth has also been reported in other groups of trauma survivors including cancer patients, refugees, and survivors of disasters.

It is important to understand that intense psychological distress does not preclude posttraumatic growth. Our findings suggest that posttraumatic growth is most likely to develop when PTSD symptoms are moderate, but not when they are too severe (Tsai *et al.*, 2015). Posttraumatic growth is also less likely in people whose PTSD symptoms are minimal. Perhaps, in order to promote growth, a traumatic experience must cause enough distress to shake the individual's view of the world and his or her place in it. Perhaps it must be disruptive enough to force individuals to reassess, revise, and rebuild fundamental aspects of their psychological, philosophical, and/or spiritual lives.

When we used the growth inventory to assess 30 former Vietnam POWs (Feder *et al.*, 2008), 93 percent described greater appreciation of life as a result of their imprisonment, 80 percent greater personal strength, and 50 percent or more described improved relationships, openness to new possibilities, and spiritual change. Among the former prisoners, there was no difference in growth inventory scores between those with PTSD and those without it. Understandably, not a single man said he would choose to repeat the experience. However, most were able, over time, to take a profoundly painful experience and make it meaningful by viewing it as a force that helped to shape their character.

Interestingly, our research also suggests that posttraumatic growth from one trauma can increase resilience to subsequent traumas (Tsai *et al.*, 2016). In a study of 1,057 US veterans followed for two years, we found that veterans who had reported gains in personal strength from a major trauma in their life were less likely to be negatively affected by a subsequent trauma, perhaps as a result of developing greater coping skills. These findings have implications for therapists and for anyone who has survived a trauma. Looking for and hopefully finding the opportunity to grow in the context of trauma may help a survivor build resilience against whatever difficulties they may face in the future.

## Your Own Meaning, Purpose, and Growth

Thinking back to our formative years, many of us were encouraged to envision and strive toward a meaningful adulthood. Our parents and teachers asked, "What do you want to be when you grow up?" Of course, life ambitions change as we grow older and more knowledgeable about the options available to us. Ideally, throughout our lives we will have the freedom to choose pursuits that allow us to use our own strengths and interests. If we are fortunate, we will have the leeway to periodically re-evaluate how we are using our skills, particularly when we encounter a setback or event that shakes our world view. It is through this process that we can, in the words of Ann Graber quoted earlier, "become more than we were before."

One example of a person who "became more than he was" before is Alejandro Abreu, who was born to poor parents in the Dominican Republic. When he was a small child, his parents brought him to New York City. His family was homeless for several years, but when he was 12 he was offered a potentially life-altering opportunity. He was invited to attend a private boarding school in Massachusetts, funded by a nonprofit program called Prep for Prep. With his father's encouragement, he accepted and thrived. He went to college with the career goal of designing video games. During his freshman year, however he became more and more captivated by English literature and creative writing; he lost interest in his computer science courses, spent too much time partying, and "felt adrift" (Abreu, 2016). When the terrorist attacks of September 11, 2001 turned the habitual American sense of national security on its head, Abreu enlisted in the US Army and was deployed to Iraq. At the time, he recalls, he wanted to "fight for my country, to avenge the dead, to free the oppressed, to make myself feel better, to give my life purpose" (Abreu, 2016).

And he did find meaning and purpose in the harsh conditions and life-or-death camaraderie of his Army experience. In 2007, he returned to college to finish his degree, now with the courage to pursue a major in English, though he "wrestled with the guilt of leaving my brothers-in-arms still fighting the war" (Abreu, 2016). He graduated college and attended law school, and along the he way got married. Since completing his law degree, he has worked as a trial attorney with the US Department of Justice in Washington, DC, and as an assistant US Attorney in Cleveland, Ohio. Abreu concluded, "Love, faith, hard work and the kindness of others raised that little boy playing outside the homeless shelter out of poverty and into a position where he can pay it forward" (Abreu, 2016).

Emily Smith, in her book, *The Power of Meaning* (2017) writes that people who believe that their lives have meaning "evaluate their lives as significant and worthwhile – as a part of something bigger. They believe their lives make sense, and they feel their lives are driven by a sense of purpose (Smith, p. 14). She also writes that "a sense of belonging clocks in as the most important driver of meaning" (Smith, p. 56). People who are socially isolated and lonely tend to feel that their lives are less meaningful.

In *Man's Search for Meaning* and *The Will to Meaning*, Viktor Frankl (1963; 1969/2014) points out that what is meaningful for one person may not be meaningful for another, or for the same person at a different point in life. For Frankl, meaning is not handed to us: We must search for it, in the concrete experiences of our daily lives.

Searching for meaning and purpose is often discussed in psychotherapy and pastoral counseling. Earlier in this chapter we described logotherapy; unlike many traditional forms of psychotherapy, logotherapy looks to the future rather than examining the past, and it focuses on the patient's areas of strength rather than solely on symptoms of psychopathology. Logotherapy uses several basic techniques: "self-distancing (learning to gain distance from and observe the self); paradoxical intention (wishing for or doing that which is feared); Socratic dialogue (interviewing designed to elicit the patient's own wisdom); and dereflection (redirecting attention from the self toward other people or meaningful goals)" (Southwick *et al.*, 2006, pp. 162–163).

Another therapy that incorporates the search for meaning and purpose is called well-being therapy, which is based on Carol Ryff's multidimensional model of well-being (Ryff & Singer, 1998; Ryff, 2012). These dimensions include autonomy, environmental mastery, personal growth, positive relations with others, purpose in life, and self-acceptance. Well-being therapy is conducted in three phases. In the first phase, the client is asked to identify moments of well-being and to describe the circumstances surrounding those positive experiences. In the second phase, the client learns to recognize how his or her own actions or thoughts may prematurely interrupt a well-being experience. Finally, in the third phase, the therapist orients the patient to Ryff's multidimensional model and discusses how each of its dimensions can be used to maximize well-being in the client's life.

But how can I search for and find meaning and purpose in my own life? Again, we turn to Frankl, whose advice grows from his profound understanding of trauma, tragedy and resilience. Frankl recommends that we search for meaning not by asking, "What is the meaning of my life?" but instead by asking, "What is life asking of me?"; not by asking, "What can I expect from life?" but rather, "What does life expect from me?" Frankl seems to be saying that none of us knows exactly how we became the person we are today, or how we arrived in this specific place, at this specific time in history. We did not choose our parents and had no say about the time or place of our birth. During our lives, of our countless experiences, we chose only some; many we did not. Nevertheless, here we are, right now, with a unique set of life experiences, skills and talents.

What is life asking of me? Everything. Everything I've got. Or, as Frankl put it (1986), life is asking me to fill the space in which I happen to have landed. My station in life, my occupation – they do not matter. What matters is what I do with what I have.

Recently, one of us (SS) had the privilege of serving as a co-therapist in a group for veterans who have been struggling with PTSD for years. The group is focused on healing through meaning and on how to help other veterans who are also struggling. One group member was a medic in Vietnam. He is confined to a wheelchair because he has a neurological disorder. He is an articulate and generous man. At the beginning of a recent group, when asked how he was doing, he replied, "I'm doing the best I can with what I've got."

# References

Abreu, A. (2016). Voice: finding beauty. *Think*, 30(1), p. 50. Retrieved from http://case.edu/think/fall2015/finding-beauty.html#.V8jfB4LrtHg

Bartone, P. T. (1989). Predictors of stress-related illness in city bus drivers. *Journal of Occupational Medicine*, 31, 657–663.

Britt, T. W., Adler, A. B. & Bartone, P. T. (2001). Deriving benefits from stressful events: The role of engagement in meaningful work and hardiness. *Journal of Occupational Health Psychology*, 6(1), 53–63.

Eggers, D. (2006). *What Is the What: The Autobiography of Valentino Achak Deng, a Novel*. New York, NY: Vintage.

Feder, A., Southwick, S. M., Goetz, R. R. *et al.* (2008). Posttraumatic growth in former Vietnam prisoners of war. *Psychiatry*, 71(4), 359–370.

Fleck, F. (2016). Don't put a tag on us: Disability is not a side issue. *Bulletin of the World Health Organization*, 94, 84–85, http://dx.doi.org/10.2471/BLT.16.030216. Retrieved from www.who.int/bulletin/volumes/94/2/16-030216/en/

Frankl, V. E. (1958). The search for meaning. *Saturday Review*, 41, September 13, p. 20.

Frankl, V. E. (1963). *Man's Search for Meaning: An Introduction to Logotherapy*. Newly revised and enlarged edn of *From Death-Camp to Existentialism*.

Translated by Ilse Lasch. Preface by Gordon W. Allport. Boston, MA: Beacon Press.

Frankl, V. (1969/2014). *The Will to Meaning: Foundations and Applications of Logotherapy*, expanded edn. New York: Plume, 2014.

Frankl, V. (1986). *The Doctor and the Soul: From Psychotherapy to Logotherapy*, revised and expanded edn. New York, NY: Vintage.

Graber, A. (2009). *The Journey Home: Preparing for Life's Ultimate Adventure.* Birmingham, AL: LogoLife Press.

Herman, J. (1997). *Trauma and Recovery: The Aftermath of Violence – From Domestic Abuse to Political Terror*, 2nd edn. New York, NY: Perseus Books.

Janoff-Bulman, R. (1992). *Shattered Assumptions: Towards a New Psychology of Trauma.* New York, NY: The Free Press.

Jung, C. G., von Franz, M-L., Henderson, J. L., Jacobi, J. & Jaffe, A. (eds.). (1968). *Man and His Symbols.* New York, NY: Random House.

King, L. A., Heintzelman, S. J. & Ward, S. J. (2016). Beyond the search for meaning: A contemporary science of the experience of meaning in life. *Current Directions in Psychological Science*, 25(4), 211–216.

Lukas, E. (2000). *Logotheraphy Textbook.* Toronto: Liberty Press.

Maddi, S. R. (1987). Hardiness training at Illinois Bell Telephone. In J. P. Opatz (ed.), *Health Promotion Evaluation*, pp. 1001–1115. Stevens Point, WI: National Wellness Institute.

Mumford, N. W. D. (2000). *Hand to Hand: From Combat to Healing.* New York, NY: Church Publishing Inc.

Pietrzak, R.H., Goldstein, M. B., Malley, J. C. *et al.* (2010). Posttraumatic growth in veterans of Operations Enduring Freedom and Iraqi Freedom. *Journal of Affective Disorders*, 126(1), 230–235.

Robison, D. (2016). Alumni profile: Ambassador gives voice to the vulnerable. *Think*, 30(2), Spring/Summer, p. 52.

Ryff, C. & Singer, B. (1998). The contours of positive human health. *Psychological Inquiry*, 9(1), 1–28.

Ryff, C. D. (2012). The role of purpose in life and personal growth in positive human health. In P. T. P. Wong (ed.), *The Human Quest for Meaning*, 2nd edn. New York, NY: Routledge Publishers.

Sheehan, C. (2006). *Peace Mom: A Mother's Journey Through Heartache to Activism.* New York, NY: Atria Books.

Smith, E. E. (2017). *The Power of Meaning: Crafting a Life That Matters.* London: Rider Books.

Southwick, S. M., Gilmartin, R., McDonough, P. & Morrissey, P. (2006). Logotherapy as an adjunctive treatment for chronic combat-related PTSD: A meaning-based intervention. *American Journal of Psychotheraphy*, 60(2), 161–174.

Tedeschi, R. G. & Calhoun, L. G. (1996). The Posttraumatic Growth Inventory: Measuring the positive legacy of trauma. *Journal of Traumatic Stress*, 9(3), 455–471.

Tsai, J., El-Gabalawy, R., Sledge, W. H., Southwick, S. M. & Pietrzak, R. H. (2015). Post-traumatic growth among veterans in the USA: results from the National Health and Resilience in Veterans Study. *Psychological Medicine*, 45(1), 165–179. DOI:10.1017/S0033291714001202

Tsai, J., Mota, N. P., Southwick, S. M. & Pietrzak, R. H. (2016). What doesn't kill you makes you stronger: A national study of U.S. military veterans. *J Affect Disord*, 189, 269–271. DOI:10.1016/j.jad.2015.08.076

Wrzesniewski, A., McCauley, C., Rozin, P. & Schwartz, B. (1997). Jobs, careers, and callings: People's relations to their work. *Journal of Research in Personality*, 31(1), 21–33.

## Re: W. Aubrey Webson, the following sources

W. Aubrey Webson / Board of Directors / [International Center for Not-for-Profit Law profile under Board of Directors] Retrieved from www.icnl.org/about/bios/webson.html

Messenger, B. (2014). Perkins International director named ambassador to United Nations: Dr. W. Aubrey Webson to represent Antigua and Barbuda. *Perkins International News*, October 2. Retrieved from www.perkins.org/stories/news/perkins-international-director-named-ambassador-to-united-nations

Dr. Webson officially appointed A&B's permanent representative to the UN (2014). *Antigua Observer*, September 29. Retrieved from http://antiguaobserver.com/dr-webson-officially-appointed-abs-permanent-representative-to-the-un/

CHAPTER 12

# The Practice of Resilience

Resilience is more than a concept. Building it requires practice. But where to begin? This is a complex question for which science does not yet have an answer. However, based on our years of experience in the fields of stress, trauma, and resilience, we believe that for most people it is best to begin by choosing one or two resilience factors that align with their personal values, feel natural to them, fit well with their lifestyle, and that seem doable. And then we recommend consistent practice and patience, because building resilience will take time and sustained effort.

Over time, you can add more resilience factors to your training. As you add factors to your practice, they may interact with one another and enhance your overall resilience. For example, people who become more optimistic often become more likeable – which in turn may open up greater access to social support. Increased social support may then provide the safety net and confidence needed to try out new, more active, creative, and effective strategies for coping with a host of challenges.

Building resilience requires the same commitment and persistence necessary to excel at a sport or succeed at following a fitness regime. The qualities and habits cultivated in athletics – persistence, drive, concentration, dogged commitment, and willingness to tolerate some pain – stand one in good stead when training to increase resilience. The Olympic gymnast Dan Millman, who went on to a career as a motivational speaker, understands that there is no way to wake up one morning transformed. Instead, he says, "Champions form the habit of doing what most people find boring or uncomfortable. The secret of success is no secret at all – it comes from sound preparation, a step-by-step process, and focused effort through the hurdles, peaks, and valleys" (1999, p. 27). *Wishing* to become more resilient is only the first step on a long path that requires sustained effort and willpower.

In the book *The Willpower Instinct: How Self-Control Works, Why It Matters, and What You Can Do to Get More of It* (2012), Kelly McGonigal points out that "Americans name lack of willpower as the number one reason they struggle to meet their goals" (p. 1). On the principle that before you change something, you need to see it as it is, McGonigal believes the best way to improve willpower is to pay attention to how and why you lose it. Do this as a nonjudgmental observer – just as the mindfulness meditation technique would recommend. The tendencies of avoidance, procrastination, and giving in to cravings are universal; we all have them to some degree in some situations. We have urges and instincts (the ancient brain) and impulse control (the modern brain), and we switch back and forth between them. Your present self wants one thing, but your future self will be better off if you do something else. McGonigal finds that willpower is not a matter of conquering the primitive impulses, but of using them in balance with our judgment and goal-directed intentions. It is a matter of training ourselves to bring our actions to consciousness and make good choices, choices that will benefit us in the long term. There is the "I will" power, the "I won't" power, and the "I want" power (i.e., staying focused on one's goal). Training ourselves to harness these three powers is what equips us to gain control over our lives and achieve our goals.

As in any training, there will be successes and failures. If one approach to training fails, try other approaches until you find one that suits you. Remember that even a "failure" doesn't mean that you are out of the race; instead, failure may be an opportunity to re-evaluate and readjust. Six-time NBA World Champion Michael Jordan emphasized this when he said, "I've missed over 9,000 shots in my career. I've lost almost 300 games. 26 times I've been trusted to take the game-winning shot and missed. I've failed over and over and over again in my life. And that is why I succeed" (Goldman & Papson, 1999, p. 49).

In his 2009 book *Got Fight? The 50 Zen Principles of Hand-to-Face Combat*, martial arts champion Forrest Griffin makes an important point: ". . . you're not meant to get everything right the first time around. If you did, it wouldn't be any fun. . . From my mistakes, I learned that I needed to pace myself better. . . I recommend not biting off more than you can chew" (Griffin & Krauss, 2009, p. 28). Instead, Griffin focuses on a long-term strategy of learning about your bad habits and then rigorously training to eliminate them, not just for weeks, but for months and years.

Part of this long-term strategy is to respect the need for recovery after stress or training. Recovery is not just about physical rest after exertion, it is also about quieting intense emotions after a stressful day or a traumatic event. In his book *Why Zebras Don't Get Ulcers* (2004), Robert Sapolsky describes what happens when a zebra is chased by a lion and narrowly escapes death. The zebra has a robust stress response with rapid activation of the sympathetic nervous system and HPA-axis. This fight–flight response allows the zebra to escape. Once the zebra is safe and out of danger, its stress response drops back to baseline rapidly. But this typically is not the case with humans because we have a highly developed prefrontal cortex that allows us to remember the past and ruminate, as well as imagine the future and anticipate. We might lay awake at night wondering, "What if I hadn't been able to escape?" "Why did I stop at that water hole without looking around for lions?" "What if it happens again?" "Will I ever be safe again?" Through this process of rumination and anticipation, humans can, and often do, keep themselves stressed day in and day out, 24/7. Sapolsky observes, "The stress response can become more damaging than the stressor itself, especially when the stress is purely psychological" (p. 13). To become resilient is to develop the ability to quiet the stress response, to return to baseline rapidly once an immediate threat is past. Finding ways to recover can be as important as successfully facing stressors in the first place.

It also helps to understand that no one can be resilient at all times and in all areas of his or her life. Psychologist Howard Gardner, author of *Extraordinary Minds* and many other books, is known for identifying various kinds of intelligence, suggesting that we all have areas of strength on which we can build. Other psychologists, notably Martin Seligman (2002), have advocated a similar approach in identifying one's "signature strengths."

Consider, for example, Lew Meyer, the firefighter who was captured in Vietnam and used physical fitness as a way to save himself and others at the Hanoi Hilton. When Meyer returned home after the war, he continued working as a firefighter; he was an expert at putting out fires. When we asked him if he ever felt afraid during a fire, he replied, "No, I love fighting fires. For me, fighting a good fire is like pitching a no-hitter." In this domain, Meyer was remarkably resilient. However, as often happens when someone is successful in a career, he was promoted to an administrative position. This post required a whole new set of skills, those needed to construct work schedules, evaluate personnel, write budgets, and enforce safety regulations. Meyer found these tasks much more difficult than putting out fires. In this domain, he no longer saw himself as resilient. Does this indicate that Meyer was flawed? Had he failed? Not at all. The point is that each of us is stronger in some areas than others.

When we engage in an activity that calls on our strengths, we may experience a state that has been called "flow." This is a term coined by psychologist Mihali Csikszentmihalyi (1990). When we experience flow, he says we are

> completely involved in an activity for its own sake. The ego falls away. Time flies. Every action, movement, and thought follows inevitably from the previous one, like playing jazz. Your whole being is involved, and you're using your skills to the utmost. (Geirland, 1996)

When Lew Meyer fought fires he often experienced something akin to flow or "being in the zone."

# How Resilience Applies to Our Modern World

In this age of convenience, it may be easier to think about resilience than to actually do what is necessary to enhance it. Here are some practical suggestions for applying the principles of resilience to everyday life in various domains.

# The Individual

Much of this book describes ten resilience factors as they relate to the individual.

- Fostering optimism,
- Facing fear,
- Solidifying moral compass,
- Practicing religion and spirituality,
- Attracting and giving social support,
- Imitating resilient role models,
- Physical training,
- Mental and emotional training,
- Enhancing cognitive and emotional flexibility,
- Finding meaning, purpose, and growth.

However, resilience is also relevant in broader contexts, such as in the family and parenting, in work and career, and even in society as a whole.

# The Family

We all need family. Ideally, it is one of our most important sources of resilience, the place where we learn what it is to feel safe, loved and accepted. It is the place where we feel protected and defended from threats, and where we are encouraged to be our best. The family is also typically the root of values. For many people, early experiences within their family form the core of what enables them to become and remain resilient.

For others, the early family experience is not so favorable. Some of us may harbor vivid childhood memories of knock-down, drag-out fights with our siblings or shouting matches with our parents. As adults, we may benefit from understanding the struggles that our parents may have faced in raising us. Perhaps they came from difficult or troubled families themselves; most likely they were doing the best they could under harsh circumstances. By trying to understand and in some cases "forgive" family members, hopefully we can open the door to rewarding and supportive relationships.

In her autobiography, *And a Voice to Sing With*, the musician Joan Baez (1987/2009) describes the rebuilding of an adult relationship with her activist younger sister, Mimi Farina, also a musician:

> We didn't have much to say to each other for some time. When we talked, the conversation was stilted, guarded, or simply fake. She seemed to be always angry, and I'm sure I just went on doing what I've been accused of doing more than once – namely, telling stories about myself. Then one day in the late seventies it dawned on us that we had not even a remnant of the close and special relationship we'd had for so many years, and we decided, mutually, to get together for lunch and "talk." We were both late, and later on, confessed that we had both taken a Valium just to be able to face each other.
>
> What I remember most about that lunch was that Mimi had no idea of her own strength and growth. When I suggested that she had often hurt my feelings, she thought I was bluffing or lying. She still saw me as powerful and untouchable, and herself as powerless and insignificant. There were lots of teary moments and righteous assertions as to who was right and who was wrong, and not much was settled, but it was an honest effort, and the beginning of the long road back to a close and honest friendship. (pp. 318–319)

This anecdote becomes more poignant with the knowledge that some 20 years after this lunch encounter, Mimi Farina died of cancer at the young age of 56.

Sadly, some families may be so toxic that reconnecting with them can only be damaging. When this is the case, it may be best to create a new "family" that provides a healthy source of strength. We may do this in marriage or a romantic relationship, with a group of friends, or colleagues at work, or with a religious congregation.

Whatever our family history contains, it is always wise to surround ourselves with allies; people who like and accept us, who treat us with kindness and respect, and who encourage us to be our best selves. In good times, these people provide a framework for sharing goodwill and resources; when troubles arise, we can count on them to "be there" for us – as we are for them.

In today's society, we often neglect a core source of family strength – ancestry. How much do you know about your parents, grandparents, and other ancestors? What were their lives like? What hardships did they face, and how did they deal with these hardships? How do their challenges compare to those that you face? The Buddhist author Thich Nhat Hanh suggests that our ancestors are within each of us. They are in our genes and in the way we were raised. They helped make us who we are. Through contemplation or simply through family storytelling, we can learn to draw on the strengths of those who lived before us. In searching for models of resilience, we needn't rely solely on famous historical figures like the "founding fathers," or Martin Luther King Jr., or Helen Keller. We can also find models of strength among our own ancestors, our grandparents, aunts, uncles, and parents, as models of strength.

Family dynamics expert Froma Walsh (2002, 2003, 2011, 2016) advocates a "family resilience framework" in therapeutic approaches to handling adversity. The Walsh Family Resilience Framework comprises nine key processes that resilient families tend to use when responding to trauma and stress. Family therapists may encourage the use of one or more of these processes when helping a family through a crisis:

- Making meaning of adversity,
- Maintaining positive outlook,
- Fostering transcendence and spirituality,
- Practicing flexibility,
- Enhancing connectedness,
- Drawing on social and economic resources,
- Achieving clarity,
- Expressing emotions openly, and
- Solving problems collaboratively.

If you have read this book from the beginning, you will notice that these resilient-family processes resemble the resilience factors we have observed among individuals in our own research. It appears that many of the principles of resilience that apply to the individual are also relevant to the well-being of the family.

# Raising Children

Will our children be prepared for the world they will face as adults? If our goal is to raise a resilient child, we must find the right balance between protecting that child and encouraging him or her to reach their full potential.

As we noted in Chapter 1, a number of social critics have written about trends toward narcissism and cynicism in today's society. In her 2007 book *Generation Me: Why Today's Young Americans Are More Confident, Assertive, Entitled – And More Miserable Than Ever Before*, psychologist Jean Twenge examines the attitudes and feelings of young people ages 18 to 25. She cites archival results of personality tests over the decades since World War II to document increases in the belief that "I am special," in the feeling that one's life is out of control, and in the need for social approval. At the same time, Twenge found that young adults had less capacity to accept criticism, to work toward a goal, and to empathize with others. For example, Twenge and her colleague

Keith Campbell (2009) observe, "On a reality TV show, a girl planning her Sweet Sixteen wants a major road blocked off so a marching band can precede her grand entrance on a red carpet" (p. 1).

In recent years, teachers and child development researchers have commented on "helicopter parenting," an overly involved style of interaction in which the parent hovers over the child and swoops in to help whenever the child encounters adversity. In a November 2009 cover story, *TIME* magazine observed:

> The insanity crept up on us slowly; we just wanted what was best for our kids. . . But in the 1990s something dramatic happened, and the needle went way past the red line. From peace and prosperity, there arose fear and anxiety; crime went down, yet parents stopped letting kids out of their sight; the percentage of kids walking or biking to school dropped from 41% in 1969 to 13% in 2001. Death by injury has dropped more than 50% since 1980, yet parents lobbied to take the jungle gyms out of playgrounds, and strollers suddenly needed the warning label "Remove Child Before Folding." Among 6-to-8-year-olds, free playtime dropped 25% from 1981 to '97, and homework more than doubled. . . By the time the frenzy had reached its peak, colleges were installing "Hi, Mom!" webcams in common areas, and employers like Ernst & Young were creating "parent packs" for recruits to give Mom and Dad, since they were involved in negotiating salary and benefits. (Gibbs, 2009)

As described in a 2008 CNN article, clinical psychologist Nancy Weisman explains why this parenting style is detrimental to resilience, referring to a sense of entitlement that kids acquire when parents rescue them every time they drop the ball. As a result, children do not learn the consequences of their behavior, how to solve their own problems, how to regulate their own emotions, how to manage stress constructively – in short, they do not learn basic coping skills. "It's important for kids to know they're not going to be rescued," Weisman says (Krache, 2008).

Middlebury College psychologist Barbara Hofer asserts that "One of the primary psychosocial tasks of the period of late adolescence and emerging adulthood is to become an autonomous individual who is self-governing and self-regulating while sustaining a healthy connection with parents" (Hofer & Moore, 2011). She surveyed more than 900 college students and their parents and found that, while the parental generation had communicated with their parents about once a week when they were in college, today's students were communicating with parents almost twice a day (13.4 times per week). Further, "nearly one in five students (19 percent) reported that parents were editing and proofing their papers".

Of course, the concern that inspires extreme over-parenting is typically well-intentioned. At the opposite end of the scale from the helicopter parent is the neglectful parent who does not have time for the child, or who withholds attention or who leaves a "latchkey" child to his or her own devices before the child has reached an appropriate level of maturity. Researchers have also expressed concern about the authoritarian parent who controls the child with threats and punishment. Educator James Loehr (1993) points out the disadvantages of this approach: "Fearful children become fearful adults. A child who is controlled by fear – fear of making mistakes, guilt, fear of failure, fear of rejection, fear of loving – will inevitably acquire nontough [non-resilient] ways of thinking and acting" (p. 219).

The British pediatrician Donald Winnicott (1958) coined the term "good-enough mother" for one who protects her infant but does not overprotect, and who fulfills the infant's needs but gradually delays gratification as the child grows older and better able to cope with adversity. This style of mothering allows the child to gradually experience and master more and more challenges. The good-enough mother does not intentionally expose the child to stress that the child cannot manage, but she does encourage ample exposure to challenges that the child can master. In this sense, the "good-enough" mother is the best mother. The same is true of good fathers, teachers, coaches, mentors, and bosses.

Journalist and mother Lenore Skenazy has written a practical guide titled *Free-Range Kids* (2010) in which she advocates allowing school-age children to experience the ups and downs of life without constant adult supervision. In her Free-Range Kids blog, Skenazy writes:

> We don't want our kids to fall off a bike. Who does? But we do want them to learn how to ride. So we have two choices: We can hold onto their handlebars... forever. That way they'll never, ever fall. Or we can wish them luck and then – let go.
>
> Chances are, if we do that, they will, at some point, fall. When they get up again, they'll have two huge things going for them:
>
> - They'll know they can fall and get back up again. If that's not a life lesson, what is?
> - They'll be learning how to actually ride a bike. (Skenazy, 2009)

Most pursuits in life take some tumbles before we get it right. In *Toughness Training for Life*, James Loehr echoes many of the same thoughts:

> Teaching children how to solve problems, how not to panic, and how to think things through clearly before acting, can make a substantial difference in their ability to control negative arousal. Kids need to know how thinking and acting impacts feelings and emotions. Being prepared for tough times simply means a code of acting and behaving that reinforces personal control. Obviously, parents who model tough [resilient] thinking and acting during tough times become the most powerful teachers... Parents who impart a love of life, a passion for living, send a powerful message to their children. No matter how tough life is, there is joy and happiness to be found. (Loehr, 1993, p. 221)

Developing personal control begins early and has an enormous impact on the overall course of life. How well children learn to control themselves will affect their psychological and physical health, their relationships, and their academic, athletic, and career success. In the 1970s, Stanford University professor Walter Mischel developed and studied the "Marshmallow Test". Four-year-olds were presented with a tray of marshmallows and told that they could eat one marshmallow now, or, if they waited until Dr. Mischel returned from an errand, they could have two marshmallows. The Marshmallow Test assesses how well a child can delay gratification. The ability to delay gratification is an essential skill for success in life. It involves tolerating the temporary discomfort of forgoing a smaller immediate reward for a larger reward in the future. Learning to delay gratification is at the heart of willpower. For example, if I cannot delay gratification and say no when someone offers me a donut, then I will never achieve my longer-term goal of reaching a healthy weight. Or, if I choose to turn off the TV in order to complete my homework, I am delaying an immediate pleasure for the longer term valued goal of succeeding in school.

Since Mischel's early research, a number of seminal studies have found that good self-control in childhood is strongly associated with later life success. For example, when adolescents who had taken the Marshmallow Test at age 4 were evaluated years later, those who had waited the longest and delayed gratification as a child handled stress more effectively as a teenager and tended to have higher grades and higher SAT scores, and be more popular.

The well-known Dunedin Multidisciplinary Health and Development Study reported similar findings. This study followed more than 1,000 children born in Dunedin, New Zealand, from birth to age 32 (Moffitt et al., 2011). One of the personal skills that the researchers assessed at intervals from age 3 to 11 was level of self-control during childhood (i.e., concentration, frustration tolerance, persistence, willpower). The research team found that higher level of childhood self-control was associated with better adult physical health, less substance dependence, higher adult socioeconomic status, better financial planning, and less frequent criminal conviction. In fact, childhood self-control was a better predictor of adult health and success than IQ, wealth of family of origin, or social class.

In the late nineteenth and early twentieth centuries, a number of organizations were founded with the goal of increasing resilience in young people. Among them were the YMCA and YWCA, the Woodcraft Indians, the Sons of Daniel Boone, and the Boy Scouts and Girl Scouts (Macleod, 1983). These organizations focused on mental, physical, social, and religious development. Even today the mission of the Boy Scouts of America is to provide "a program for young people that builds character, trains them in the responsibilities of participating citizenship, and develops personal fitness," and the mission of Girl Scouts of America is to "build girls of courage, confidence, and character, who make the world a better place."

Other programs promote specific aspects of resilience in children. One example is the Penn Resiliency Project (www.ppc.sas.upenn.edu/prpsum.htm)

for teachers in elementary and middle school. Headed by Jane Gillham and Karen Reivich, this project offers a series of lesson plans designed to help students challenge negative beliefs and learn "assertiveness, negotiation, decision-making, social problem-solving, and relaxation." As another example, in their book *Raising Resilient Children,* Robert Brooks and Sam Goldstein (2001) describe a classroom exercise that any teacher can use to encourage cognitive flexibility. Teachers ask the class on the first day, "Who feels they are going to make a mistake or not understand something in class this year?" (p. 279). Then, before any students raise their hands, teachers raise their own hands, and they begin a class discussion about the value of making mistakes and learning from them. A third example of a program that can enhance resilience in children is the Giraffe Project, which we described in Chapter 4 on moral compass. The Giraffe Project asks each child to "stick your neck out" to do what is right.

# Work and Career

Many of us have faced – or will face – difficult situations at work – receiving a negative performance review, being passed over for a promotion, or even losing our job. In the book *Firing Back: How Great Leaders Rebound After Career Disasters*, Jeffrey Sonnenfeld and Andrew Ward (2007) acknowledge that "...career distress can be one of the greatest sources of life stress. Being fired, for example, has been ranked... among the most stressful events in life, just after death of family members, jail, and personal injury or illness" (p. 6). However, as devastating as job loss can be, the authors recommend facing up to the reality of what has happened, and using it as a platform for recovery. "Leaders should not be measured by how they bask in the gratification of their accomplishments," they argue. "Rather, they should be measured by how they respond when fate deflates the joys and hard-earned triumphs. How well do they pick themselves up and get back in the race?" (p. 3).

Sonnenfeld and Ward also point out that business leaders who are now household names, like Michael Bloomberg and Steve Jobs, were fired from firms before they started their own enterprises; and that Jimmy Carter, despite failing to be re-elected in 1980, "...continued tirelessly in his humanitarian, public health, and diplomacy missions, heavily promoting democratic reform around the world and was eventually recognized as a Nobel laureate for peace" (p. 3).

While not everyone can be a Steve Jobs or a Jimmy Carter, most of us can bolster our careers by learning to face fear, cultivate realistic optimism, learn from role models, and give and receive social support. The work environment is sometimes viewed as a dog-eat-dog world where one has to "go along to get along," but resilience comes from staying true to one's values and moral compass, even if it means passing up an opportunity for career advancement. And surely cognitive flexibility, humor, and finding meaning and purpose are as valuable at work as they are in personal life.

Indeed, many researchers and business experts have recognized the importance of finding meaning in tasks performed at work, no matter how humble. As an example, The GoodWork Project was developed by psychologists Mihaly Csikszentmihalyi, William Damon, and Howard Gardner in order to advocate and promote "work that is excellent in quality, socially responsible, and meaningful to its practitioners" (Harvard Project Zero, 2017). Employees who understand the significance of their mission at work are more likely to give their full effort, to "go the extra mile." This was the finding of organizational behavior researchers Michael Cole, Heike Bruch, and Bernd Vogel (2006); workers were less cynical and more resistant to the stresses of organizational crises if their supervisor helped them to understand the significance of their efforts.

There are many fine books about career success that incorporate a variety of the resilience factors we have identified. Among these are *The Seven Habits of Highly Effective People* by Steven Covey, and *The Pyramid of Success: Building Blocks for a Better Life* by the famed UCLA basketball coach John Wooden. Wooden was a renowned and beloved basketball player and coach who was inducted into the Basketball Hall of Fame as both player and coach. With Wooden as head coach, the UCLA men's team won seven consecutive NCAA national championships and ten championships in 12 years. Wooden based his formula for success on fundamental building blocks that he described in his Seven Point Creed and his Pyramid of Success. He was given the Seven Point Creed by his father, Joshua, when he graduated from grammar school:

- Be true to yourself.
- Make each day your masterpiece.
- Help others.
- Drink deeply from good books, especially the Bible.
- Make friendship a fine art.
- Build a shelter against a rainy day.
- Pray for guidance and give thanks for your blessings every day.

(Wooden & Tobin, 2004, p. 25)

Wooden spent over a decade constructing his Pyramid of Success. He believed that real strength began with building a strong foundation. In his words, "The first two blocks of the pyramid are the two cornerstones because to be strong, you have to have a strong foundation. The cornerstones of success to me, in anything, are hard work and enjoy what you are doing. So, one cornerstone is industriousness and the other is enthusiasm. The other elements of the pyramid include: Friendship, Loyalty, Cooperation, Self-Control, Alertness, Initiative, Intentness, Condition, Skill, Team Spirit, Poise, Confidence, Competitive Greatness" (Wooden, 2011).

# Society on the Large Scale: Community Resilience

Most of us live in communities where we share with others a wide variety of resources and services. As noted by Dartmouth professor Fran Norris, community members are dependent on one another both in good times and in bad. For example, some traumatic events, such as natural disasters or wars, are experienced simultaneously by a large number of people. Norris writes,

> . . . we must recognize that survivors are connected and dependent upon one another's coping strategies. . . They help each other but also compete for scarce resources. Household preparedness is vital, but one household can no more prepare for disaster than it could, on its own, protect itself from crime or disease, educate its children, or keep the roads safe. Thus an individual's resilience is inextricably linked to the community's ability to prepare for, respond to, and adapt to adverse conditions. Simply put, when problems are shared, so must be solutions. (Norris, Sherrieb & Pfefferbaum, 2010, p. 1)

Norris believes that community resilience relies on effective sharing of resources. In her model, community resilience depends on four primary resources: economic development, social capital, information and communication, and community competence. The first resource, economic development, is influenced by the diversity and distribution of resources in addition to the volume of resources. Communities are more vulnerable and less resilient when they rely on a narrow range of resources (e.g., a city dependent on one large automobile plant) or when distribution of community resources is markedly unequal (e.g., the poorest neighborhood may suffer the most in natural disasters).

Social capital refers, in part, to relationships between the individual and his/her neighborhood, community organizations, and community at large. Elements of social capital that foster community resilience include citizen participation, emotional connection to the community mutual concerns and shared values, and the receiving and giving of social support.

Community resilience also depends on communication and the effective sharing of information. For example, during emergencies, information that is shared accurately to community members can save lives. Finally, Norris describes the need for meaningful intentional action. Resilient communities work together with creativity and flexibility to solve problems.

# Applying Resilience Factors: The Case of Fred Southwick

One of the authors (SS) has a brother who, like Jerry White (mentioned in Chapters 7, 10, and 11), has undergone a leg amputation. On July 4, 2012, Fred Southwick was standing on his paddleboard at Jack's Beach in Ponte Vedra, Florida, when his left leg buckled beneath him in response to a sudden and intense cramp. Later that month, while he was warming up for a Master's rowing race – one of three in which he was to compete that day – the gripping pain returned. As a lifelong athlete, Fred was accustomed to pushing through pain, so he finished all three races despite near-crippling discomfort. One week later, Fred noticed that his left foot had turned white. As a professor of medicine at the University of Florida, he knew this was serious. This was no minor athletic injury; this was ischemic artery disease. His calf and foot had been screaming with pain because they were not getting the blood and oxygen they needed. Fred could not believe what he was seeing.

During his first visit to the vascular surgeon, Fred felt relieved when he learned that a simple arterial bypass would likely solve the problem. However, when the surgeon reviewed Fred's angiogram, he was surprised to find no functional arteries in the lower left limb.

"Fred, I'm sorry, but there just aren't any healthy vessels in your leg that we can use for bypass. I don't know how this happened. Let's admit you to the hospital to explore the area and I'll go in and see if there are any clots we can clean up." Although no one used the word *amputation*, Fred knew what the angiogram meant. He agreed to the exploratory operation but understood it was a long shot.

As Fred expected, the procedure did not improve blood flow, but it did confirm that all the major vessels in his left lower leg were totally blocked, resembling ribbons of calcified stone. The intense pain he had been feeling was the vise-like crushing sensation that patients with angina describe when their cardiac muscle is deprived of oxygen.

After taking time to consider the decision, Fred met with his surgeon and asked him to amputate his left leg. Fred saw no other way, and he refused to live a restricted life in which he was in constant, severe pain and could walk no farther than a block or so without stopping to recuperate. He understood that his life would be different, but he also believed that a below-the-knee amputation would not slow him down all that much. He could still go out at dawn to row on Lake Santa Fe or ride his bike with the Gainesville bike club.

Several days later, his surgeon performed a below-the-knee amputation. Afterward Fred remembers looking down and seeing half a leg and no foot. "It was hard to believe, very strange, almost like I was dreaming."

Fred tried his best to maintain a sense of humor. "This has been a very efficient way to diet. I lost 10 pounds in one day."

At home, the pain continued even with intermittent infusions of the pain medication pivocain. Then, a few days after the surgery, while changing the dressing on his leg, Fred noticed a dark brown jelly-like substance oozing from the wound. Fred suspected that his knee was dying and that he would need another operation to remove the necrotic tissue. He would need a "revision"; an above-the-knee amputation. As a doctor, Fred also knew that above-the-knee amputees face much greater challenges than below-the-knee amputees. Without the knee, there is no place for the large hamstring and quadriceps muscles to attach, and that means that it is very difficult to move an artificial limb. But in his present condition he was a high risk for a life-threatening infection from the necrotic tissue. A second surgery was imperative.

Fred was admitted to the hospital and underwent the revision. Soon he was back home with no knee. For days Fred did not have the energy or the inclination to do anything other than watch television. After 40 episodes of the HBO series *Prison Break*, he wondered whether he might spend the rest of his life sitting on the couch. Fred began to ask himself, "Who am I? Will I ever be able to work again? Will I be able to row again? What will people think of me?" And he remembers getting sick and tired of hearing well-intentioned people say, "Fred, if anyone can get through this, it's you. You will be a real inspiration for others."

Even though Fred disliked it when people told him that he would get through it, they were correct. Within one year, Fred was back at work full-time and competing in rowing races. Fred made it through by using many of the resilience-enhancing strategies that we have described in this book. These include: realistic optimism, facing fears, accepting that which cannot be changed, cognitive reappraisal of the negative and looking for opportunity in the midst of adversity, reaching out for social support, imitating resilient role models, physical fitness and a healthy lifestyle, cognitive flexibility, and searching for and finding meaning and purpose in the context of adversity.

Fred has always approached life from an optimistic but realistic viewpoint. In his words, "You have to look on the bright side whenever you can. Too much negative thinking will sink you. What good does it do to constantly focus on what went wrong or what could go wrong? I won't pretend that I haven't had lots of doubt and plenty of negative feelings, but I never let them stick around for too long. I've been like this since grade school."

Fred also confronted his fears. During the diagnostic process, when his doctors were determining the extent of his injury, Fred was worried. But, when he found out that he needed an amputation, worry turned to fear and disbelief. "How could this be?" he wondered. At the time, Fred did not fully understand that many more fears lay ahead.

At each step of his recovery, Fred faced his fear by learning what he needed to know and what he needed to do in order to achieve his goal. He recalls:

> I was terrified, going to the airport and flying for the first time after the surgery, going to work, starting as an attending on the wards. I was really worried; would my limb hurt too much, would I really be able to function? Would I be able to walk my daughter Ashley down the aisle and dance the father–daughter dance with her at her wedding? So what I did with each new activity was focus on the goal, what I wanted to achieve. I did not focus on what could go wrong because if you focus on what goes wrong, then you will be afraid to do it. I just looked at the goal and thought, "Wouldn't it be nice if I can do this." I didn't say "I can do this," I said, "I hope I can do this."

Eighteen months after his amputation, Fred did walk Ashley down the aisle and dance with her at her wedding.

Fred is someone who embraces a strong moral code. He was raised in a family where stoicism was the name of the game. "What's done is done." Looking back with regret was discouraged. "No sense crying over spilled milk." Instead, the idea was to let go and accept things we are powerless to change. However, in Fred's case, letting go and accepting what he could not change was especially challenging because the loss of his leg may have been due to a previous surgical error. Understandably, Fred felt a great deal of frustration, but he also knew that whatever may have gone wrong was an honest mistake, and that his medical team was highly competent. The right thing to do, he believed, was to get on with his life as best he could; to control what he could control and not complain about what was beyond his control. Of course, this was not easy. Whenever Fred felt sorry for himself or angry about his situation, he summoned up the courage to productively move forward with his life.

While many people turn to religion and spirituality to deal with adversity, Fred did not specifically do so.

> I know that in recovery God can be a partner to lighten the load. I did not use religion in that sense, and that's just me. I did practice my own version of mindfulness and I really did look at my injury from every angle. I didn't avoid it, I looked at what this meant, it was my misfortune, and I accepted it for what it was. I realized there must be a reason why this happened to me and I tried to remain open to the question of where this loss will take me.

For Fred, the most important resilience factor was social support.

> Kathie, my wife, had to wheel me to all my appointments, she had to change the dressings, she had to do everything for what was an incredibly tough year. You really do test your partner when things go bad, and Kathie passed with flying colors. My daughter Ashley, she's a nurse practitioner. She was there with me at every surgery, and she came and helped as a caregiver at the house. My brother flew to Florida to be with me during some of the hardest times. And the group that was just

incredible was my recovery team. They've been amazing in every way. They, and so many of my friends and colleagues, have been very sensitive, concerned and open. They tried to help in any way they could. Resilience is a team sport. You cannot do this on your own; reaching out is critical.

After a few months I began walking without a cane, and I had gone back to work, but with limitations. It was a big hurdle when I actually served as the medical attending for two weeks on the wards, which means being on your feet for hours at a stretch. I was able to attend and I actually had no problem although the Chief, Michael Lauzardo, came with me the first three days of rounds and said, "Look Fred, if you can't do it, I'll take care of it."

Fred also benefited from strong role models.

My father was an orthopedic surgeon. He is 92 now. I remember as a kid, whenever we got hurt he would say, "Oh, it will get better, don't worry about it. You're fine." One time in high school, I sprained my ankle and my football coach told me to ask my father what I should do to treat it. Dad said, "Don't walk on it." And my mother is the ultimate stoic. Even when she was having a serious health crisis, her assessment was, "Well, it's just part of life. I'm getting old." So I learned my stoicism from my mother and my father.

As someone who had competed in sports all his life, Fred was highly motivated to begin physical training as soon as possible after his surgeries. At first, he needed physical therapy to address the healing and functioning of his leg. "It was pretty discouraging compared to what I'd been doing before; here I was with no leg and using a walker." However, physical therapy was just the beginning of Fred's journey.

I realized I had to get my muscle back, so I went to Gainesville Health and Fitness, but with my walker I just could not exercise. I tried to bench press and I almost fell to the floor. I said, "Wow, I need a trainer!" So I went to the person who picks trainers and she said, "I have the perfect person for you." This trainer, Bryon, had played fullback for the University of Florida football team. He got me going the first day. But by the end of the workout the pain in my limb was so intense that I fainted. Everyone was freaking out. [However, over time,] he built me up, I gained back the 20 pounds I had lost. I'm stronger than I was before this all happened.

I was very excited when I got the Genium, which is a high-tech prosthesis with microprocessors and a gyroscope. It actually senses when I'm pushing off, it knows the rate I'm going. What a difference. It's like an ultra-bionic leg. One day I was walking into Gainesville Health and Fitness and someone said, "Wow that looks really cool." I am not sure I'd agree, but anyway she was trying to be nice. I was so pleased when I came home with the Genium, I decided to go to the lake and walk in the grass. Well, it turned out I had the setting wrong and it was releasing the knee too quickly. I stubbed my toe on the grass and fell flat on my face and pulled a muscle in my back. Wow, was I discouraged. I never even made it to the lake. It was really a big low.

I know athletics provides meaningful feedback. You can actually judge objectively whether you're reaching your goals. I really wanted to get back into rowing, but rowing turned out to be a little trickier than you might imagine. When it came to actually rowing, initially I had to use flotations so I wouldn't drown from flipping the boat over because these boats are only a foot and a half wide. If you put the oar in wrong, you flip. Then my prosthesis specialist made a special prosthesis for rowing that has a simple free knee joint. What that allows me to do with my gluteus muscles is actually drive down and straighten the knee so I can get power. With this, I went into competition in the Head of the Chattahoochee race, and I rowed the stroke seat. We covered 3 miles in 17 minutes and 30 seconds and we were in the middle of the pack. I was very proud of our boat. In the midst of it, I was concentrating so hard I just forgot I had a problem with my leg.

Later on, the team wanted me to row in an ergometer [indoor rowing machine] race called the Southern Sprints of Melbourne. The world record for 1,000 meters with an above-the-knee amputation is 3 minutes 45 seconds and they were hoping that I might be able to break that record. My trainer Bryon put in a great training system and I worked through two months of training for this race. So here I am in the race, I've got pretty good bend in my knee, I'm getting good flexion, good drive. By the last 200, I'm not feeling good, it really hurts. Lactic acid like you just cannot even believe. Everyone was cheering me on, hoping I'm going to break a record, but I knew I wasn't, but still I wanted to do it as fast as I could. I ended up finishing in 3 minutes and 53 seconds. So, here I am 70 years old and I'm only 8 seconds off the world record for all ages of above the knee amputees, though I'm not sure I want to do this again, quite frankly.

Fred also talked about the need to be flexible. In his words:

Life equals change. I've been handed a major change and I've accepted that. I knew life would be different; I really did envision it as a challenge and it certainly has been. In medicine, I work in the area of quality improvement, which is kind of ironic. Quality improvement requires that all physicians, all caregivers, all personnel change how they do things. So I'm actually using that in my life as well as my work. I frame my loss as a new athletic challenge. Just as you learn how to cross country ski, I see learning how to walk on a prosthesis as a sport. One of the ways that I determine if I'm being successful is how much people stare at me when I walk by. If I don't see stares, then I did pretty well today and if I see stares then oh darn, my gait isn't as good as I thought.

Finally, Fred has gradually found meaning and purpose in his misfortune. He has gradually developed a survivor mission.

Even though there many many amputees out there, there is not a good network, at least not in Gainesville. There are websites, but I really wanted to ask people, "What did you go through?" and I could not find many other amputees. I realized there are large numbers of patients out there who have been injured and really have no voice. I began organizing patients to give them more of a voice in our health systems so they are treated more fairly and equitably. I've created a website where I've shared my experience and that of other patients who have been injured. And what it's done for me, I can tell you, having experienced warmth, empathy and caring from others has made me far more empathetic as a physician in my care of patients. Furthermore, I can tell that my patients sense this. I don't even know what I'm doing, but they know I understand and I really don't sweat the small stuff.

# Activities That Incorporate Multiple Resilience Factors: A Few Examples

As we have pointed out earlier, resilience factors tend to build upon one another and sometimes operate synergistically. Here are just a few examples.

# Become a Volunteer

Volunteering to join with others in the pursuit of a worthy goal has many potential benefits. First and foremost, it can provide aid to an organization, to a cause, or to people in need. But it can also strengthen the volunteer, him- or herself, by enhancing one or more resilience factors.

After giving a talk on resilience to a Yale Medical School Alumni group, one of us (SS) was approached by a board member from the Hole in the Wall Gang Camp, a no-fee outdoor retreat for children with cancer and other serious illnesses that was founded by the actor and philanthropist Paul Newman. The board member felt that the principles of resilience were strongly related to the camp's mission. The following summer I volunteered to serve for a week as a camp counselor at The Hole in the Wall Gang Camp in Ashford, Connecticut. Following the success of the Ashford camp, other sister camps have opened throughout the United States and overseas, all serving children with serious illnesses.

As I drove to Ashford, I didn't know exactly what to expect. I had been a camp counselor at age 20, but that was a long time ago, and the kids I counseled were not sick. I did know that I would be sleeping on a bunk bed in a cabin with 12-year-old boys.

Entering the grounds, I was impressed with the beauty of the place: a compound of sturdy, well designed but rustic looking buildings set near a pristine New England lake. The camp was equipped with an infirmary staffed by expert medical personnel, a theater where the kids had a chance to perform, a building devoted to arts and crafts, a boathouse, a horseback riding stable, a gymnasium, and a grand hexagonal dining hall that resembled a huge American Indian lodge with multicolored banners hanging from its vaulted ceiling.

During the weekly orientation for new volunteers, I was introduced to my two new bosses, college-age counselors, who had both worked at the camp for several years. They made me feel right at home.

When I first walked into the cabin, six or seven boys were playing a game of some sort, and one of the counselors was helping another boy unpack his clothes. I said hello and was directed to one of the upper bunks, which had my name taped on it. I unpacked my gear and then stepped into the bathroom. Looking into the mirror, I was startled to see this old guy with white hair staring back. "That can't be me," I thought. I must look like a frail grandfather to these kids. Somehow, before coming to the camp, I had convinced myself that I was still that "cool" 20-year-old counselor who loved to challenge campers to running races and games of basketball, and who was up on the latest in pop culture and hip music. Now I began to wonder if the Hole in the Wall Gang campers would have any interest in listening to the cassette tapes of The Byrds, Three Dog Night, and Peter, Paul and Mary. I began to feel uneasy, a little anxious, pretty irrelevant.

Now what? Why would these kids want to hang out with an old guy like me? Maybe signing up to be a volunteer counselor wasn't such a good idea.

Just then, one of the boys walked up to me and asked, "Steve, would you like to be on my team?"

"Sure," I replied. "But I don't know the rules, and I don't know if I will be any good at it."

"Don't worry," he said. "We'll teach you. You'll be OK. It's not that hard."

And, indeed, with his invitation, I was now OK. I was now a member of the team. The mission of the Hole in the Wall Gang Camp is to give children suffering from major medical illnesses the chance to spend time in a rural setting where they can just plain have fun. That's what Paul Newman wanted for all children, no matter how ill. He wanted them to have a relatively carefree week of fun.

Even though all of the kids had a serious medical illness, and in some cases a major physical disability, they knew how to have fun; they invented games, cracked jokes, and made friends in a matter of minutes. They were not entitled, narcissistic, Me-generation types. Instead, they were fun-loving, generous and kind. Over the course of the week, I don't remember hearing a single complaint from any of the kids about his illness.

When I look back on this week and think about resilience, a number of factors stand out. Serving as a volunteer counselor helped – and at times forced – me to step out of my comfort zone, increase my flexibility, contribute to a worthy goal, receive and give social support, and look more closely at my own purpose and mission in life. However, the most powerful boost to my own resilience came in the form of role models: the devoted, sturdy and selfless men and women on the staff, and, most important, the boys in my cabin. I continue to be impressed by the degree of resilience, bravery, and grace that I witnessed in these young gentlemen, and try my best to imitate them. There are an unlimited number of ways to volunteer your time and energy. You can serve at a soup kitchen, join a choir, tutor a child, teach an adult to read, help build a house for the homeless, clean up a neighborhood park, or work for world peace. As an example, our friend Martha is a retired nurse who volunteers with the Red Cross in her community. One weekend a month, she is on call. If an event such as a fire, a flood, a water main break or a gas leak occurs in her community and people need to be evacuated, Martha is the nurse on duty at the Red Cross evacuation site. Another friend, Paul, is an experienced businessman who volunteers with Service Corps of Retired Executives (SCORE) to help people prepare tax returns. Gladys, who has always enjoyed painting and sewing, volunteers at her local senior center by teaching classes in fabric painting. Dorothy, who was widowed several years ago, volunteers with a local hospice by facilitating a weekly grief support group. And George, a junior in college, started a drop-in tutoring service for students who needed help with their course work.

Depending on the organization, volunteering may also provide us with opportunities to deepen our religious or spiritual practice (e.g., participating in a religious-based mission), to exercise moral courage (e.g., joining a group that fights against a perceived injustice), to improve physical health (e.g., participating in a bike ride to raise funds for cancer research), and/or to boost brain fitness (e.g., becoming a tutor or volunteer consultant). And for anyone, the experience may foster cognitive and emotional flexibility. This results, in part, because volunteering typically involves stepping out of one's normal routine and sometimes out of one's social, geographic, or cultural comfort zone. In addition, volunteer organizations often bring together a heterogeneous group of individuals from different work and family backgrounds, and they typically operate within a structure or hierarchy that differs from the one the volunteer is accustomed to at work or at home.

# Athletic Competition

Physical exercise, as we have described in Chapter 8, is associated with both physical and emotional resilience. Although we can build resilience by exercising alone, exercising with a friend adds social support, and by joining a competition we actively seek to challenge and test ourselves. Even better, competition involving team sports provides us with camaraderie and opportunities to find new role models. Finally, competing for a cause – for example, a 10 kilometer run for cancer – adds the dimension of altruism. Whether consciously or not, we may put to work at least five resilience factors by participating in such an event. Opportunities abound: as just one of countless possible examples, the Team in Training (TNT) program organizes marathons, half-marathons, bike rides, ski marathons, and other athletic events to raise money for the Leukemia & Lymphoma Society.

In the United States today, some teachers and parents believe that competition is destructive to the emotional well-being of children, and they try to create an alternate world where everyone is a winner, where everyone wins a trophy. However, competition is unavoidable. It permeates modern life: we compete in athletics, for entrance into college, for jobs, even for mates. Sometimes we win and sometimes we lose.

Jeff Gruen, the father of Deborah, the remarkable young woman born with a potentially disabling condition whom we met earlier in the book, learned about the value of competition from both of his daughters. Until his daughters joined the local swim club, Gruen believed that competition was bad, that it undermined confidence, camaraderie, and the sheer joy of learning. To protect his children, he enrolled them in a "kinder" and "gentler" alternative private school.

> Competition is bad. That was my basic premise in life. We sent our kids to a little hippie school where there was no competition. They would have gym class but they wouldn't keep score, that kind of stuff, and I ate that up. I thought, "Yeah, that's the way kids should live."

But Jeff's older daughter, Michele, didn't see it that way.

> When Michele was about seven or eight, she started swimming more competitively, and one day we were driving home from a meet, she couldn't have been more than first or second grade, and she says, "Well, how did I do, Dad?"
> Honestly, she did terribly. She came in dead last. But I said, "You did fine."
> "No Dad, how did I do?"
> "You did very well. Your time was really very good."
> "No Dad, did I beat that other girl? Did I come in third?"
> And I remember thinking, "Wow, I don't get this. I send you to hippie school where they have no competitive sports and you ask, 'How did I do, Dad? I want to know. I have a right to know.'" I just wasn't getting it at all.

Gradually both Michele and her sister Deborah taught their father to rethink competition. Later, their example proved helpful to Gruen as he came to understand the value of tolerating and even embracing competition at the medical school.

> I learned an incredible amount about how to professionally survive [as a pediatric researcher] and about my academic career through their sports. Part of the reason I didn't do sports growing up was that I didn't understand them. If I can't win, I don't want to play, and that was really my attitude for years and years. And with my children, [they weren't big winners] but they loved it. It took me a long, long time to learn that they didn't have to win the race to be happy. . . For them, their P.B., their personal best, became really important, and I didn't understand it. If I couldn't get the big paper published, do the big experiment, get the big grant, it made me very angry and very upset, which is a tough way to conduct a professional career, especially if you are constantly comparing yourself with people at Yale, which we all naturally do. So it took me a long time to learn this.

Many of the resilient people we interviewed like to compete in various ways. They recognize that competition, when kept in perspective, can bolster feelings of self-efficacy and bring out our best. It can enhance performance and propel us to heights that we would not otherwise reach.

## Become a Mentor

Mentoring takes the concept of role models and turns it around. As a mentor, you serve as a model for someone who needs skill building and encouragement. In the process, you also develop your own skills, because when we teach we learn. In addition, mentors typically embrace an optimistic outlook (believing that their mentee's life will get better), practice altruism (giving of their time and talents), give and receive social support (from program coordinators, fellow mentors, and their mentee), and so forth.

Perhaps the most widely known mentoring program is Big Brothers Big Sisters of America (BBBS; www.bigsnyc.org/v-stories.php#annette), which matches children ages 6 through 18 with adult mentors. BBBS also has programs devoted to special populations such as children whose parents are in the military or in prison. The minimum time commitment is one hour per week. Volunteers can meet their little "brother" or "sister" in the community or at school, and the emphasis is on friendship. In an impact study published in 2000, Joseph P. Tierney and colleagues found that, compared to a control group, children who had been BBBS mentees for at least 18 months were less likely to start using drugs and alcohol and less likely to hit someone; they also showed improved school attendance and performance, improved attitudes toward completing schoolwork; and better relationships with peers and family members.

While Big Brothers Big Sisters mentoring is structured as a long-term relationship – many BBBS pairs stay together for five years or more – other programs provide opportunities for mentoring that are one-time commitments. The National Foundation for Teaching Entrepreneurship (NFTE), for example, teaches low-income high school students how to start a business. Adults with business experience present a lesson in their areas of expertise, take students on a field trip, or sit on a panel that evaluates students' business plans.

## Survivor Mission: Go Ahead, Be a Bob Woodruff or a Jerry White

In Chapter 9, on mental and emotional training, we told the story of Bob Woodruff, the ABC journalist who suffered a traumatic brain injury when he was wounded by a roadside bomb in Iraq. With his wife, Lee, Bob co-wrote the book *In an Instant: A Family's Journey of Love and Healing* (2007) chronicling his injury and the process of rehabilitation.

The Woodruffs also founded The Bob Woodruff Foundation to help other survivors of combat-related injuries. According to its website, ReMind.org, the foundation "provides resources and support to service members, veterans and their families to successfully reintegrate into their communities so they may thrive physically, psychologically, socially and economically." Like Jerry White, who founded the International Landmine Survivor Network, Bob and Lee Woodruff have chosen to use their traumatic experience as a platform for helping others.

One need not be wealthy or famous to embrace a survivor mission. Just look at Valentino Achak Deng and his Lost Boys Foundation, or remember the women who started Mothers Against Drunk Drivers. While funding can certainly help, passion, a clear mission, and persistence are essential.

# Resilience: It's Your Responsibility

Ultimately, resilience is about understanding the difference between fate and freedom, and learning to take responsibility for one's own life. Human beings are free, but with freedom comes responsibility, the responsibility to find and imitate resilient role models; to cultivate positive emotions and optimism; to face our fears; to confront rather than avoid problems; to learn from failure; to constructively reframe unpleasant, stressful, and traumatic events; to seek out and to attract social support; to keep our bodies in the best physical shape possible through exercise, good nutrition, and sleep; to use whatever strengths we have and to cultivate those strengths; to devote time and energy to spirituality and religion for those so inclined; to assist others who are in need; to search for, extract and create meaning; to acquire the knowledge and skills necessary to achieve goals through training; to accept that achievement rarely comes without enormous work and hardship; to build strength of character with a moral and ethical core; to find and embrace a survivor mission when appropriate; to persist when it would be easier to give up; to search for opportunity in adversity; to accept what cannot be changed; to try our best to bear unavoidable physical and psychological pain with grace and dignity; to learn and to grow from the hand that fate deals us, even when that hand is a bad one; and to do the best we can with what we've got. These are the choices that each of us faces, repetitively, throughout life. For some, of course, the burden is much greater than for others.

"When should I begin to train?" you might ask. The answer: now. As John McCain writes in *Why Courage Matters*,

> If you do the things you think you cannot do, you'll feel your resistance, your hope, your dignity, your courage, grow stronger every time you prove it. You will someday face

harder choices that very well might require more courage. You're getting ready for them. (McCain & Salter, 2008, p. 205)

Next you might ask, "How will I know if I have succeeded in my training?" Who should I compare myself to? Forrest Griffin in his book *Got Fight?* has a good answer.

Although it can be depressing to admit to yourself that you will never be the best, it is liberating at the same time. Instead of trying to be better than everyone else, which is existentially arrogant, you can focus on being the best that *you* can be... you can take pride in the fact that you did the most you possibly could with what you were given. You can take pride in every accomplishment. What more can you ask for? (Griffin & Krauss, 2009, p. 84)

Our friend Willie tells us of his experience volunteering with the Special Olympics, the competitive athletics program for those with intellectual disabilities. Willie has been a volunteer for the past 16 years because he likes to "see all those smiling faces. Everybody tries so hard. They don't hold back."

Willie remembers one contestant in particular. He was a small teenager who wore a metal brace on his right leg. Willie first noticed him because he was wearing a blue-and-gold uniform, the same colors that Willie himself had worn years earlier when he played saxophone in his high school band. As Willie watched the young man hobble to the starting line with six other contestants, he wondered why these Special Olympians were so eager to compete. What drove them to push themselves to their limit? And Willie also worried about the young man with the leg brace. How in the world could he compete with the other contestants? Would he even have the strength and coordination to complete the 100-yard race?

When the starting pistol fired, everyone began to shout and cheer: the crowd, the parents, the coaches, the contestants. The excitement again reminded Willie of his high school days when the fans erupted with excitement as his band marched onto the football field for their half-time show. Now the cheers were for these Special Olympians. A tall, lean, red-headed girl came in first, followed by a short muscular boy with Down syndrome. As the others finished one by one, Willie noticed that the young man with the braces was far behind the pack. His neurological disorder made his body movements appear spastic and irregular. He swerved from right to left and from left from right as he slowly made his way down the track.

Eventually the young man joined the other racers at the finish line. His coach immediately shook his hand and patted him on the shoulder, a job well done. Then, one of the other contestants, a petite teenage girl, approached the young man, and in a loud voice said, "You came in last."

"Tha, tha, that's OK," he stuttered, as he faced the girl and looked her in the eye. "I came in."

And perhaps that is the essence of this book: we need not be the swiftest or the strongest. What counts instead is that we "come in" – that we develop our talents, put forth our best effort, and commit ourselves to a life of purpose, growth, and resilience.

# References

Baez, J. (1987, 2009). *And a Voice to Sing With: A Memoir.* New York, NY: Simon & Schuster.

Batista, E. (2014, September 15). The Marshmallow Test for grownups. *Harvard Business Review.* Retrieved from https://hbr.org/2014/09/the-marshmallow-test-for-grownups

Boy Scouts of America (2010). Statement at www.scouting.org/ Accessed November 1, 2010.

Brooks, R. & Goldstein, S. (2001). *Raising Resilient Children: Fostering Strength, Hope, and Optimism in Your Child.* New York, NY: McGraw-Hill.

Casey, B. J., Somerville, L. H., Gotlib, I. H. *et al.* (2011). Behavioral and neural correlates of delay of gratification 40 years later. *Proceedings of the National Academy of Sciences USA,* 108(36), 14998.

Cole, M. S., Bruch, H. & Vogel, B. (2006). Emotion as mediators of the relations between perceived supervisor support and psychological hardiness on employee cynicism. *Journal of Organizational Behavior,* 27(4), 463–484.

Csikszentmihalyi, M. (1990). *Flow: The Psychology of Optimal Experience.* New York, NY: Harper and Row.

Geirland, J. (1996). Go with the flow. *Wired* magazine, September, Issue 4.09. Accessed May 7, 2010 at www.wired.com/wired/archive/4.09/czik_pr.html

Gibbs, N. (2009). The growing backlash against overparenting. *TIME* Magazine, November 20. Accessed July 2, 2010 at www.time.com/time/nation/article/0,8599,1940395,00.html

Griffin, F. & Krauss, E. (2009). *Got fight? The 50 Zen Principles of Hand-to-Face Combat.* New York, NY: William Morrow.

Goldman, R. & Papson, S. (1999). *Nike Culture: The Sign of the Swoosh.* Thousand Oaks, CA: Sage.

Harvard Project Zero (2017). Goodwork Project. Harvard Graduate School of Education. Retrieved from http://thegoodproject.org/projects/the-good-work-project/

Hofer, B. K. & Moore, A. S. (2011). *The iConnected Parent: Staying Close to Your Kids in College (and Beyond) While Letting Them Grow Up.* New York, NY: Atria Books.

Krache, D. (2008). How to ground a "helicopter parent". CNN online article, August 19. Accessed July 2, 2010 at www.cnn.com/2008/LIVING/personal/08/13/helicopter.parents/index.html

Lehrer, J. (2009). Don't! The secret of self-control. *New Yorker*, January 01, 26–32.

Loehr, J. (1993). *Toughness Training for Life: A Revolutionary Program for Maximizing Health, Happiness and Productivity*. New York, NY: Dutton.

Macleod, D. L. (1983). *Building Character in the American Boy: The Boy Scouts, YMCA and Their Forerunners, 1870–1920*. Madison, WI: University of Wisconsin Press.

McCain, J. & Salter, M. (2008). *Why Courage Matters: The Way to a Braver Life*. New York, NY: Ballantine Books.

McGonigal, K. (2012). *The Willpower Instinct: How Self-Control Works, Why It Matters, and What You Can Do to Get More of It*. New York, NY: Penguin Group.

Millman, D. (1999). *Body Mind Mastery: Training for Sport and Life*, 3rd edn. Novato, CA: New World Library.

Mischel, W., Ayduk, O., Berman, M. G. *et al.* (2011). 'Willpower' over the life span: Decomposing self-regulation. *Social Cognitive and Affective Neuroscience*, 6(2), 252–256.

Moffitt, T. E., Arseneault, L., Belsky, D. *et al.* (2011). A gradient of childhood self-control predicts health, wealth, and public safety. *Proceedings of the National Academy of Sciences USA*, 108(7), 2693.

National Foundation for Teaching Entrepreneurship (NFTE). Available at www.nfte.com/Volunteer/

Norris, F. H., Sherrieb, K. & Pfefferbaum, B. (2010). Community resilience: Concepts, assessment, and implications for intervention. In Southwick, S., Charney, D., Friedman, M. & Litz, B. (eds.), *Resilience: Responding to Challenges Across the Lifespan*. Cambridge: Cambridge University Press.

Sapolsky, R. M. (2004). *Why Zebras Don't Get Ulcers*. New York, NY: Henry Holt and Company.

Sasse, B. E. (2017). *The Vanishing American Adult: Our Coming-of-Age Crisis – And How to Rebuild a Culture of Self-Reliance*. New York, NY: St. Martin's Press.

Schlam, T. R., Wilson, N. L., Shoda, Y., Mischel, W. & Ayduk, O. (2013). Preschoolers' delay of gratification predicts their body mass 30 years later. *Journal of Pediatrics*, 162(1), 90–93.

Seligman, M. E. P. (2002). *Authentic Happiness: Using the New Positive Psychology to Realize Your Potential for Lasting Fulfillment*. New York, NY: Free Press.

Silvers, J. A., Insel, C., Powers, A. *et al.* (2016). vlPFC-vmPFC-amygdala interactions underlie age-related differences in cognitive regulation of emotion. *Cerebral Cortex*, 27(7), 3502–3514.

Silvers, J. A., Insel, C., Powers, A. *et al.* (2017). The transition from childhood to adolescence is marked by a general decrease in amygdala reactivity and an affect-specific ventral-to-dorsal shift in medial prefrontal recruitment. *Developmental Cognitive Neuroscience*, 25, 128–137.

Skenazy, L. (2009). Free-Range Kids blog post. Accessed July 2, 2010 at http://freerangekids.wordpress.com/faq/#7

Skenazy, L. (2010). *Free-Range Kids: How to Raise Safe, Self-Reliant Children (Without Going Nuts with Worry)*. Hoboken, NJ: Jossey-Bass.

Sonnenfeld, J. & Ward, A. (2007). *Firing Back: How Great Leaders Rebound After Career Disasters*. Cambridge, MA: Harvard Business Press.

The GoodWork Project: Excellence, ethics, and engagement in the professions. www.goodworkproject.org/

Tierney, J. P. & Grossman, J. B., with Resch, N. L. (2000). *Making a Difference: An Impact Study of Big Brothers Big Sisters*. Philadelphia, PA: Public/Private Ventures.

Twenge, J. M. (2007). *Generation Me: Why Today's Young Americans Are More Confident, Assertive, Entitled – And More Miserable Than Ever Before*. New York, NY: Free Press.

Twenge, J. & Campbell, W. K. (2009). *The Narcissism Epidemic: Living in the Age of Entitlement*. New York, NY: Free Press.

Walsh, F. (2002). A family resilience framework: Innovative practice applications. *Family Relations*, 51(2), 130–137.

Walsh, F. (ed.) (2003). *Normal Family Processes: Growing Diversity and Complexity*, 3rd edn. New York, NY: Guilford Press.

Walsh, F. (2011). Family resilience: A collaborative approach in response to stressful life challenges. In S. M. Southwick, B. T. Litz, D. Charney *et al.* (eds.), *Resilience and Mental Health: Challenges Across the Lifespan*, pp. 149–161. New York, NY: Cambridge University Press.

Walsh, F. (2016). *Strengthening Family Resilience*, 2nd edn. New York, NY: Guilford Press.

Winnicott, D. W (1958). Mind and its relation to the psyche-soma. In *Collected Papers, Through Paediatrics to Psychoanalysis*, pp. 243–254. London: Tavistock Publications. (Reprinted from *British Journal of Medical Psychology*, 27 (1954), 201–209.)

Wooden, J. The pyramid of success. Accessed April 4, 2011 at www.coachwooden .com/index2.html. See also http://sports.espn.go.com/espn/eticket/story? page=wooden

Wooden, J. & Tobin, J. (2004). *They Call Me Coach*. New York, NY: McGraw-Hill.

Woodruff, L. & Woodruff, B. (2007). *In an Instant: A Family's Journey of Love and Healing*. New York, NY: Random House.

# APPENDIX 1

# Further Information About Posttraumatic Stress Disorder

For those desiring further information, we offer these additional details about posttraumatic stress disorder (PTSD).

## What Is Posttraumatic Stress Disorder?

Although PTSD has existed throughout human history and can be found in all cultures throughout the world, it has only been formally recognized in the medical and psychological professions since the 1980s. Initially it was primarily associated with Vietnam combat veterans, but soon many other categories of trauma were recognized as potential causes of PTSD, including (but not limited to) rape, sexual molestation, robbery and other violent crimes, accidents, terrorism and torture, natural disasters, and witnessing the same.

Survivors who suffer with PTSD re-experience their traumatic event again and again in the form of intrusive and distressing memories, nightmares and flashbacks (i.e. acting or feeling as if the traumatic event is occurring again in the present). And many become psychologically distressed and/or physiologically aroused when they are reminded of the event. PTSD is also characterized by avoidance of people, places, activities, conversations, feelings and thoughts that remind the survivor of the trauma. A detachment from others and a restriction of emotions is common. Finally, individuals with PTSD typically complain of increased arousal, marked by hypervigilance, difficulty sleeping, irritability, exaggerated startle, and in some cases outbursts of anger (American Psychological Association, 2010).

Guilt, shame, and the inability to trust others are not formally part of the PTSD diagnosis but are common among trauma sufferers. Survivors often feel guilty for having lived when others died and/or believe that they could have or should have done more to prevent the trauma or to help others during the event – even when intervening was not possible. For example, several of Jimmy Dunne's colleagues at Sandler O'Neill spoke of feeling "haunted, wondering who else they could have saved. 'I feel guilty because I left... Why didn't I tell them to get out? I should have told them to leave'" (Brooker, 2002, p. 60). Feelings of self-blame can become overpowering, sometimes to the point that the individual contemplates suicide. Indeed, along with a rise in PTSD among military veterans, there has been increasing concern about suicides of active duty personnel deployed in Iraq and Afghanistan (Dao, 2010).

Feelings of powerlessness and of being permanently changed by the trauma are also common. Human rights worker Sister Dianna Ortiz quotes a torture survivor who expresses how the memory of trauma continues to permeate daily living:

> Once I was safe, I thought I was free of my torturers. I actually believed that I would never see them again, that I would never have to smell them or hear their voices. But what I soon realized was that they were within me; they literally had made their home inside my soul. . . . I felt so dirty, so contaminated by evil. (Ortiz, 2001, pp. 18–19)

To deal with their symptoms, survivors with PTSD often self-medicate with substances of abuse hoping to calm their hyperactive nervous system, improve sleep, and suppress traumatic memories. Those who become exhausted from night after night of sleeplessness and nightmares may experiment with whatever substances they can obtain. Alcohol, benzodiazapines (Valium, Xanax, Ativan), and opiates (codeine, heroin) each suppress the central nervous system and have a quieting effect that counters the hypervigilance typical of PTSD. These substances can be so effective that survivors with PTSD may develop a substance abuse disorder (Jacobsen, Southwick & Costen, 2001). In fact, nearly 50 percent of PTSD patients meet criteria for alcohol dependence at some point during their life (Jacobsen, Southwick & Costen, 2001). In addition, trauma survivors may develop one or more related psychological disorders, such as major depression or panic disorder. In-depth descriptions of these related disorders are beyond the scope of this book, but we mention them to underscore the complexity of psychological reactions to trauma.

It is easy to see how PTSD symptoms can be debilitating and can interfere dramatically with daily life. These symptoms can derail careers, marriages, family relationships and friendships. In a 1999 study, Mary L. Malik and colleagues found that PTSD impaired quality of life more severely than either major depression or obsessive-compulsive disorder (Malik *et al.*, 1999).

# How Is PTSD Assessed?

Researchers have developed a number of instruments to assess PTSD; these include the Clinician-Administered PTSD Scale (CAPS), the Posttraumatic Stress Diagnostic Scale (PDS), and the PTSD Checklist (PCL), among others (see Blake *et al.*, 1995; Foa, 1995, 1997; Friedman *et al.*, 2007; Weathers *et al.*, 1993). The CAPS is administered by a trained mental health professional; it focuses on two factors: frequency of symptoms and intensity of symptoms. Sample CAPS questions are, "Have you ever had unwanted memories of [the traumatic event]? What were they like? What did you remember?" and "How much distress or discomfort did these memories cause you? Were you able to put them out of your mind and think about something else? How hard did you have to try? How much did they interfere with your life?" The PDS and the PCL similarly assess the symptoms listed by the American Psychiatric Association, but are in the form of self-report scales in which patients rate their own level of symptoms and distress. The PCL comes in several versions, including one for military personnel and one for civilians. Like the CAPS, it asks patients to rate the level to which they were bothered in the past month by phenomena such as "Suddenly acting or feeling as if a stressful experience were happening again (as if you were reliving it)"; "Having physical reactions (e.g. heart pounding, trouble breathing, sweating) when something reminded you of a stressful experience"; and "Feeling emotionally numb or being unable to have loving feelings for those close to you."

## How Prevalent Is PTSD?

Estimates vary as to the prevalence of PTSD (Friedman, Keane & Resick, 2007). A well-designed study in 2013 found that roughly 8 percent of all Americans experience PTSD at some point in their life, with 5.7 percent of men and 12.8 percent of women meeting criteria for the disorder. Survivors of certain kinds of trauma are more likely than others to be affected. About 12 percent of accident survivors experience PTSD and among combat veterans the rate is 10–30 percent (National Center for PTSD, 2009) (Kilpatrick *et al.*, 2013). There are varied estimates of the rate of PTSD in US veterans returning from Iraq and Afghanistan. The World Health Organization (2006) reported 11.2–17.1 percent, compared with a baseline rate of 5 percent before deployment. A Rand Corporation study in 2008 found that 19 percent of these veterans experienced symptoms of either PTSD or major depression (Alvarez, 2008).

As we have said earlier in this book, most people who undergo a trauma will not develop PTSD; of course, the more intense, severe and overwhelming the trauma, the more likely it is that symptoms of PTSD will follow. Fortunately, treatment techniques that can be effective in helping individuals to recover from PTSD and other anxiety-related problems are now widely in use. Some of these techniques have been briefly discussed at various junctures in the book.

## References

Alvarez, L. (2008). Nearly a fifth of war veterans report mental disorders, a private study finds. *New York Times,* April 18. Accessed February 15, 2010 at www.nytimes.com/2008/04/18/us/18vets.html

American Psychiatric Association (2013). *Diagnostic and Statistical Manual of Mental Disorders*, 5th edn. Arlington, VA: American Psychiatric Association.

American Psychological Association (2010). *The Road to Resilience*. Washington, DC: American Psychological Association. Accessed June 25, 2010 at www.apa .org/helpcenter/road-resilience.aspx

Blake, D. D., Weathers, F. W., Nagy,L. M. *et al.* (1995). The development of a clinician-administered PTSD scale. *Journal of Traumatic Stress*, 8, 75–90.

Brooker, K. (2002). Starting over. *Fortune*, January 21, 50–68.

Dao,J. (2010). At War: Notes from the front lines: Presidential condolences and troop suicides. *New York Times*, February 1. Accessed February 15, 2010 at http://atwar.blogs.nytimes.com/2010/02/01/presidential-condolences-and-troop-suicides/

Foa, E. B. (1995). *The Posttraumatic Diagnostic Scale (PDS) Manual*. Minneapolis, MN: National Computer Systems.

Foa, E. B. (1997). Psychological processes related to recovery from a trauma and an effective treatment for PTSD. In R. Yehuda & A. McFarlane (eds.), *Psychobiology of Post-Traumatic Stress Disorder*, pp. 410–424. New York, NY: New York Academy of Science.

Friedman, M. J., Keane, T. M., Resick, P. R. (eds.) (2007). *Handbook of PTSD: Science and Practice*. New York, NY: The Guilford Press.

Jacobsen,L. K., Southwick, S. M. & Kosten, T. R. (2001). Substance use disorders in patients with posttraumatic stress disorder: A review of the literature. *American Journal of Psychiatry*, 158 (August), 1184–1190.

Kilpatrick, D. G., Resnick, H.S., Milanak, M. E. *et al.* (2013). National estimates of exposure to traumatic events and PTSD prevalence using DSM-IV and DSM-5 criteria. *Journal of Traumatic Stress*, 26(5), 537–547.

Litz, B. T. (2005). Has resilience to severe trauma been underestimated? *American Psychologist*, 60, 262.

Luthar, S.S. (2006). Resilience in development: A synthesis of research across five decades. In D. Cicchetti & D. J. Cohen (eds.), *Developmental Psychopathology* Vol. 3: *Risk Disorder, and Adaptation*, 2nd edn, pp. 740–795. New York, NY: Wiley.

Maguen, S., Lucenko, B. A., Reger, M. A. *et al.* (2010). The impact of reported direct and indirect killing on mental health symptoms in Iraq War veterans. *Journal of Traumatic Stress*, 23(1), 86–90.

Malik, M. L., Connor, K. M., Sutherland, S. M. *et al.* (1999). Quality of life and posttraumatic stress disorder: A pilot study assessing changes in sf-36 scores before and after treatment in a placebo-controlled trial of Fluoxetine. *Journal of Traumatic Stress*, 12(2), April, 387–393.

McEwen, B.S. (2007). Physiology and neurobiology of stress and adaptation: Central role of the brain. *Physiological Reviews*, 87, 873–904.

National Center for PTSD, Department of Veterans Affairs (2009). How common is PTSD? Accessed January 2009 at www.ptsd.va.gov/

Norris, F. H., & Slone, L. B. (2007). The epidemiology of trauma and PTSD. In M. J., Friedman, T. M. Keane, & P. A. Resick, (eds.), *Handbook of PTSD*, pp. 78–98. New York, NY: Guilford Press.

Ortiz, D. (2001). The survivor's perspective: Voices from the center. In E. Gerrity, T. M. Keane, & F. Turna, (eds.), *The Mental Health Consequences of Torture*. New York, NY: Kluwer Academic/Plenum Publishers.

Weathers, F. W., Litz, B. T., Herman, D. S., Huska, J. A. & Keane, T. M. (1993). The PTSD Checklist (PCL): Reliability, validity, and diagnostic utility. Paper presented at the Annual Meeting of International Society for Traumatic Stress Studies, San Antonio, TX, October, 1993.

World Health Organization (2006). Report of a workshop on tracking health performance and humanitarian outcomes. Accessed November 22, 2009 at www.who.int/hac/events/benchmarkmeeting/en/index.html

# Community Resilience

Throughout this book, we have focused primarily on resilience in the individual. However, it is important to emphasize that our own personal resilience is influenced by the resilience of those around us and by what resources are available to us. That is, our own resilience is strongly influenced by the resilience of family, friends and colleagues, organizations that we belong to, and by the strength of our communities.

## What Is Community Resilience?

A panel of scientists at Oak Ridge National Laboratory defined community resilience as the "capability to prepare for, respond to, and recover from significant multi-hazard threats with minimum damage to public safety and health, the economy, and national security" (Wilbanks, 2007, p. 2). In an interdisciplinary study aptly titled "Community resilience as a metaphor, theory, set of capacities, and strategy for disaster readiness," Fran Norris and colleagues describe attributes such as economic development, social capital, adaptation and wellness that serve as a safety net for communities (Norris *et al.*, 2008).

Judith Rodin, president of the Rockefeller Foundation, notes in her book *The Resilience Dividend: Being Strong in a World Where Things Go Wrong* (Rodin, 2014) that our world has always been beset by major disruptions, but in modern times these disruptions can have greater impact because of urbanization, climate change, and globalization. As the world's population becomes increasingly concentrated in urban settings, disruptions such as extreme weather events, drought, poor air quality, spread of disease, and infrastructure failure (e.g., electrical outage) can have rapid and devastating effects on large numbers of people. Similarly, globalization and near instantaneous worldwide communication via modern technology means increased economic and political volatility. In Rodin's view, because "everything is interconnected – a massive system of systems – a single disruption often triggers another, which exacerbates the effects of the first, so that the original shock becomes a cascade of crises" (p. 5).

In the financial crisis of 2008, for example, a high-risk pattern of subprime lending at the consumer level, derivatives trading at the Wall Street level, and increasingly lax regulation at the government level had been developing for a decade. When a few hedge funds found themselves lacking the necessary liquidity to continue trading, global markets reacted with sell-offs, sending small investors running for the exits. Then Lehman Brothers, one of the world's largest investment banks, was forced to declare bankruptcy and liquidate its assets, a failure that grabbed headlines the world over and sent stock prices plummeting. Suddenly, millions of middle-class workers saw their life savings lose up to half their value – as the joke went, "My 401(k) is now just a 4(k)." As mortgage lenders tightened their practices, millions of homeowners were threatened with foreclosure and many would-be buyers were suddenly unable to qualify for loans. Thousands of companies cut their staff, leaving millions of workers unemployed. Fears of a worsening recession stopped consumers from spending on big-ticket items, especially cars, which in turn sent the automobile industry into a crisis. These cascading problems could only be stopped by a multifaceted effort on the part of private enterprise, government at multiple levels, and smaller community-based organizations.

In examining community resilience, our task is to ask what could have been done differently to prevent such a crisis, or to mitigate its severity, or to speed recovery. To that end, Rodin proposes a useful framework of five characteristics of community resilience. In Rodin's framework, the resilient community is aware, diverse, integrated, self-regulating, and adaptive. What do these attributes mean?

The *aware* community continually monitors potential threats and accurately assesses its resources, strengths, weaknesses, and vulnerabilities during times of both disruption and relative calm. It is human nature to worry about problems only when they occur, but here is where community resilience comes in: just as individuals need to train and challenge in order to become resilient, so communities need to plan, conduct drills, and anticipate what could go wrong. For example, when planning for or responding to crises, it is critical to have an accurate accounting of available resources.

The *diverse* community embraces different capacities and a range of ideas, opinions, attitudes, information sources, and technical elements. When one or more of its major components fails, it can enlist alternative or redundant resources and capacities to serve as back-ups.

In the *integrated* community, people, groups, organizations, resources, and activities are well coordinated, making it possible to effectively share information, prepare for potential disruptions, respond to adversity, learn from the process, and ideally grow stronger. Integration can be enhanced by incorporating feedback loops that continuously gather relevant information, analyze that information, and inform the community so that appropriate adjustments can be made.

When the *self-regulating* community is jolted by a major disruption, the community has the capacity to contain that failure – to fail safely – and thus limit the damage and prevent a cascade of further failures. This allows the community to bounce back more rapidly.

The *adaptive* community adjusts to changing circumstances. It is capable of making changes proactively to prevent disaster, develop new plans, modify behaviors, and apply existing resources to new purposes. To remain strong in today's rapidly changing world, communities must have the flexibility to adapt to a broad range of fluid environmental, economic, and political circumstances.

Rodin's framework echoes a central message of this book: that resilience is not about stability, but rather knowing how to react to change; better yet, embracing change. Sustainability does not mean remaining the same, but rather being able to adapt and grow; to remain viable through a broad range of changes and challenges over time. Systems naturally resist change, but by being rigid they become highly vulnerable to disruption, decay, and dysfunction. Although structure and hierarchy are important – without them there would be chaos – flexibility is key to survival.

Preparation includes good coordination among disparate elements. When department heads and others in leadership positions are well acquainted with each other and have developed mutually respectful, constructive relationships, they can put those relationships to good use when disaster strikes. As with the other kinds of resilience that we have discussed throughout this book, community resilience takes time and practice. Community leaders must prepare for challenges by anticipating what can go wrong. No community will anticipate all possibilities, but the more practice it has in dealing with a variety of potential disruptions, the better prepared it will be. In a crisis there will be failures, but, with enough preparation, communities are likely to fail more safely.

# Responding to Disaster

A resilient community might be described as a strong group of informed and motivated people who care about each other and are willing to work together. Ideally, leadership provides direction and sets priorities, but in the absence of existing leadership hopefully someone will step forward and make decisions. That is what happened in the summer of 2011 when the small Massachusetts town of Monson was hit by a tornado – a rare occurrence in New England, and something for which the town was completely unprepared. Two college students, sisters Caitria and Morgan O'Neill, found themselves at the center of a recovery effort because the town's police and fire headquarters had suffered direct hits, and the church across from the O'Neill home became the default community gathering place. Seeing that everyone wanted to help but no one knew what to do, the sisters began inventorying donations. They created a Google Voice number as a hotline that townspeople could call for information and help, set up a Facebook page, printed informational flyers, and spoke to news reporters to get the word out. "We had to learn how to answer questions quickly and to solve problems in about a minute or less because otherwise something more urgent would come up and it just wouldn't get done," said Caitria. Morgan added, "We didn't get our authority from the Board of Selectmen or the emergency management director or the United Way. We just started making decisions because someone, anyone, had to" (O'Neill & O'Neill, 2012, at 3:30). In the midst of their exhaustion after several 17-hour days at their makeshift command post, the sisters came to the realization that "it shouldn't be this hard." As they were harnessing communications technology to build a recovery infrastructure, they thought, why not make it available ahead of time, so that when a community is hit by a disaster it would not have to start from scratch?

The result was the software framework recovers.org which empowers organizations to manage local resources and coordinate community recovery efforts, provides a central coordinating point for information and materials, and enables residents to offer and request help (https://recovers.org/about 2016; O'Neill, 2012). Cities, towns, and communities can enroll and access the software when a disaster occurs.

In some cultures, the idea that communities work together during times of adversity may come more naturally. When a massive tsunami struck southeast Asia on December 25, 2004, it spread a swath of destruction for thousands of miles from Indonesia to Africa. How did individuals, families, and communities cope and recover? Northwestern University health psychologist Greg Miller (2005) conducted a post-event study of mental health in the affected areas and concluded that "Asian culture, with its emphasis on group welfare over individual self-reliance, seems to have been a powerful, positive influence" (p. 1031). One of Miller's informants was Athula Sumathipala, a Sri Lankan psychiatrist who worked with tsunami survivors. Sumathipala observed that "People came together to support each other and look after the necessities. . . A man who lost his own son would care for someone else's son" (quoted in Miller, 2005, p. 1031). In such cases, community resilience was bolstered by individuals who demonstrated compassion and willingness to look beyond their own interests to contribute to the common good.

In recent decades, politicians and media have often referred to "Rust Belt" cities in the American heartland that fell into economic and social decline as industrial manufacturing jobs were gradually phased out by automation and robotics, outsourcing, and globalization. Cities like Detroit, Youngstown, Peoria, and Pittsburgh thrived during the twentieth century largely on single industries: automobile manufacturing, coal mining and processing, heavy equipment manufacturing, and steel mills, respectively. A lack of economic diversity can mean that a community also relies on a narrow range of skills, perspectives, and ideas, leaving it without the resources it will need to change with the times and remain viable.

Pittsburgh is an example of a Rust Belt city that, over the years, has successfully transitioned from a single-industry economy to an economy supported by a variety of industries, including advanced technology and robotics, healthcare and biomedical sciences, engineering, and finance. Accompanying this economic revitalization, there has been a renewal of cultural and social activity, an active base of charities and philanthropies, a low crime rate, a young workforce, high rates of literacy and higher-than-average intelligence scores. Rankings of the most livable US cities by the *Economist*, *Forbes*, and the *Places Rated Almanac* have listed Pittsburgh at or near the top six times in the years 2000 to 2015. The Grosvenor property group named it as the fifth most resilient city in the world (Vennare, 2016).

In addition to the slow economic and social downturn experienced by neighborhoods, cities or even relatively large geographical regions may be struck by sudden and overwhelming disasters. Such was the case for New Orleans and the surrounding region. In 2005, when Hurricane Katrina's storm surge breached the levees, flood walls, and drainage canals that kept much of the city's land above water, some 80 percent of the city was flooded, and its infrastructure – electrical, water, and sewer utilities, not to mention transportation – was knocked out of commission. More than 1,800 lives were lost, and the monetary cost of damage was estimated at $153 billion (Ross, 2015). Although the Coast Guard was well prepared (Rodin 2014), the overall assessments of the response by public and private organizations were uniformly critical.

Hurricane Katrina struck a city plagued by poverty, crime, failing schools, and racial inequality. Nearly a quarter of Orleans Parish residents lived below the federal poverty line, and some 30 percent did not own a car; these percentages were significantly greater when applied to the city's African American population (Katz, 2006; Ross, 2015). One can well imagine that a family with such limited resources would not have the option to evacuate out of town and rent a motel room until it was safe to return. Instead, thousands of residents were stranded for days on rooftops, highway overpasses, and patches of high ground without access to food or potable water. The Louisiana Superdome and the New Orleans Convention Center, declared shelters for those with nowhere else to go, were soon packed with upwards of 45,000 people – nearly one-tenth of the city's entire population ('Desperate SOS', 2005; Hurricane Katrina, 2005).

Sadly, thousands of residents lost their homes – disproportionately African Americans. Many were offered incentives to relocate to other parts of the United States as far away as Michigan, Oregon, and Georgia. Others found housing in mobile homes provided by the Federal Emergency Management Agency (FEMA), a program intended to be temporary but ultimately lasting several years and in many cases only delaying, not avoiding, the occupants' need to move away from southern Louisiana rather than return to their familiar neighborhoods. This response shredded the social fabric of the community, not only reducing the population but also removing families who had lived in New Orleans for generations and making it all but impossible for friends and neighbors to stay in touch with one another. (Seidenberg, 2005; Robertson, 2015).

In February 2006, less than six months after Hurricane Katrina, the Assistant to the President for Homeland Security and Counterterrorism issued a White House report assessing the federal response (Townsend, 2006). Viewed against Judith Rodin's community resilience factors, the report identifies problems in virtually every area, starting with a serious lack of what Rodin calls integration:

Command centers in the Department of Homeland Security (DHS) and elsewhere in the Federal government had unclear, and often overlapping, roles and responsibilities that were exposed as flawed during this disaster. . . State and local authorities understood the devastation was serious but, due to the destruction of infrastructure and response capabilities, lacked the ability to communicate with each other and coordinate a response. . . Far too often, the process required numerous time consuming approval signatures and data processing steps prior to any action, delaying the response. As a result, many agencies took action under their own independent authorities while also responding to mission assignments from the Federal Emergency Management Agency (FEMA), creating further process confusion and potential duplication of efforts (p. 2).

Eight months after the storm, the United States Senate issued a report (2006, May) that echoed and elaborated on the assessments of the White House report, identifying glaring problems in the following areas.

- Lack of awareness and preparedness: "None of the relevant government agencies had a plan for responding to a levee breach" (p. 17); "staggeringly, the City of New Orleans Fire Department owned no boats, and the New Orleans Police Department owned five" (p. 9).
- Lack of integration and self-regulation: The report cited "FEMA's lack of financial controls. . . poor contracting practices" (p. 18); "flaws in the structure of FEMA and DHS that are too substantial to mend" (p. 18).
- Lack of adaptation and flexibility: Key officials followed established protocols to delay decision-making until a full "ground truth" assessment could be made; they "did not grasp the need to act on the less-than-complete information that is to be expected in a disaster" (p. 9).

The Senate report concluded that "one would hardly characterize the region's reaction as resilient, although some elements of resilience were in place before the storm and there has been a determined effort to bring about a full-fledged recovery that reflects a resilient spirit, if not a resilient social and physical infrastructure" (p. 2).

Three years after Katrina, a report authored by a group of scientists with Oak Ridge National Laboratory, working in a federally funded program called the Community and Regional Resilience Initiative (CARRI), endeavored to apply the lessons of New Orleans to a community resilience framework

(Colten, Kates & Laska, 2008). The CARRI approach moves chronologically by advising that a community develop the ability to anticipate multi-hazard threats, then to respond to hazard events, subsequently to recover, and finally to reduce its vulnerability to future threats. As part of this four-step framework, CARRI notes that "recovery takes longer than expected" and "surprises should be expected" (p. ix). The report concludes: "We hope this assessment of resilience before, during, and after Katrina and into the future will offer guidance for implementing a more comprehensive, effective, and equitable approach to dealing with hurricanes and other hazard events and that Katrina will become a lesson that remains deeply ingrained in the social memory of the city's citizens" (p. 25).

*New York Times* reporter Gary Rivlin (2015) traced the response from the first days of the Katrina flood through the ensuing decade. Focusing on the social dimensions of New Orleans and its residents, Rivlin examined the political and business maneuvering, and the issues of culture, race, and class, that came into play as different sections of the city, and different segments of its population, struggled to survive and revive after Katrina. He reported that although a host of grants were bestowed upon New Orleans, residents and well-meaning outsiders often picked and chose winners and losers, jockeying to implement one favored project at the expense of another. While many neighborhoods were rebuilt, ten years after Katrina the impoverished and predominantly black Lower Ninth Ward remained largely a ghost town, and the percentage of Orleans Parish residents living below the poverty line was greater in 2015 than in 2005 (Robertson, 2015; Ross, 2015). By 2015, although the levees were repaired and strengthened, the city remained vulnerable to another flood in the future because it still lacked the necessary coordination of services and cohesiveness of people.

# A Framework for Applying Community Resilience

What would it take to turn around a city with such deeply entrenched challenges as those that New Orleans continues to face? Clearly there is no sure-fire solution, and any attempts to outline a method of tackling such multifaceted problems might well prove inadequate when applied in the all-too-real world. Nevertheless, at a theoretical level we can at least identify concrete steps to increase a community's level of resilience. Returning to Judith Rodin's conceptualization of resilient communities, Rodin offers a "3 Rs" framework for building such resilience comprising readiness, responsiveness, and revitalization.

## Readiness

Rodin describes readiness as beginning at the political level, as the community's governing bodies need to exercise leadership and support for the initiative. It is also a largely governmental role to activate and coordinate readiness among police, fire, and public works first responders – although private institutions such as healthcare facilities also need to participate. A key to readiness is identifying likely disasters and ensuring the capacity to scale up during an emergency. Readiness also requires hands-on drills in which community members practice responding to what can go wrong based on various scenarios. (To this last point, it should be noted that FEMA actually held a hurricane drill in New Orleans in 2004. However, the recommendations that the drill produced were not implemented. Moreover, the administration had previously discontinued a FEMA program called Project Impact that helped communities prepare for possible disasters [Rivlin, 2015].)

## Responsiveness

In this stage of the framework, the community has practiced drills sufficiently to make responses automatic. When responsiveness is achieved, leaders are able to maintain rational decision-making and not be ruled by emotions. All five attributes of community resilience – awareness, diversity, integration, self-regulation, and adaptation – come into play and are drawn on. Synergy is exhibited as the community's response becomes more than the sum of its parts.

## Revitalization

This third stage is reached in the aftermath of a disaster, and is characterized by the quality of social cohesion. Community members have a strong sense of identity: They are proud of belonging to this place, this community, and they collectively commemorate the adversity they have faced, painful though it may be. The opportunity to tell their stories and listen to each other is one meaningful step on the pathway to recovery. Finally, revitalization includes incorporating the lessons learned from the experience so that the community emerges stronger and better prepared to meet the challenges of a future disaster.

Volunteers Ian Breckenridge-Jackson and Caroline Heldman were in New Orleans helping with the Lower Ninth Ward's recovery when they observed that "there was nowhere people could go to just hear those stories" (Chang, 2016, p. 15). To address this need, they were instrumental in developing an oral history project and co-founding the Lower Ninth Ward Living Museum, which opened its doors in 2011. The museum celebrates the area's history through stories and exhibits, and serves as a center for arts and cultural events, tutoring and homework coaching, sports and other community activities.

Communication scholars Michael S. Bowman and Ruth Laurion Bowman (2010) affirmed the need of those who lived through Hurricane Katrina to tell their stories, and pointed to a willing audience of onlookers fascinated by the drama of this horrific disaster (as evidenced by the popular "disaster tours" offered to New Orleans vacationers in the years after Katrina). Yet, they identified several problems inherent in this storytelling. First, they observed that America was quick to forget about southern Louisiana's trauma as the hard work of recovery dragged on year after year. The excitement of a hurricane and epic flood was one thing; the grinding tedium of reassembling a city and a society was quite another. Second, they questioned how to achieve a "consensus on what 'our' story should be" (p. 457), given that an audience of Gulf Coast residents would have a very different understanding of events and conditions than would an audience of outsiders. Who was doing the telling, who was doing the listening, and what difference did it make? Third, they observed the "banality, commodification, and spectacle of today's media culture" (p. 458) as a milieu in which stories will inevitably be heard. Acknowledging these problems, they advocated full engagement in storytelling as a catalyst for change, as a means of creating "the conditions for something to happen" (p. 460). In this way, storytelling can make a valuable contribution to revitalization.

## Community Resilience Rests on Active Compassion

Putting compassion into practice – going out of one's way to actively help the next person – is the linchpin of community resilience, for community members need to not only care about one another but also take action to help. An interesting example involves Amy Peake, a British yoga instructor and mother of three. Peake had not been through a trauma herself, but a chance incident in 2014 evoked compassion and moved her to start a project to help Syrian refugees. Peake happened to see a news photograph of a vast crowd of refugees waiting to receive food in a camp near the Syrian border, where basic necessities like food and toilet paper are scarce. She reports thinking, "What if I were there? How would I cope with no food, no water, no shelter, no access to medicine?. . . How would I deal with all of this – and then on top have my period with no sanitary towels?" (Loving Humanity, 2016). Imagining herself in someone else's place led her to to take action regarding a necessary product that is rarely spoken of.

Through research, Peake learned that although the refugees occasionally received sanitary pads from aid organizations, there were not enough to go around. Women and their daughters often had to use rags and other unsanitary materials, or trade their meager food money to buy sanitary pads from a shop in the camp. Furthermore, many families had had ill, elderly or disabled members who needed incontinence pads because they could not walk the distance to the camp's communal toilets.

It came to Peake's attention that an inventor in India had developed a hand-powered machine to turn wood pulp into sanitary pad material. "That machine should be in the refugee camps and if isn't perhaps I should take it there," she thought (Matharu, 2015). Soon Peake solicited donations from her local Rotary Club, founded a charity called Loving Humanity, and traveled to India to meet with the inventor and others who were using a similar machine in a rural village. Several refinements later, she had enlisted the participation of the UN High Commission for Refugees and started a pilot program in the Za'atari refugee camp near the Jordanian-Syrian border, where 80,000 to 100,000 Syrians were living (Venema, 2015).

The machines would employ women, providing them with a means to earn income; and the operation would be modified according to user feedback to ensure that the raw materials, machinery, process, and finished products were meeting their intended needs. Larger plans for scaling the program up to more camps and other communities were also being developed Authorities on women's issues in the developing world have long acknowledged that the more adolescent girls have access to sanitary pads, the longer they are able to stay in school, thus boosting the educational level of their families and communities.

Amy Peake knew she could not save the world, but she harnessed her compassion to make a difference in a specific way for a specific community. She zeroed in on a specific and neglected necessity of life for people who had been forced to flee their homes. She researched what could be done to fill that need. She put it into action, not only by giving refugees the needed items but by teaching them and securing the equipment and materials for the community to produce them.

## Conclusions and Future Directions

Examining resilience as a community attribute provides additional ways of understanding how we – as individuals and as members of a social unit – can better cope with the stressors and traumas that are bound to confront us at one time or another. When we think about how to become more resilient, or embark upon a plan to challenge ourselves to build greater resilience, we can expand our intentions to include our neighbors and associates. In this way, we can all help and encourage each other in times of adversity. Fran Norris and colleagues (2007) described this as a two-way chain reaction, such that if I as an individual am resilient, I can help my community, and if my community is resilient, it can help me. The interdependence goes up and down the chain, serving as a well-functioning ecosystem.

Yet we must also conclude that it is often more difficult for a community to achieve resilience than it is for an individual. By definition, communities encompass large and complex networks of people, infrastructure, economic and cultural interests, political factions, and the like. The aforementioned examples of Rust Belt cities and New Orleans demonstrate some of the challenges and obstacles that communities may have to confront if they are to build their resilience.

Further, we echo Judith Rodin's (2014) observation that communities tend to be acutely focused on resilience when a threat is imminent, present, or recent – but to lapse into an "out of sight, out of mind" complacency once the threat is past. Great plans for a resiliency program may be developed in the wake of a disaster, but then set on a shelf for lack of funding or political will. Leaders or grassroots citizens may point out the need to be prepared against one vulnerability or another, only to be ignored or characterized as alarmists. Thus, a key challenge for community resilience is to awaken public opinion so that building resilience is seen as a worthwhile investment that will, over time, pay off in economic and social dividends.

This discussion only scratches the surface of the topic of community resilience. Future research could take many different directions and identifies numerous factors that influence community resilience, each of which might merit further study.

There are also a number of published sources that might serve as springboards for further study. Some include the following, which we list in bibliographic format with our annotations.

Chandra, A. & Acosta, J. D. (2013). *Building Resilient Communities: An Online Training. User's Guide and Audio Transcript.* Santa Monica, CA: RAND Corporation. Prepared by the RAND Corporation's Investment in People and Ideas program, this training resource covers principles of resilience, contrasts resilience against emergency preparedness, and identifies action items for organizations and for entire communities.

Dealing with disasters (2005). *Science*, 309(5737), 973–1136. This special issue of *Science* focuses on the Indian Ocean tsunami of December 2004 and the societal, psychological, and economic responses observed in affected communities and in recovery efforts from around the globe.

Hall, J. S. & Zautra, A. J. (2010). Indicators of community resilience: What are they, why bother? In J. W. Reich, A. J. Zautra & J. S. Hall, *Handbook of Adult Resilience* Chapter 17, pp. 350–371. New York, NY: Guilford Press. The authors call for a CRI (Community Resilience Index). "In essence a community is defined by the presence of sustained and substantial positive social interaction among people who share common ground" (p. 351).

Resilient personality of cities could help in a recession (2015). Press release. Society for Personality and Social Psychology, September 29. Retrieved from www.spsp .org/press_release/city-personality-resiliency . The press release summarizes findings from a study by Obschonka, Stuetzer, Audretsch, Rentfrow, Potter & Gosling (2015) that assessed macro-psychological factors associated with regional economic resilience.

Wulff, K., Donato, D. & Lurie, N. (2015). What is health resilience and how can we build it? *Annual Review of Public Health*, 36, 361–374. The authors advocate a community resilience paradigm as a means of helping "communities and individuals not just to mitigate damage and heal, but to thrive" (p. 361). They define community resilience as the "ability to withstand a disaster with efforts to strengthen day-to-day systems to improve the public's health and vitality" (p. 362).

# References

Bowman, M. S. & Bowman, R. L. (2010). Telling Katrina stories: Problems and opportunities in engaging disaster. *Quarterly Journal of Speech*, 96(4), 455–461.

Colten, C. E., Kates, R. W. & Laska, S. B. (2008). Community Resilience: Lessons from New Orleans and Hurricane Katrina. CARRI Research Report 3. Oak Ridge National Laboratory: Community & Regional Resilience Initiative. www.resilientUS.org

'Desperate SOS' for New Orleans (2005). BBC News, September 2. Retrieved from http://news.bbc.co.uk/2/hi/americas/4206620.stm

Gates,C. (2015, August 30). Council designer regrets Share an Idea didn't go further. *Stuff*. Retrieved from www.stuff.co.nz/the-press/71573351/Council-designer-regrets-Share-an-Idea-didn-t-go-further

Girl, 10, used geography lesson to save lives (2005). *The Telegraph*, January 1. Retrieved from www.telegraph.co.uk/news/1480192/Girl-10-used-geography-lesson-to-save-lives.html

Hurricane Katrina: Photos and video from Day Four interactive feature (2005). *New York Times*, September 2. Retrieved from www.nytimes.com/packages/khtml/2005/09/02/national/20050902_STORM_FEATURE.html

Kaiser Family Foundation (2015). New Orleans ten years after the storm: African Americans and whites live differing realities. [infographic]. Retrieved from http://kff.org/infographic/new-orleans-ten-years-after-the-storm-african-americans-and-whites-live-differing-realities/

Katz, B. (2006). Op-Ed: Concentrated poverty in New Orleans and other American cities. Blog post, Brookings Institution, August 4. Retrieved from www.brookings.edu/opinions/concentrated-poverty-in-new-orleans-and-other-american-cities/

Loving Humanity (2016). About us. Retrieved from http://lovinghumanity.org.uk/aboutus/

Matharu, H. (2015). The 'sanitary pad missionary' bringing dignity and jobs to Syria's female refugees. *The Independent*, December 4. Retrieved from www.independent.co.uk/news/uk/the-sanitary-pad-missionary-bringing-dignity-and-employment-to-syrias-female-refugees-a6760741.html

Miller, G. (2005). The tsunami's psychological aftermath. *Science*, 308, 1030–1033.

Norris, F. H., Stevens, S. P., Pfefferbaum, B., Wyche, K. F. & Pfefferbaum, R. L. (2008). Community resilience as a metaphor, theory, set of capacities, and strategy for disaster readiness. *American Journal of Community Psychology*, 41, 127–150.

O'Neill, C. & O'Neill, M. (2012). How to step up in the face of disaster. TEDxBoston 2012. Filmed June 2012. Retrieved from www.ted.com/talks/caitria_and_morgan_o_neill_how_to_step_up_in_the_face_of_disaster?language=en

O'Neill, C. (2012). How communities bounce back from disaster. *CNN*, September 2. Retrieved from http://edition.cnn.com/2012/09/02/opinion/oneill-disaster-recovery/index.html

Recovers.org (2016). Retrieved from https://recovers.org/about

Rivlin, G. (2015). *Katrina: After the Flood*. New York, NY: Simon & Schuster.

Robertson, C. (2015). Racially disparate views of New Orleans's recovery after Hurricane Katrina. *New York Times*, August 24. Retrieved from www.nytimes.com/2015/08/25/us/hurricane-katrina-new-orleans-recovery-ten-years-opinion.html

Rodin, J. (2014). *The Resilience Dividend: Being Strong in a World Where Things Go Wrong*, 1st edn. New York, NY: PublicAffairs.

Roig-Franzia, M. (2015). A 'resilience lab': An influx of capital and newcomers has triggered changes in New Orleans. *The Washington Post*, August 22. Retrieved from www.washingtonpost.com/sf/national/2015/08/22/a-resilience-lab/?tid=HP_more

Ross, J. (2015). Katrina may be a metaphor to some, but it's still a reality to New Orleans: 10 years after Katrina. *The Washington Post*, August 27. Retrieved from www.washingtonpost.com/national/katrina-may-be-a-metaphor-to-some-but-its-still-a-reality-to-new-orleans/2015/08/27/f53bfaa6-4b69-11e5-902f-39e9219e574b_story.html

Seidenberg, J. (2005). Cultural competency in disaster recovery: Lessons learned from the Hurricane Katrina: Experience for better serving marginalized communities. Unpublished report, UC Berkeley School of Law. Retrieved from www.law.berkeley.edu/library/resources/disasters/Seidenberg.pdf

Townsend, F. F. (2006). Chapter Five: Lessons Learned. In F. F. Townsend, *The Federal Response to Hurricane Katrina: Lessons Learned*. Retrieved from http://georgewbush-whitehouse.archives.gov/reports/katrina-lessons-learned/chapter5.html

US Senate (2006). Hurricane Katrina: A nation still unprepared. Report of the Senate Committee on Homeland Security and Governmental Affairs: Executive Summary. Senate Report 109-322. 109th Congress (2005–2006). Washington, DC: US Government Publishing Office. Retrieved from www.congress.gov/congressional-report/109th-congress/senate-report/322/1

Venema, V. (2015). The unlikely sanitary pad missionary. *BBC World Service*, December 3. Retrieved from www.bbc.com/news/magazine-34925238

Vennare, J. (2016). 26 rankings that prove Pittsburgh is better than every other city. FITT, presented by UPMC Health Plan. Retrieved from https://fitt.co/pittsburgh/pittsburgh-best-city/

Wilbanks, T. J., Leiby, P., Perlack,R. Ensminger, J. T. & Wright, S. B. (2007). Toward an integrated analysis of mitigation and adaptation: Some preliminary findings. Oak Ridge, TN, USA: Environmental Sciences Division, Oak Ridge National Laboratory. Retrieved from http://citeseerx.ist.psu.edu/viewdoc/download? doi=10.1.1.132.1271&rep=rep1&type=pdf

Wilson, K. (2015). Stamford teen wins Girl Scout Gold Award for creating Stepping Stone exhibit. *The Hour*, July 24. Retrieved from www.thehour.com/norwalk/article/Stamford-teen-earns-Girl-Scout-Gold-Award-for-8102478.php

# Index